Occupational Therapy: Perspectives and Processes

For Churchill Livingstone:

Editorial director: Mary Law
Project editor: Valerie Bain
Project manager: Valerie Burgess
Project controller: Pat Miller
Indexer: Jill Halliday
Design direction: Judith Wright
Sales promotion executive: Maria O'Connor

Occupational Therapy: Perspectives and Processes

Rosemary Hagedorn DipCOT SROT DipTCDHEd
Practising Occupational Therapist, formerly Occupational Therapy Course Director,
Crawley College, Crawley, UK

CHURCHILL LIVINGSTONE
EDINBURGH HONG KONG LONDON MADRID MELBOURNE NEW YORK AND TOKYO 1995

CHURCHILL LIVINGSTONE
Medical Division of Pearson Professional Limited

Distributed in the United States of America by Churchill
Livingstone, 650 Avenue of the Americas, New York, N.Y.
10011, and by associated companies, branches and
representatives throughout the world.

First published 1995

ISBN 0 443 04978 5

British Library Cataloguing in Publication Data
A catalogue record for this book is available from the British
Library.

Library of Congress Cataloging in Publication Data
A catalog record for this book is available from the Library of
Congress.

The
publisher's
policy is to use
**paper manufactured
from sustainable forests**

Printed in the United States of America

Contents

Preface

This book is the result of a personal journey through the profession of occupational therapy over the past 30 years, in which I have visited various aspects of practice, management and education.

The content was evolved, in the language of qualitative research, through a process of heuristic enquiry and inward reflection, by means of which I have attempted to define and communicate a set of ideas, beliefs, values, assumptions and methods of practice.

The personal nature of this search is emphasized at the start because most textbooks on occupational therapy are edited compilations, using many expert sources. These texts give an overview of professional practice at a point in time, and use collective experience to provide a comprehensive and balanced view of accepted theory and practice.

My own professional journey has been informed and influenced by the work of other writers and researchers who have provided important maps and signposts, but my description of occupational therapy is inevitably partial – in both senses. There are, in professional terms, places I have not been, and there are aspects of practice about which I am positively or negatively biased. It is important to recognize that the journey continues, that there is no fixed route or final destination, and that travellers may have different experiences, even on the same path.

I do believe, however, that there is room for the individual perspective, and I hope that this book will be of use to both students and more experienced practitioners, and that it may stimulate others to evaluate their own practice, to conduct further research and to reflect on the nature of their own professional journeys.

The main content is arranged in two parts, 'Perspectives' and 'Processes.' In the first part, Perspectives, various views of occupational therapy are discussed, and some new ideas are introduced concerning the core of the profession, the nature of occupations, the theoretical basis for practice, and the nature of humans as 'occupational beings'.

In the second part, Processes, the problem-based case management process is described, together with six generic processes of occupational therapy. Appendix 1 contains some experiential or reflective exercises connected with these processes, which the reader may like to try.

The material in Part 2 is likely to be more familiar, even to the extent of restating things which are obvious to the more experienced practitioner. Stating the obvious is sometimes necessary, however, simply because it is often taken for granted and because, at some points in one's professional development, it may not be obvious at all. While any isolated process may appear simple, it is the synthesis of these processes in relation to the unique circumstances affecting each individual patient or client that transmutes the basic techniques gained by the student into the expert, apparently intuitive, practice of the experienced occupational therapist.

You will discover, as you read, that words are important to me. I am fascinated by their duality, by their use as descriptive tools and precise units of information, and by their symbolism, which reflects the richness of human experience.

Occupational therapy is both science and art. But what kind of art? Constructive arts, such as painting or sculpture, do not seem to provide the required metaphor. If the therapist is the artist, does the patient become the subject of the painting, or even the paint and canvas? Clay or stone are passive in the sculptor's hands. These art forms seem to place the therapist in a controlling, directive, interpretive, relationship with the patient.

For me, therapy is more akin to poetry. The therapist, like the poet, uses words as tools, is concerned with communication, with describing and finding meaning in the phenomena of life, and with storytelling. He or she must seek to see past the overt surface textures of things to the covert, multilayered symbols and emotions which lie beneath and yet, like the poet, remain detached enough to observe, describe and analyse these things.

The patient may be the co-poet, the subject of the poem, the reader of it, and perhaps all these things. A poem seldom seeks to provide total answers or any kind of finite solution, it is only a part of a story. Today's poem may be different from yesterday's; tomorrow's will be different again.

To be a poet, one must be well acquainted with rules, forms, techniques: the basic science which both constrains and promotes the making of a poem. Yet this is not enough; technique alone cannot provide inspiration. A good poem, like 'good therapy' is far more than the sum of its parts. The poet must be inspired to create, but even with inspiration the struggle 'to make it work' remains.

The reader is seldom aware of the full wastepaper basket or the hours spent trying to find the right word, the exact phrase; similarly, the patient remains largely unaware of the struggles of the therapist on his or her behalf. Gifted poets are born as much as made; I suspect that gifted therapists are also.

Arundel 1995   R.H.

Perspectives

PART CONTENTS

Occupational Therapy: A Retrospective

THE RELEVANCE OF HISTORY

THE EARLY YEARS

Many texts on occupational therapy begin with a summary of the genesis and history of the profession. The need to show historical lineage is an interesting phenomenon. Why is the profession so anxious to prove a respectable and legitimate genealogy, often stretching back 2500 years or more with references to Hippocrates, Galen, Plato and Aristotle?

It is true that the ideas and practices of innovative thinkers resonate down the centuries, but much of the early practice of medicine was based on magico-religious thinking which would be totally alien to us now, depending as it did on an imperfect understanding of the human body and beliefs in sympathetic and ritual magic, myth and the intervention of the gods. If participation in dance, theatre or other creative occupations was used for curative purposes, the underlying intentions and perceptions of it were often far removed from those of occupational therapy.

An analogy can be drawn with the use of herbal remedies: a plant might have been chosen because the shape of its leaves suggested an affinity with a particular organ of the body. The effects may or may not have been beneficial, but if it seemed effective the remedy was likely to be continued, even though the cause and effect were incompatible in scientific terms. Similarly, dancing might be seen to cause emotional catharsis, but might well have been used to induce trance, drive out an evil spirit or placate a god; very probably these distinctions were, in any case, blurred and irrelevant to the participants.

Thinkers such as Plato and Aristotle were geniuses far ahead of their own times and Hippocrates was a very advanced medical practitioner for his day, but even if some early philosophical ideas and enlightened medical practices are relevant, these were wiped out and repressed during the centuries in which knowledge was lost, much scientific research was banned as heretical, surgery was literally 'barbarous', and therapy owned more to superstition and alchemical mysteries than to reason.

Persian and Chinese medicine became highly sophisticated but remained virtually unknown in the West. Much essential knowledge was destroyed in the burning of ancient libraries during wars or by the intentional destruction of books regarded as heretical. It was not until the classical revival in the 18th century that the ideas of ancient Greek philosophers once again became influential in mainstream western philosophical thinking, and scientific research became acceptable.

Attempts to relate occupational therapy to ancient ideas and practices are therefore correct in tracing 'modern' scientific practice and philosophical thought back to the remote past, but are optimistic in suggesting more than tenuous similarities with contemporary occupational therapy practices.

THE 19TH CENTURY

Despite some notable if tentative and isolated gestures in Britain and France during the 18th century, e.g. Pinel, Tuke, Tissot and Buchan, occupational therapy did not begin to evolve in a recognizable form until the latter part of the 19th century. By that time the 'age of enlightenment' had instigated the scientific revolutions which have shaped the present century. During the late 19th and early 20th centuries scientific researchers, writers and philosophers exploded cherished beliefs with new, challenging and often atheistic or political explanations of the human condition. Scientific enquiry snowballed and

fundamental changes occurred in views of the nature of humanity, human rights, the duties of the state, and the individual's contribution to society.

The early 19th century produced developments in health care which kindled those which revolutionized medicine and surgery in the 20th century. In addition the socioeconomic conditions of western Europe and America at the end of the 19th century were finally, if briefly, sufficiently stable to permit evolutions in health care resulting in the treatment of 'the sick' as individuals. The legacy of hospitals, asylums, and workhouses in Britain, all dating from this period, is an example of social concern and philanthropy, but also of the largely paternalistic view of such provision.

By the end of the 19th century it is possible to see in place the ideas which have shaped the scientific basis, philosophy, value and practice of occupational therapy. These are derived directly from the thinking and conditions at this time, and could not have been put widely into practice any earlier due to the absence of the necessary attitudes, concepts and knowledge, and of a sufficient infrastructure for health care.

The American pioneers of occupational therapy came from a variety of professions. They include psychiatrists (Adolf Meyer and William Rush Dunton Jnr) a doctor (Herbert Hall), a nurse (Susan Tracey), a teacher of design (Susan Cox Johnson), a social worker (Eleanor Clark Slagle) and two architects (George Barton and Thomas Bessell Kidner) (Reed & Sanderson 1983). This diversity may well be the basis of the uniquely wide-ranging body of knowledge claimed by the profession, which is both our strength and our problem.

What lay behind the focus on occupations as curative agents? Some of the fundamental reasons are discussed in later chapters, but to a large extent this thinking is also a product of its period. In the late 18th, and throughout the 19th century the tenet that work is 'good' – in the sense of both being morally superior to idleness, and producing desirable outcomes for the individual and society – was strongly held. Work was regarded as an economic and social necessity for the State, and the individual had an obligation to provide labour if possible.

Empirical observation in psychiatric hospitals in several countries had already established that patients who had an occupation often made better progress than those who did not. However patients could be exploited by being obliged to perform monotonous uncreative tasks without reference to their medical condition. It was a short step to the concept that whilst all occupation was good, some forms might be more appropriate than others, and that patients deprived of occupation should be enabled by the interventions of those who cared for them, to engage in it.

THE 20th CENTURY

There are many good reviews of the development of the profession between the two World Wars to which readers may refer for more detail (e.g. Reed 1993, Creek 1990, Jay et al 1992). Ironically, it was the need to return people to combat or productive war work which spurred on many of the developments in therapy and, indeed, in medicine and surgery. Milestones in the development of occupational therapy in the USA and UK are given in Box 1.1.

The above outline of the development of the profession demonstrates that the driving forces have been environmental on one hand (the political, cultural, socioeconomic, scientific, technical and philosophical changes which have occurred during the past 90 years or so) and personal on the other hand (the thoughts, knowledge, values, ideas, personal creativity and imagination of committed individuals). This should come as no surprise to therapists believing in the dynamics of person – environment – occupation interactions.

Occupational therapy has inevitably changed in the last 90 years and , if it is to remain relevant, it must continue to evolve. The ever-important question is how far can we adapt while retaining our essential core of identity? That in itself raises the fundamental question of whether there *is* an essential core, and if so, whether or not it is

Box 1.1	
1914	George Barton coined the term 'occupational therapy'
1915	William Dunton Jnr produced first textbook on occupational therapy; Eleanor Clark Slagle organized first occupational therapy school in Chicago
1917	National Society for the Promotion of occupational therapy founded in USA
1925	First American-trained occupational therapist employed in UK, in Aberdeen
1930	Dr Elizabeth Casson set up Dorset House, first occupational therapy training school in UK, in Bristol (later transferred to Oxford)
1931	National Registry of occupational therapists set up in USA
1932	Scottish Association of occupational therapy founded
1936	English Association of occupational therapy founded
1938	British Journal of occupational therapy first published
1952	World Federation of occupational therapy founded
1962	Council for Professions Supplementary to Medicine introduced State Registration for UK occupational therapists
1974	Scottish and English Associations of occupational therapy combined to form British Association of Occupational Therapists

mutable. What may we let go, and what must we fight to retain?

The profession is undoubtedly influenced, sometimes unduly, by new frames of reference or new 'fashions' which affect practice. It may be questioned whether our rejection or acceptance of these is based on objective evidence. On the other hand many of our current concepts and the basic definition of the profession are clearly similar to the ideas of our founders. This may be an encouraging indication that there is a core, but it could equally be argued that we are simply resistive to change.

A historical perspective is able sometimes to demonstrate continuity and to illuminate the difference between fundamental and peripheral changes. A brief review of the changes in practice and philosophy in Britain in the past 40 years as influenced by changes in health care and social policy, and by frames of reference and models of practice may therefore be informative.

This is, admittedly, an insular view; inevitably, environmental influences have led to local variations in the profession. I believe that the exploration of such variations, and the extent to which occupational therapy retains similarities in different countries or areas of practice can considerably enhance our understanding of the core philosophy and processes. If we fail to recognize this, we lose sight of the core and are in danger of fragmentation.

OCCUPATIONAL THERAPY IN BRITAIN SINCE 1950

1950–1959

Social policy

The majority of occupational therapists worked for the new National Health Service (NHS). Most hospitals were managed by their own Boards, working with a Medical Director and a Matron. Occupational therapists practised in large tuberculosis (TB) sanatoria, in mental hospitals and mental subnormality hospitals, in large 'manor house' physical rehabilitation centres and in the larger general hospitals. There was still a postwar shortage of qualified staff and services were irregular. Helpers and assistants were employed to extend the services provided by qualified staff. Care in the community was the province of a miscellany of charities and local welfare departments.

Health care

Restricted diet and special health care policies, such as dietary supplements for mothers and babies during the war years had, ironically, contributed to the health of the nation. The need to attend to war injuries hastened the development of prosthetics, orthotics, plastic surgery and other forms of surgery.

Antibiotics were coming into common use and immunization was routine. Many serious epidemic diseases, especially TB, continued to present a major problem. Extended stays in hospital during recovery from illness or trauma were commonplace. Epidemics of polio left many adults and children with serious permanent disabilities.

Philosophy and practice

Therapy was viewed as requiring close medical supervision and was strongly influenced by the medical model. Rehabilitation for work and normal life was important, but therapy for maintenance and diversional occupation was common in both psychiatric and physical fields. Traditional craftwork was used extensively and crafts were held to have intrinsic therapeutic qualities, e.g. 'sedative' and 'stimulating' (O'Sullivan 1955). However, industrial therapy and group work using analytical frames of reference were introduced in psychiatry towards the end of this decade. In physical rehabilitation long periods of hospitalization provided the opportunity for extensive and complex programmes of graded therapy based on biomechanical principles.

Education

Most occupational therapy schools were privately run, although some had links with hospitals. The 3-year training course was standardized nationally and included extended training in a range of traditional craft skills. Medical and biological sciences were taught in a highly traditional manner with the emphasis on 'learning the facts'. Clinical practice included extended placements in general or psychiatric settings. The final diploma examinations entitled practitioners to join the Association of Occupational Therapists (or Scottish Association) and to use the letters MAOT.

1960–1969

Social policy

The welfare state was securely established, and this newly-confident decade marked a period of consolidation rather than innovation as Britain shed the restrictions of the postwar years. Improvement in the economy allowed some hospital building and renovation schemes to commence. Occupational therapists remained largely hospital-based and medical directors of occupational therapy services ensured adherence to medical models of management and therapy. State registration for therapists affirmed their professional identity and provided the public with protection against malpractice.

Health care

Developments in all branches of medicine continued, most notably in chemotherapy, and especially in the field of psychiatry where new drugs revolutionized the control of symptoms and behaviours and made it possible to include previously disturbed patients in therapy. Physically-based treatments still predominated in psychiatry; electroconvulsant therapy was much used. In addition, group therapy and various forms of analysis were gaining ground, as was behaviourism. In physical medicine major advances in surgical techniques were made, replacement joints were invented, and TB finally reached the point of near-extinction in the UK. Day hospitals for elderly people and psychiatric patients were pioneered. In Scotland in 1968, therapists began to work in collaboration with community social services departments.

Philosophy and practice

The second half of this decade witnessed an adverse reaction to craftwork and a desire to be viewed by other professions as more scientific. Rehabilitation became the dominant model, and the rehabilitation team became important in physical rehabilitation. Increased emphasis was placed on assessment and specific restoration of function, and more sophisticated physical rehabilitation equipment was developed.

In psychiatric practice, group therapy began to be used by therapists; behavioural psychology was also very influential, leading to token economies and behavioural modification programmes. Craftwork was still used extensively in psychiatry, but was decreasing in favour of domestic training, social skills training and industrial therapy.

Education

Although some new schools were developed in response to the growing demand for therapists, there was little change in the national pattern of education; indeed, the existing craft-based curriculum became somewhat out of step with the leading edge of practice by the end of the decade.

1970–1979

Social policy

Notwithstanding some interruptions due to crises in funding, the national hospital building programme led to the creation of well-equipped rehabilitation departments and day hospitals in district general hospitals. The large manor house rehabilitation centres closed, as a combination of improved local facilities and surgical techniques reduced the need for prolonged rehabilitation. The increasing number of elderly people meant that gerontology became an important occupational therapy specialty. Most psychiatric care was still located in large out-of-town institutions, and psychiatry and mental handicap remained 'Cinderella services', lacking investment.

The reorganization of the NHS in 1974 provided a new national management structure (differing slightly in Scotland and Wales) with geographical divisions into regions, areas and districts, and when social services consequently split from the NHS, community occupational therapists developed their own pay and managerial structures – by the end of the decade around 20% of therapists worked in the community.

Health care

In surgery and in chemotherapy further rapid advances were made in diagnostic techniques using sophisticated investigative equipment. Hospital stays became ever shorter. The optimism about the potential of chemotherapy to prevent acute psychiatric patients becoming 'chronic' diminished in the face of the realization that by now a group of patients was becoming 'the new long-stay'. Nonetheless, the management of acute psychiatric episodes in the community, was becoming more widespread and effective by means of domiciliary support, day hospitals or short admissions to local units.

Philosophy and practice

In physical practice there was a further move away from craftwork, until, in some cases, productive activities were dropped entirely in favour of remedial games, biomechanical exercises using adapted equipment and sensorimotor neurodevelopmental techniques, following the work of Ayres, Rood and Bobath (Trombly 1989, Ayres 1972).

Shortening admission times, due to medical and surgical advances, meant that there was no longer time to undertake a full graded treatment programme, and therapy focused increasingly on providing immediate solutions to functional problems. Activities of daily living (ADL) assessment remained important but this too became condensed into a tighter timeframe, and facilitating discharge from hospital became the prime objective.

In psychiatry, following developments in psychotherapy, group work took over from most other forms of Occupational Therapy. Industrial therapy was decreasing, partly in response to external industrial changes, but use of creative therapies increased. By the end of the decade the diminution of long-stay psychiatric hospitals was becoming apparent, and the move towards community care was taking root. Cognitive therapy began to exert its influence.

Professional literature during this decade was frequently soul-searching and introspective, questioning the direction of the profession, but this discussion lacked the conceptual and intellectual depth of the equivalent debate in the USA. Medical influence on the profession was still apparent, as evidenced by the number of articles published in the British Journal of

Occupational Therapy written by medical practitioners rather than therapists.

In general, the search for professional validity tended to draw therapists into borrowing from or emulating other professions (physiotherapists, psychologists, psychotherapists, counsellors, social workers or doctors) rather than stimulating development and evaluation of the professional core.

Education

The general uncertainty permeating the profession was felt also in education, curricula were in danger of becoming either fossilized or fragmented. This problem affected other professions too, and in the late 1970s the Council for Professions Supplementary to Medicine (CPSM) appointed an experienced occupational therapist as Educational Research Officer to investigate and report on professional training.

The move from private, rather isolated, occupational therapy schools into higher education had begun and by the end of this decade it became clear that a radical review of the curriculum was necessary. Some schools had already evolved new curricula and the constraints of a nationally standardized scheme were recognized. New guidelines for professional education were developed; a formal training scheme for helpers was initiated, and in 1979 an innovative 4-year inservice diploma to enable helpers and technicians to qualify as therapists was piloted in Essex.

1980–1989
Social policy

The NHS was influenced strongly by Government policy – financial constraints, health care priorities, Care in the Community initiatives and the Griffiths Management Review all affected occupational therapy practice and management.

Following the removal of the area tier of management in England and Wales, district health authorities assumed managerial responsibility for groups of hospitals. District occupational therapists gradually took over the management of occupational therapy services, and by the end of the decade a group of managerial therapists was wholly responsible for a client group and for multidisciplinary management.

The move of psychiatric care into the community began to impinge on public consciousness and became belatedly controversial as many large hospitals closed towards the end of the decade, raising a heated debate over whether Victorian paternalism had been replaced by a vacuum rather than by the package of socially concerned community care which was intended.

By the late 1980s, changes in working patterns, especially the increased employment of women, and changes in social and family structures and values, which had begun in the 1960s, had made their mark on everyday life and social and occupational roles.

Health care

Improved techniques in surgery and medicine enabled severely disabled or very elderly individuals to live longer, and required the development of specialized rehabilitation techniques. Services were developed to assist disabled people in the community but these failed to match the turnover in the acute areas of general hospitals. The need to maintain and support elderly dementing individuals became pressing, and the integration of people with mental illness and learning disabilities in the community provided a further incentive to develop innovative services.

The 1980s also saw a shift in focus towards health education and prevention, still tentative and under-resourced but at least a movement towards social medicine and a true 'health' service, as opposed to the traditional model of a reactive 'sickness service'. Occupational therapists moved cautiously into this new field.

Philosophy and practice

In the area of mental handicap and mental health, the prospective closure of large hospitals and the move to the community increased the demand for occupational therapy services and made therapists re-examine their own role in relation to other professions. Therapists were frequently at the forefront of community initiatives; new psychiatric units in district general hospitals or the community were built or planned; hostels and group homes were built for discharged clients and day centres and 'drop in' centres were created to support them.

In physical occupational therapy care of the elderly continued to be important; acute admissions passed through the service more rapidly, leaving even less time for therapy, and in some cases reducing the role of therapists to that of 'discharge technicians'.

There were serious staff shortages in all fields of occupational therapy. Helpers were valued as assistants, and development of their skills was encouraged, but there was also professional anxiety that such workers were being placed in positions of greater responsibility for therapy than was desirable.

Awareness that occupational therapy skills are particularly valuable in care in the community led to a considerable expansion in such posts, placing further strains on the understaffed NHS.

As a means of focusing political and public attention on the profession an independent commission was set up by the College of Occupational Therapists to produce a report on the profession, which identified both its important role in health care and the acute shortage of therapists (Blom Cooper 1989).

Interest in, and awareness of, models of practice and frames of reference grew. The ideas of Reed & Sanderson (1983) and of Kielhofner (1985) were particularly influential, leading to a review of how therapists actually used occupations. Creative and constructive activities once again became acceptable and occupational therapy, which ceased to have an occupational focus, was increasingly questioned. There was a new emphasis on 'problem solving' and human–environment interactions; new developmental, cognitive and humanistic approaches and techniques were used, while biomechanical and neuro-developmental approaches continued in the physical field.

Education

At the start of the decade the old diploma syllabus was phased out and a new curriculum, Diploma '81, was introduced, which was influential in freeing occupational therapy schools from the constraints of national examinations. By the end of the decade the new impetus in education and the implementation of Diploma '81 had forced educationalists to review curricula and in the process to become more aware of the philosophical debates within the profession in the USA. Theory and conceptual debate and analysis began to permeate through courses and management education was recognized as an essential component of basic training.

The increasing academic content of courses took its toll on both clinical experience and practical skills, and a tension developed between those educationalists who stressed the need for the student to acquire specific competencies and those who emphasized the importance of a sound scientific and theoretical basis for practice and research.

As the need for improved research was acknowledged, pressure grew to create a graduate level in the profession. At the same time, the decreasing number of school leavers and the continuing pressure to train more therapists led to diversification in occupational therapy education, and a deliberate move towards widening access to it. The first two degree courses commenced in 1986, and in 1988 an accelerated course for graduates was introduced at the London Medical College.

THE 1990s

Social policy

In the current decade, the restructuring of health authorities and the development of NHS Trusts, the provider/purchaser system of budgeting and service provision, and the escalating costs of acute treatment have put pressure on resources and therapeutic practice. This pressure, along with a tendency to criticise the negative aspects of 'professionalism' have coincided with an increased demand within the profession for specific standards and the implementation of formal quality management systems.

Following these management changes in the NHS a less secure career structure exists at managerial level with the loss of many district therapist posts; however, there is more multidisciplinary management and greater opportunities for therapists to move into other areas of management. Therapists are still a scarce resource.

It is too early to predict the long-term effect of these managerial changes, but the overall impact seems to be destabilizing. One already observable result is a move away from the consistency of provision achieved during the 1980s towards more uneven service provision and standards. Variations occur from one health service trust to another, due less to local need than to the efficacy of local therapists in marketing, budgeting and bargaining on behalf of their services, and the willingness of local managers to take account of their professional opinions and expertise. It must be hoped that this is a temporary phase, and not a return to the patterns of service which were found during the 1950s and early 1960s when good services were improved but under-resourced or ineffective services were starved out of existence.

The transition of people with learning disabilities and mental health conditions into normal life in the community continues, and few large institutional-style hospitals remain open. The Care in the Community initiative has created more changes in working and managerial practices affecting social services and occupational therapists but practical resources and services still lag behind the demand for care generated by relocation of patients and pressures for early discharge. The important developments in primary health care here created new roles for occupational therapists in the community.

The speed of continuing change both in social policy and society as a whole has left many health care workers feeling insecure, threatened and generally overwhelmed, with no opportunity to consolidate after each new 'knock' from the system. Occupational therapists are not immune from, or alone in, these perceptions.

Health care

This last decade of the 20th century is the age of technology: computers, scanners, microsurgery, replacement parts for almost everything and the prospect of genetic therapy. Most of these advances, although welcome, are either irrelevant to therapists or have served mainly to remove some traditional areas of concern in occupational therapy, by eliminating either the need or the time for intervention. Adaptive as ever, therapists have also exploited new technologies for their therapeutic and managerial advantages.

On the other hand, in some ways more individuals are in need of occupational therapy than ever before. There is a predominantly ageing population, living longer and requiring more services; people become severely disabled through accident or illness and survive, whereas a decade ago they would have died. People with learning disabilities and chronic psychiatric problems are now regarded as priorities. The stresses of life have not lessened; neither have stress-related illnesses nor mental disorders. In fact, health education could be a growth area for therapists.

Supporting people in the community is undoubtedly a key role for the occupational therapist who, however, is obliged increasingly to 'market' services in competition with other professions, many of which, also faced by changing, and in some cases diminishing, roles are laying claim to areas of expertise which occupational therapists have traditionally seen as 'theirs'.

Philosophy and practice

Practice is being refocused on the occupational needs and competencies of the individual. There is increasing interest in theory, models of practice, research, and the processes of clinical and ethical reasoning and reflective practice as applied by occupational therapists. There has also been a welcome increase in the publication of books and articles dealing with occupational therapy theory and competencies by UK authors.

Having now become reasonably literate in such topics, therapists are becoming interested

in putting the theories into practice, and this new, reflective attitude should promote professional development and research.

Practice generally follows the trends set in the late 1980s, and it is too soon to predict how market forces, and other sociomedical changes will affect occupational therapy.

Education

Most 'paramedical' professions have now completed the move to graduate status and in occupational therapy the transition towards a wholly graduate profession has been achieved. All courses are now located in or linked to universities. Courses leading to degrees such as a BSc or an MSc in occupational therapy are available in many universities, and postgraduate educational opportunities covering a variety of health-related and educational degrees are now offered. The first UK Professor of Occupational Therapy has been appointed in Edinburgh.

CONCLUSION

Some important trends emerge from the preceding description of occupational therapy in the UK since the Second World War. Clearly, the NHS seems to have had more than its fair share of political and economical change. Also obvious is the change caused by improvements in medical and surgical techniques, particularly in the location of care, and in the restrictions on time available for delivery of therapy in hospital. Equally important are the substantial sociocultural changes which have altered environments, roles and patterns of occupation over the past 40 years. As occupational therapists we must pay particular heed to these changes, to avoid the risk of applying outdated theories and values to our clients.

No health care profession practises in a vacuum. The 'technological revolution' of this century has produced dramatic worldwide changes of as much significance as those wrought by the industrial and agrarian revolutions of the past. Occupational therapists have been obliged to react to these major changes. In Britain the profession, being adaptive and concerned with management issues, has managed, on the whole, to take a reasonably positive and at times, pro-active approach to these changes, jettisoning some 'traditional' techniques and acquiring new skills. An analysis of all these factors and the profession's responses is interesting, but requires research beyond the scope of this book.

I find of considerable interest the continuing tension and dialogue – almost at times an argument – between the two elements of our profession, the 'art' and the 'science'. It is almost as if during the late 1960s and early 1970s we became so diffident and apologetic over the use of our art that we almost abandoned it in an attempt to become totally, provably, scientific, borrowing the technical wizardry and dazzling theories of other professions for our own benefit, while omitting to develop our own theories and relevant research base.

During the last decade we seem to have become more aware of the dangers of this piecemeal approach, and more concerned with defining and developing the unique core skills of the occupational therapist. This must be beneficial, subject to the recognition that the reductionist research techniques of pure science are largely incompatible with the organic and highly indivi-dual art of therapy.

2

Definitions

WORDS ARE IMPORTANT

As well as studying the *history* of occupational therapy (Ch. 1), it is possible also to trace the developments in the *definition* of occupation and occupational therapy in order to obtain insight into the methods, purposes and concerns of the profession.

When discussing definitions it is all too easy to sink into a quagmire of semantics, expending time and energy in a pedantic search for meaning. An understandable reaction to this is to dismiss arguments over the meanings of words as time-wasting and irrelevant.

Neither of these approaches is helpful. Words are important; they are the tools of scientific and academic communication. They also carry the subtleties of thought and the overlays of emotion, values or attitudes which the user, intentionally or otherwise, conveys. Precision in language is necessary, and it is essential for a profession to have an agreed vocabulary, avoiding the use of jargon.

There are two central debates: what is meant by occupation, and what is occupational therapy? Since occupation is the central focus of occupational therapy it is entirely to be expected that much of the literature is devoted to explaining the essential role played by occupation in human life, the results of failures in occupational performance and the remedial potential of occupations.

There is, however, a difficulty. We are occupational therapists, yet we speak and write mainly about participation in and use of *activities*. The words 'occupation' and 'activity' are frequently used interchangeably within the profession. There is little doubt that therapists and those outside the profession do not interpret the two words in the same way, which leads to misunderstanding. What, then, is occupation? Is it, or is it not the same thing as activity? And does any of this matter?

The profession may be in danger of altering the meanings of language in order to make practice fit an idealized, all-encompassing notion of 'occupation'. However, it has to be accepted that living language is not stable – meanings change and evolve, and regular reappraisal is necessary.

It is not surprising that therapists tend to find it difficult to put the complexities of human performance and occupational therapy practice into words (Creek 1992). Many therapists have become so bored by the labyrinthine complexities of what they see as a fruitless debate that the suggestion that occupational therapists should change their title as a means of avoiding further discussion has been made more than once. Yet it is important for occupational therapists to understand clearly the key concepts of their profession.

DEFINITIONS OF OCCUPATION

Kielhofner (1993) gives the following definition:

Occupation is the dominant activity of human beings that includes serious, productive pursuits and playful, creative and festive behaviours. It is the result of evolutionary processes culminating in biological, psychological and social need for both playful and productive activity.

Within the framework of the model of human occupation, Kielhofner and his associates give a closely-argued description of the genesis, scope and nature of occupations, stressing the importance of person–environment interactions, and the role of personal volition and choice in motivating action.

Alternatively, Reed & Sanderson (1980) propose that occupation is:

Purposeful behaviour designed to achieve a desired goal. A specific action, function or sphere of action that involves learning or doing by direct experience.

In the glossary of the second edition (1983), however, this is simplified to:

Activities or tasks which engage a person's resources of time and energy, specifically, self-maintenance, productivity and leisure.

Like Kielhofner, Reed & Sanderson describe very precisely the features of occupations and their relationship with the environment.

All occupations are determined by the environment. That is, occupations are developed and exist because of the physical, individual or collective environment. Occupations which fulfil needs to deal with the environment continue to exist (and) . . . are developed.

In a subsequent book, Reed (1984) lists the role of occupations in human life:

1. Occupation is fundamental to human existence and health because it maintains and provides for the life-support systems and because it gives meaning to life.
2. Occupation is performed as a holism or gestalt in which the whole is different from the sum of its parts.
3. Occupation is a dynamic process which changes in form and complexity over time and in different places.
4. Occupation is influenced, altered and changed by the physical, biological and sociocultural environments in which an individual lives.
5. Occupation can be used to facilitate adaptation to the environment or facilitate the deliberate manipulation of the environment.

She lists problems in occupations as follows:

1. Occupations may become non-adaptive or maladaptive when certain alterations or changes occur in the physical, biological, or sociocultural environments.
2. Certain occupations may hinder adaptation to the environment of hinder the deliberate manipulation of the environment.
3. Lack of adaptive occupation affects health adversely.

Reed uses occupation as an umbrella term for all human performance and emphasizes the adaptive and changing nature of human performance within the environment.

Creek (1990) states that an occupation is:

Any goal directed activity that has meaning for the individual and is composed of skills and values.

Cynkin & Robinson (1990) do not use the word occupation at all, and substitute activity. Their list of assumptions concerning activity may be compared with those of Reed given above:

Activities of many kinds are characteristic of and define human existence.

Activities are socioculturally regulated by a system of values, beliefs and customs and are thus defined by and in turn define, acceptable norms of behaviour.

Change in activities related behaviour can move in a direction from dysfunctional to functional.

They later add that 'activities of every-day living can be regarded as external representations of a state of humanness'. They do not offer an explanation for the rejection of the term 'occupation'.

Kielhofner (1993) defines the difference between occupation and activity as follows:

Occupation refers to human activity; however, not all activity is occupation: humans engage in survival, sexual, spiritual and social activities in addition to those activities that are specifically occupational in nature.

Some activities, therefore, are occupations, (work, daily living tasks and play) but some are not (survival, sexual and spiritual activities). However, there is little guidance on how one can separate these two types of activity. Kielhofner adds later in the same text that:

Placing certain activities into spheres of human activity is not meant to suggest that all human activities can be neatly categorized into these areas.

Significantly Kielhofner proceeds to state that:

Occupational therapy is not concerned with all forms of activity: it focuses on that which is occupational in human life.

However, if the relationship between the occupational and non-occupational elements of human action is so entangled and interrelated, how can the therapist separate out the legitimate concerns from those which are beyond the scope of occupational therapy? Are we to deal only with 'occupations' and to exclude activities, or must we expand our definition of occupation to be all-inclusive?

Mocellin (1992a) in a critical review of the influence of American theorizing on occupational therapy draws attention to:

The liberal and over-inclusive definition of occupation (which) incorporates activities which have to do with bodily function.

I do not think that he is suggesting here that we should not be concerned with basic ADL, but that we should not describe occupations as encompassing basic self-care. He adds:

The issue is not only with the inclusion of activities but also with how these relate to occupational roles and how occupational therapists may assist in the restoration of these roles.

Allen (1985) states that:

it is assumed that purposeful activity is occupational therapy's treatment method.

However, most of her text deals with tasks:

Routine tasks are the activities that a person does on a daily basis. Routine tasks usually involve food, clothing, shelter, transportation, general health precautions and money management. Routine tasks are commonly referred to as activities of daily living.

These examples show the freedom with which the words occupation, activity and task are used and interchanged. This raises a number of questions: are the words true synonyms? Do they require more definition? Are there, as implied by some writers, differing levels of performance, and if so, where do these key words fit?

Young & Quinn (1992), confronted by the same problem, comment that the interchangeable use of words 'is a pity, as each has its own meaning'. They state that:

Occupation refers to that which occupies us between birth and death and is sometimes, for convenience, classified into occupations related to play, leisure, work, and self-maintenance. Activity is (quoting Chambers) 'the quality or state of being active' and also 'essential for the maintenance and continuance of life.' Tasks 'can be seen as segments of an activity, a sequence of tasks combining to form an activity'.

There has been an energetic debate over whether the basic study of human occupations – occupational science – should be separated from, or remain a part of occupational therapy (Mosey 1992, Clark et al 1993).

In a discussion of the development of occupational science Clark & Larson (1993) note:

Yerxa et al have provisionally defined occupation as the specific 'chunks' of activity within the on-going stream of human behaviour which are named in the lexicon of the culture.

The concept of an occupation having a name is significant, as will be discussed shortly. This definition still uses activity as a synonym for occupation, but seems to employ the definition of activity given by Reed (1983):

A specific action, function or sphere of action that involves learning or doing by direct experience.

Later in the same text the author quotes a paper (at that time unpublished) by the philosopher Aaron Ben Ze'ev, entitled 'What is an occupational activity?' His definition is:

A repeated complex pattern of actions whose value is not limited to the value of its external results.

This is interesting as Ben Ze'ev implies, as does Kielhofner, that some basic and utilitarian activities are 'non-occupational'.

This debate may be of great academic interest, but it is confusing to the practitioner in need of working definitions. Flexibility of language is, as already noted, the province of the poet rather than of the researcher. The lack of specificity does not become a problem in general discussion, but it can present difficulties when attempting to develop coherent theories or tools for the analysis of occupations, which is the special area of expertise claimed by occupational therapists.

If we do not, as a profession, have a common understanding of terminology, it becomes harder to explore and develop concepts using these words. Creek (1992) draws attention to another dilemma – our actions may be affected by the words we use to describe them. Words which define may also restrict. If we do not use words, our non-linguistic schemata (which Schon (1983) describes as 'knowing more than we can say') come into play; this may be beneficial.

A similar difficulty occurs when discussing theory. The cognitive schemata of theories are conveyed and understood through words, but since most definitions are proposed on the basis of a particular model or frame of reference, they are limited by the author's perspective. It is hard to find a neutral, generic definition with words which are neither theory-specific nor, in some way, value-laden.

The debate about occupations and activities is not simple; it is a debate not only about semantics, but also about professional identity and 'the legitimate tools' of the profession (Mosey 1986).

Are we *occupational* therapists or *activity* therapists? Are all activities and tasks part of our concern, or is there some non-occupational area of human performance which should be excluded? These questions have been asked for many decades, and may well continue to excite passionate opinions for several more before a real consensus is achieved. In the meantime, the practising members of the profession need a generally accepted means of continuing to describe what they do.

DEFINITIONS OF OCCUPATIONAL THERAPY

The definition of occupational therapy also poses a problem. Inevitably definitions spring from personal perspectives and frames of reference, use the language derived from these, and have sometimes given rise to dissent between practitioners holding differing views – or, quite often, between those who hold the same views but express them differently.

It is interesting to delve into archival material and reference books to compare the early definitions of occupational therapy, but it seems unnecessary to repeat these here, except to note that they are, on the whole, reassuringly recognizable. The first formal definition was written in the USA in 1992, significantly, by a doctor, H A Pattison. This states that occupational therapy is:

Any activity, mental or physical, definitely prescribed and guided for the distinct purpose of contributing to, and hastening the recovery from, disease or injury. (Reed & Sanderson 1983)

More relevant, perhaps, are the views expressed in the past decade, since these have directed current thinking. An analysis of commonly used words and concepts can indicate shared themes and point towards a generally agreed view of occupational therapy.

Mosey (1981), in her review of the profession, devotes a chapter to definition and commences with the view that:

Occupational therapy is defined as the art and science of using selected theories from a variety of disciplines and professions as a guide for collaborating with the client in order to assess that individual's ability to perform life tasks and, if necessary, to assist the individual in acquiring knowledge, skills and attitudes necessary to perform life tasks.

Clients are described as:

Individuals whose abilities to cope with tasks of daily living are threatened or impaired by biological, psychological or sociological stress, trauma or deficit.

Mosey adds that 'Fundamental . . . is the concern for and use of the non-human environment', and that practice 'concurrently requires execution of personal interactions on the part of the therapist'.

The idea that therapists draw their theories from other disciplines and professions is interesting: as noted, the founders came from a variety of professions. Is there, then, no theoretical basis 'owned' by occupational therapy? There can be no doubt that most frames of reference are derivative, stemming from the various explanations of human motivation, behaviour and learning.

The development of models of practice specific to occupational therapy during the last decade has been motivated at least in part by the desire to define a model which is 'ours'. It is ironic that some of these models (Kielhofner's model of human occupation; Reed's biopsychosocial adaptation through occupations) are now in turn being 'borrowed' by professions such as nursing.

In 1983 Reed & Sanderson also began their book with a semantic analysis of the component words 'occupation' and 'therapy' and concluded:

The name occupational therapy is meant to convey that the practice involves the treatment of illness or disability through the analysis and use of the occupations which fill up a person's time and space and engage the individual in activity.

Later in the same text they state that:

Occupational therapy . . . is the use of directed, purposeful occupations to influence positively a person's state of well-being and thus the state of a person's health.

They suggest that criteria for definition of a profession should include:

- unique features
- goals or purposes
- population served
- programmes offered
- process model used to deliver service
- means through which results are achieved

and they complete an analysis using these headings.

The 1981 American Association of Occupational Therapists (AOTA) definition of occupational therapy follows Reed's principles and begins:

Occupational therapy is the use of purposeful activity with individuals who are limited by physical injury or illness, psychosocial dysfunction, developmental or learning disabilities, poverty and cultural differences or the aging process in order to maximise independence, prevent disability and maintain health. The practice encompasses evaluation, treatment and consultation.'

The definition proceeds to list the practices and services provided.

Turner (1981) offers:

Occupational therapy is the treatment of the whole individual by his active participation in purposeful living.

In her second edition (1992) she undertook a review of past definitions and quoted several recent ones including the following:

Occupational therapists assess and treat people using purposeful activity to prevent disability and develop independent function. (BJOT 1989)

Occupational therapy is the treatment of physical and psychiatric conditions through specific activities to help people to reach their maximum level of function and independence in all aspects of daily life. (WFOT 1989)

Creek (1990) suggested:

The restoration of optimum functional independence and life satisfaction through the analysis and use of selected occupations that enable the individual to develop the adaptive skills required to support life roles.

Young & Quinn (1992) quote Mocellin (1984):

Occupational therapy is the health profession which teaches competent behaviour in the area of living, learning and working to individuals experiencing illness, developmental deficits and/or physical and psychosocial dysfunction.

My own contribution (Hagedorn 1992) was:

The prescription of occupations, interactions and environmental adaptations to enable the individual to regain, develop or retain the occupational skills and roles required to maintain personal well-being and to achieve meaningful personal goals and relationships appropriate to the relevant social and cultural setting.

In 1994 the College of Occupational Therapists issued a position statement on core skills and a conceptual foundation for practice (COT 1994). This adopts the WFOT definition quoted above, adding the following explanation of the role of the occupational therapist:

The occupational therapist assesses the physical, psychological and social functions of the individual, identifies areas of dysfunction and involves the individual in a structured programme of activity to overcome disability. The activities selected will relate to the consumer's personal, social, cultural and economic needs and will reflect the environmental factors which govern his/her life.

The statement also offers the definition provided by the Committee of Occupational Therapists for the European Communities (COTEC):

Occupational therapists assess and treat people using purposeful activity to prevent disability and develop independent function.

These are a few examples selected from a long list. In a profession as diverse and complex as occupational therapy there will always be difficulties in defining practice concisely. In recognition of this, many authors move on from definition to make general statements of shared beliefs, values, or actions, in relation to the therapeutic nature of occupations or the goals of therapy.

In attempting to define what is unique about occupational therapy, Reed (1984) writes that occupational therapy can help people to:

Learn or re-learn the performance of occupations necessary to adapt to daily life. (and) To organise and

balance the sequence of activity within their occupational performance.

and that therapists can:

Provide suggestions for adaptive ways of performing occupations which may facilitate performance for those with disability.

Provide the resources for practising and trying out different ways of performing occupations for those with disabilities.

Identify areas of dysfunction in the total performance of occupations.

Provide specialised equipment to assist in the performance of daily occupations for those with disabilities.

The Canadian Association of Occupational Therapists Task Force (1983) in developing the guidelines for the client-based practice of occupational therapy, based on the model of occupational performance, state the following beliefs as important to the practice of therapy (Law et al 1990):

The individual client is an essential part of occupational therapy practice; the client should be treated in an holistic manner; activity analysis and adaptation may be used to effect change in the individual's performance; an important consideration . . . is the client's developmental stage; role expectations must be taken into consideration in assessing a client's performance.

Turner (1992) also proposes fundamental beliefs' and concludes that:

Occupational therapists believe that:

- Occupation (purposeful activity) is central to normal human existence and that its absence or disruption is a threat to health.
- When health is disrupted, selected occupation is an effective means of recouping normal behaviour and function.
- There is inherent value in activity: experiencing the doing' process is what brings results. This involves active participation and effort on behalf of the individual and selection of the appropriate activity, occupation or task by the therapist.
- All individuals have value. Each individual has his own skills, problems, needs and motives, and social and cultural heritage. The individual needs to work with the therapist in determining the priorities for the restoration of function.

Taken together, the above definitions give various views of occupational therapy including:

- descriptions of the individual requiring therapy
- the reasons for therapy to be provided
- the benefits of occupation
- the areas of human life (occupations, roles, environment) with which therapy is concerned;
- the means whereby therapy is provided
- the goals of therapy
- the services provided by the therapist
- the values which the therapist should hold

Despite the differences in terminology and the nuances of inclusion or exclusion, there are recognizable themes running through these definitions, e.g. use of activity for prophylaxis, education, development and rehabilitation; focus on the individual as valuable and capable of positive change. However, a definition can only indicate the headlines, and the subtext is complex.

WHAT DO OCCUPATIONAL THERAPISTS DO?

What do therapists actually do when they treat patients, or intervene on behalf of a client? Because of the scope and variety of practice it becomes difficult to give a concise explanation, and short ones tend to degenerate into lists. Many authors have given descriptions of occupational therapy interventions. The AOTA describes such intervention (Hopkins & Smith 1993) in general terms as follows: occupational therapy:

Addresses function and uses specific procedures and activities to
a) develop, maintain, improve and/or restore the performance of necessary functions
b) compensate for dysfunction
c) minimize or prevent debilitation and/or
d) promote health and wellness.

There follows a long list of functional areas and skills with which a therapist may be concerned, but no real explanation of what the therapist *does*.

Reed (1984) lists six outcomes of therapy:
The person will, as a result of intervention:

1. Be able to perform or have performed, those occupations which meet the individual's needs and are acceptable to the person and society.
2. Have the necessary performance skills for the individual's repertoire of self-maintenance, productivity and leisure.
3. Achieve a balance of occupations thus attaining a maximum degree of actualization, autonomy and achievement.
4. Be able to adapt the environment or adapt to it.
5. Meet both deficiency needs and growth needs.
6. If unable to function independently, be provided with assistive devices or environmental adaptation.

(Adapted from Reed 1984)

This is a useful description of 'what', but again avoids stating 'how'; but Reed follows this up with a chart which lists intervention strategies or tools under the headings illustrated in Box 2.1.

This is a more useful list in identifying actual interventions, but the listings under each heading lack coherence.

Mosey (1986) defines the profession's philosophical assumptions, ethical code, body of knowledge, domain of concern, nature and principles of practice, and then lists the legitimate tools of therapy. These are:

- the non-human environment
- conscious use of self
- the teaching learning process

Box 2.1 Intervention strategies	
Media or agents	People, living things, and activities
Modalities	Areas of work, recreation, ADL, etc
Teaching methods	Various
Therapeutic approaches	Use of occupational and environmental analysis, adaptation and various specific techniques derived from frames of reference
Specialized techniques	More adaptive and specialized techniques.

- purposeful activities
- activity groups
- activity analysis and synthesis.

Turner (1992) writing on physical dysfunction, includes chapter headings on occupational therapy interventions in the areas of life skills, mobility skills, workshop activities and orthotics, and further describes interventions for specific physical conditions.

Creek (1990) similarly lists occupational therapy media and methods relevant to work in mental health, including:

- developing physical fitness
- sensory integration
- cognitive approaches
- group psychotherapy
- drama
- social skills training
- play therapy
- computers.

She, like Turner, then describes interventions for client groups. It seems therefore, that the nature of intervention may be described by:

1. defining the concerns or purposes of occupational therapy
2. describing the areas of human life subject to intervention
3. describing core processes used by the therapist
4. listing functional skills which the therapist seeks to improve
5. describing treatment aims for a specific condition or group of clients
6. listing techniques derived from frames of reference (e.g. cognitive, biomechanical, psychotherapeutic)

7. describing treatment methods for a specific condition
8. listing specialized techniques, skills and procedures
9. listing agents and media used to provide therapy
10. defining the outcomes of intervention.

The first three of these statements concern the general philosophy and processes of therapy; points 4 and 5 refer to the aims of therapy; points 6–9 describe the methods used to carry out therapy; and point 10 deals with the outcomes of therapy.

Each of the above needs to be considered separately in order to achieve a global description of occupational therapy. Such a description will be generalized, to avoid the risk of becoming of longwinded.

There is a further complication: in recent literature much emphasis has been placed on the use of models of practice and frames of reference to coordinate and structure therapy. There is a risk of conceptual confusion between the fundamental and relatively unchanging principles and practice of the profession, and the ways in which these may legitimately be altered in particular contexts, using theoretical models. What one does depends on which model is being used: each model brings a new definition. Is there one entity called 'occupational therapy' – or many?

The following chapters are concerned with identifying whether or not there are constants – core elements which, however they may be altered by particular forms of practice, are essential components without which the profession ceases to have an identity and integrity.

3

In search of the core

Over the past decade new terminology has been adopted in discussions of the theoretical and philosophical foundations of occupational therapy. Expressions such as *paradigm*, *model* and *frame of reference* have filtered down from the academic heights to cause varying degrees of interest, argument, confusion and consternation among both practitioners and educationalists.

It would be wrong to reject this terminology as simple jargon, for it indicates an effort to come to grips with two related questions of fundamental importance to the profession: first, the existence of an occupational therapy paradigm, and secondly, an understanding of the relationships between philosophy, theory and practice.

The basic questions are deceptively simple: is there a stable core at the heart of the profession, and if so, of what does it consist, and how does it relate to other important, but perhaps more changeable elements?

AN OCCUPATIONAL THERAPY PARADIGM

In the last decade much, rather esoteric, debate has taken place about whether or not it is legitimate for a practice-based profession such as occupational therapy to own a paradigm. Opinions on this are divided, not least because it seems that there are differing views of what a paradigm constitutes.

Some theorists use the word to mean an example or pattern (the dictionary definition) while others use it in the scientific sense, following Kuhn (1970), Kuhn himself has given various explanations of the term, but generally uses it to mean accepted examples of scientific practice including law, theory appreciation and instrumentation which, when the paradigm becomes accepted, represent a radically new conceptualization of phenomena.

Fundamental to this view is the idea that a paradigm exists and is challenged, then a crisis occurs and the old paradigm is replaced by something quite new and different – a paradigm shift. In science this is relatively simple to observe, e.g. the paradigm shift which occurred when physics leapt from relativity to quantum theory, which has left physicists in the uncomfortable position of having competing and incompatible paradigms which they feel compelled to resolve.

Four books published between 1990 and 1992 deal in various ways with the concept of a professional core. Interestingly, although these books were written at about the same time, the authors were working independently, in different locations.

Creek (1990) produced a paradigm containing philosophy, content, theory and process of practice. She describes feedback between this core and the practice of occupational therapy, and between the profession and the environment in which it exists (Fig. 3.1).

Kielhofner (1992) explored the concept of paradigm in some depth. He uses the term to mean both 'a conceptual perspective ... defining the nature and purpose of the field', and 'a cultural core' (sharing common beliefs and perspectives which enable therapists to understand what they are doing and how they should practice). He characterizes the occupational therapy paradigm as including 'three components; core assumptions (what members of the profession fundamentally know and believe about their field and their practice), a focal viewpoint (a commonly shared view of phenomena with which members are interested – 'a map of the territory') and values (deeply held convictions pertaining to the rights of those served and the obligations of the practitioner).'

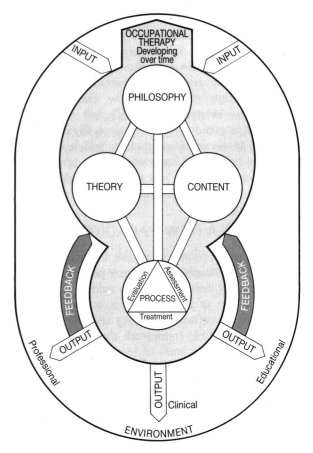

Figure 3.1 A paradigm of occupational therapy. (Reproduced from Creek 1990 Occupational therapy and mental health, with permission.)

This core is surrounded by a layer of conceptual practice models. 'The paradigm is a global vision, and the models are practical attempts to implement that vision in practice.' The paradigm and practice models interact, but the paradigm is relatively stable, the models being continually mutable. An outer sphere of related knowledge surrounds the whole and feeds into the practice models (Fig. 3.2). Kielhofner also describes a paradigm shift, which will be explained shortly.

This view of a professional paradigm is echoed by Young and Quinn (1992) who propose an inner 'hard core' for the profession, composed of professional knowledge, values, authority, limits, and nature of practice. This is surrounded by the

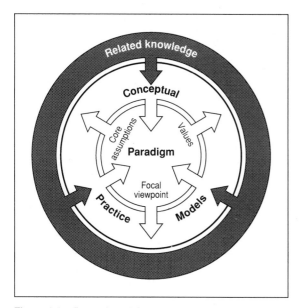

Figure 3.2 Dynamics of the knowledge base. (Adapted from Kielhofner 1992 Conceptual foundations of occupational therapy, with permission.)

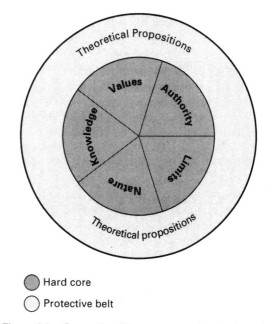

Figure 3.3 Occupational therapy core and protective belt. (Reproduced from Young & Quinn 1992 Theories and practice of occupational therapy, with permission.)

changeable theoretical propositions which inform practice and which are gradually tested, accepted or discarded (Fig. 3.3).

In a review of basic theoretical structures (Hagedorn 1992) I illustrated the relationships between the core of the profession, its theoretical concepts, the environment affecting client, therapist and service delivery, and the elements which feed the development of new ideas or practice (Fig. 3.4).

It is clear that we are all trying, in our own way, to express the same concept; that of a central core (or paradigm) surrounded by a belt of frames of reference or models, informed by related knowledge, research, values and experience, and responsive to or adapted by the environment of professional practice. Thus there does seem to be an emerging academic concensus that there is a core – but is the content of this core stable or evolving, and should it be described as a paradigm?

Kielhofner (1992) takes a Kuhnian view and argues that we have passed through two paradigm shifts in the history of the profession and are engaged in a third. The first paradigm

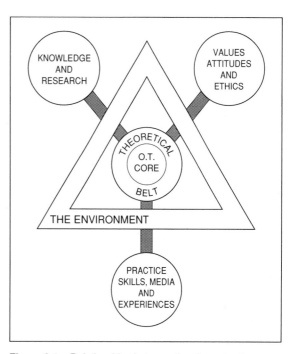

Figure 3.4 Relationships between the elements of professional practice.

was that of occupation, focusing on its central importance to human life and health and the potentially remedial effects of engagement in selected occupations. The second paradigm was mechanistic, in which occupational therapy was effectively subverted by the medical model, adopted a largely reductionist approach and attempted to become scientific.

Following the crisis during which this was rejected the evolving paradigm returned to the occupational basis of the profession, but with a more sophisticated understanding of the links between environment and occupation, and between occupational meanings and personal actualization and well-being.

Mocellin (1992b) is critical of this view and writes:

There are problems in applying the Kuhnian notion of paradigm to occupational therapy . . . The conservatism and tunnel vision essential to adherence to a paradigm conflict with the extreme flexibility of occupational therapy, both in its beliefs and theoretical choices and in the use of these in education and clinical practice.

He points to the evolutionary, syncretist nature of the development of occupational therapy practice and theory; this is incompatible with the idea of paradigm shift which is, by definition, a sudden and total change.

Having practised throughout most of the period during which Kielhofner describes these shifts as occurring, I accept that these changes did occur, as described in Chapter 1. However, like Mocellin, I remain unconvinced that we have really seen two paradigm shifts in such a comparatively short space of time. I am also uncomfortable with the very prescriptive idea of a scientific paradigm; indeed the urge to borrow this concept seems to be the academic equivalent of the urge to find 'validity' which led to the mechanistic versions of practice which Kielhofner rejects. My own hypothesis is that we do have a stable core of philosophy and practice, but that this is a paradigm only (if at all) in the less prescriptive sense of being a pattern.

I view this core as organic in nature, and therefore able to evolve. It is organic because it reflects the ideas, values and culture of the societies in which therapists practise, and of therapists who are themselves changing organisms. The core is not sealed. Like a cell, it has selectively permeable boundaries, which define the area of enclosure and permit the entrance and exit of material.

In a scientific paradigm the boundary is impermeable. Once punctured the whole structure disintegrates to be replaced by another. In the case of the occupational therapy core, there is an inner philosophical nucleus which contains, the 'genetic pattern' of occupational therapy: its central components and concerns. This changes only very slowly, if at all. The outer rings contain the principles, purposes and processes of therapy, and these can more readily accept material from the theoretical belt outside the core.

When there is a balance of pressures on each side of the boundary, i.e. when the contents of the core and of the belt are in harmony, there is little transmission of material across the boundaries. However, pressure tends to build up on the outside of a barrier, in the form of a strong new idea or theory, a new discovery, a change in knowledge or new practice.

Once this pressure is strong enough, a new idea is able to filter through. Such new material first enters the theoretical belt and then, if the pressure is sufficient, progresses through the outer layers of the core. The selective quality of the boundary usually ensures that only relevant and compatible material is allowed to enter. However, occupational therapists are notorious for accepting and including new ideas and methods in their practice, which may imply that the present boundary 'membrane' is a rather crude and insufficiently discriminating filter. Therapists are also reluctant to throw anything away, be it an object or a concept, in case it 'comes in useful'; this has resulted in some parts of the core becoming unduly cluttered.

Sometimes the new material fits so neatly with the core that it becomes totally integrated, and we may feel that it has always been there, reinterpreting former ideas in the light of new knowledge; humanistic and cognitive psychology are good examples. At other times the material is recognized as 'foreign' to the occupational therapy organism and is expelled, as a cell might eject an unwelcome bacterium, as was the case with the invasion of strong mechanistic ideology during the 1970s.

An inherited problem which makes the core of occupational therapy vulnerable to unwanted inclusions is that the core was imperfectly described from the outset, leading to uncertainties concerning its boundaries.

During the 1970s the belt was invaded by some powerful medical model and scientific concepts which in turn moved into the core. These concepts were not universally accepted, however, and they were ultimately questioned and rejected by therapists who sought to restore the boundaries.

This coincided with yet another invasion from the periphery during the 1980s, which concerned the profession's need for a sound academic basis and defined paradigm. At the same time in the USA there was a call for a return to 'the original thinking'.

The knowledge that the cause of uncertainty stems from the failure to define the original core has now led to efforts to redefine it; inevitably, these incorporate current language and concepts. It is certainly possible to detect theoretical oscillation but, if we are to use the word paradigm, perhaps what occurred was a 'paradigm wobble' rather than a paradigm shift, which would demand the replacement of the entire structure.

By viewing the core as organic and capable of change by inclusion or expulsion we are able to see the profession as capable of evolution and development in a continuous cycle, rather than through a series of abrupt crises. There is, however, a more subtle, but equally fundamental change in perspective implicit in this whole process. As an occupational therapy student in the early 1960s, I was taught facts, procedures, skills and techniques. I was trained primarily to 'do' – to perform as a therapist. Neither I nor my contemporaries recall being required to 'think', to criticise, reflect or challenge the received wisdom and practices; indeed, I retain an impression that this was discouraged!

Students currently receiving degree-level professional education, while still acquiring competencies are now actively encouraged to think about what they are doing, and to take a critical approach to both personal practice and the theoretical basis of the profession.

It has become accepted that therapists write books exploring the philosophy, theories and fundamental principles of occupational therapy, and not simply the application of techniques to specific disorders. It is easy to forget that this approach was extremely rare in Britain before 1980, and to overlook the very important and complex underlying changes in professional attitudes and practices.

I am uncertain whether this is a shift in professional education or in practice as a whole, but it does seem highly significant, and it reflects the creation of a model of education which is so radically different that it might even qualify as a paradigm shift. Indeed educators, like physicists, were left at the end of the 1980s with competing paradigms.

Perhaps this is another example of the invasion of the core by strongly defined ideas, stemming originally from the field of education, but now filtering through to affect practice. There has been an undeniable change in perspective from the performance of practice skills to the exploration of the rationale of the profession, and the coincidence of views from independent authors described earlier lends weight to the idea of an active, but incomplete, attempt to redefine the core.

If the result of this process is that we can, finally, 'say what we do' and make our boundaries clearer and more selectively permeable, it would be welcomed by both the profession and its users and colleagues. If, on the other hand, the result is further contemplation and obscure academic writing, it will be counterproductive; we would be better engaged in providing therapy and conducting research until a full understanding is achieved.

THE CONTENT OF THE CORE

In my recent explorations, which began with a desire to become familiar with the content of the theoretical belt, I have found myself drawn inexorably away from this periphery and towards an examination of the content of the core; particularly of the ways in which the core and belt interact in practice through the medium of clinical reasoning.

The consensus of opinion on core content currently includes the elements listed in Box 3.1.

Of the elements in Box 3.1, the core components seem the most significant, for they define the philosophy of the profession and the territory to which the remaining elements relate. Values concerning these elements influence strongly the nature of practice and mould the formation of core assumptions. These then draw relevant knowledge into the core, and lead to the purposes of therapy. These principles and purposes produce processes whereby the goals of occupational therapy may be achieved. Each element of the core reacts with every other element in a continual and dynamic dialogue.

There is plainly much work to be done in defining these core elements, for the practical and academic life of the profession cannot progress in a continuing conceptual haze. This book is an attempt to share my personal explorations and hypotheses, with especial reference to core components and core processes.

THE CORE COMPONENTS OF OCCUPATIONAL THERAPY

In order for therapy to take place, four central components are required: the person in need of therapy, the therapist providing it, the occupational focus of it, and a suitable environment relating to each of these components.

These core elements remain constant, despite the changes in perspective and emphasis offered by the various models and frames of reference contained in the belt. These are, to return to the simile of the cell, the 'genetic pattern' for occupational therapy contained in the 'nucleus' of the core. If any part of the core is to be considered a paradigm, it is this central nucleus.

Stewart (1992) proposed a saltire-shaped model to illustrate this point (Fig. 3.5), and stated:

The key components of the occupational therapy process are first of all the client with his or her needs, abilities and aspirations; secondly the therapist, who, through establishing rapport and applying professional judgement selects and modifies as necessary the third element – the activities which form part of the programme of intervention . . . fourthly . . . the influences of the environment, both physical and human have to be taken into account.

She continues:

We end up with a very simple diagram of what in reality is a complicated interaction between these four components . . . The mission is simple, let us not be apologetic about it. The means of achieving it are infinitely varied, which is perhaps why occupational therapists find it so hard to describe what they do.

Polatajko (1992) lists 'the three essential elements of the discipline: the individual, human life and occupations', and adds that 'individuals are social beings and are shaped by their environment'.

Box 3.1	The core of occupational therapy
Core components	The central content of practice and a definition of its goals, concerns and limits
Core values	The fundamental values and ethics
Core assumptions	The fundamental beliefs and premises
Core knowledge	The academic and research basis of the profession
Core purposes	The general objectives and intentions of therapy
Core processes	The means whereby occupational therapy is organized and provided to an individual and the framework for the development of core skills.

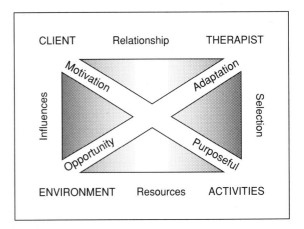

Figure 3.5 A model of practice. (Adapted from Stewart 1992, with permission.)

She uses the three dimensions of individual, occupation and environment in her occupational competence model. Vercruysse (1994) similarly constructs a central triad consisting of the person, the therapist and the medium.

This is another example of parallel development of theory, for Polatajko's ideas resemble closely several of my own which I had been working on since 1991. The subject of Vercruysse's presentation at the World Federation of Occupational Therapists (WFOT) Congress in 1994 also bore a remarkable resemblance to the central triad which I had already defined (Hagedorn 1992). I had concluded that the central relationship in occupational therapy is not a dyad, but a *triad*, 'person, therapist, occupation', which operates within an environment.

The core content of the profession must, therefore, relate to these four elements. Occupational therapy can be conceptualized as a dynamic entity which occurs at the interface of these elements, *and only when all are present* (Fig. 3.7).

In terms of symbolism it may be worth noting that the triad is globally acknowledged as more complete and more powerful than the dyad. Dyads are a primitive symbol of intense emotion, of either love or, more often, dualistic conflict or confrontation. Triads, on the other hand, symbolize power and completeness, a dynamic balance of forces whether complementary or opposite (Father, Son and Holy Spirit; Brahma, Vishnu, Shiva; maiden, mother, crone; child, parent, adult). The occupational therapy triadic interaction can be more complete and balanced than a dyadic one, the occupational element balancing the dyadic interaction.

When the three central elements are placed in an interactive environment, this dynamic, triadic, relationship begins; this is the unique feature of occupational therapy. As in a chemical reaction, all three elements must be present for occupational therapy to occur, the therapist is the catalyst which binds the other elements into the reaction.

Most significantly, if one of these elements is removed, occupational therapy cannot happen. It is of course obvious that one must have both a person in need of therapy and a therapist. Some kind of environment is bound to be present – nothing occurs in a vacuum – the important

feature of therapy is how the environment is viewed, used or adapted. However, what of the occupation? I assert that if this element is removed, whatever is happening may still be therapy, but *it is not occupational therapy*. Put simply, occupational therapy is like a three-legged stool; take one leg away and the stool falls over and ceases to be a stool (Fig. 3.6).

This does not mean that occupation must always be applied as a therapy in which the patient is actively engaged. It is sometimes better to describe the therapist as providing or facilitating 'intervention' (action on behalf of or with the client) rather than 'therapy' (treatment of the patient). However, the dialogue with the person (patient/client) must include occupational concerns, explore relevant occupational difficulties and competencies, and relate to that person as a performer of occupations in a particular physical and sociocultural environment. In addition, the occupational elements must remain in focus during the whole process of therapy.

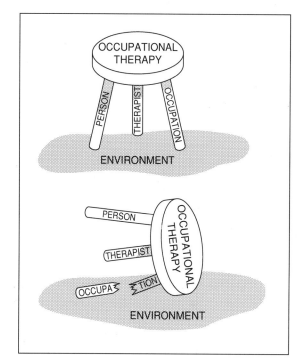

Figure 3.6 The 'occupational therapy stool' and the stool broken.

Therefore, occupational therapists *who spend the majority of their time* utilizing skills which are not occupationally referenced, such as counselling, non-activity related group work, facilitatory positioning without subsequent functional performance, activities which provide exercise but which lack productivity or purpose, *are not working within the terms of reference of the profession for which they trained.* I am happy to accept a definition of 'activity' that includes subjective and experiential elements, not just objective 'products', but I firmly reject the notion of an optional 'occupational frame of reference' located externally to the core within the theoretical belt. 'Occupation' belongs within the central core, it is not an optional extra.

Whether or not you are prepared to accept this controversial statement, it is made as a necessary justification of the way in which the content of the following chapters are arranged; they provide an exploration of past and current perspectives on the four elements already described, and, of these, occupations will receive the largest share of attention.

As shown in Figure 3.7, the central core on which the philosophy of therapy is based can be presented as a triangle linking the person, occupation and therapist, surrounded by environment, which affects all three.

This triangle has three axes. On the base of the triangle is person/environment/therapist (P–E–T). This indicates the importance of the therapeutic relationship within a suitable environment. It also deals with relationships between people within the environment. The focus of this axis is interaction.

On the left of the figure the axis links person/environment/occupation. This relates to the central importance of the person as an active agent within the environment, adapting and using it by means of occupations and activities, and in return being shaped by both environment and occupations. The focus of this axis is competence.

On the right of the figure the axis links therapist/environment/occupation. This represents the focus on the therapist's use of occupations, activities and environments to provide therapy, and on the therapist's intervention in these areas.

The core thus represents three statements concerning the central philosophy of occupational therapy:

1. Occupational therapy involves a therapist and a patient in a dynamic interaction which has an occupational focus within a given environment.

2. A person is a unique individual, interactive with, and influenced by, the social and physical environment. A person attains competence in a range of roles, occupations and activities. Through competent performance the person experiences identity and effects changes in the environment for her personal health, satisfaction, and well-being. The environment affects the nature of and necessity for the performance of roles, occupations and activities.

3. The therapist can, by using or adapting roles, occupations, activities or environments, intervene to enable or enhance a person's performance, to remove or minimize dysfunction, to empower personal autonomy and to enable the person to achieve an enhanced sense of well-being, positive meaning, and quality of life.

The four core components in turn give rise to associated core values, assumptions and knowledge – the principles of the profession.

CORE PRINCIPLES: VALUES, ASSUMPTIONS AND KNOWLEDGE

The central triad extends its influence outwards through the core. Each axis gives rise to a segment in which the primary themes are developed and expanded, and finally translated into action.

The core values, assumptions and knowledge of the profession relate to people, occupations, environments, therapists and therapy. Together these represent the guiding principles of the profession (see centre of Fig. 3.10 on page 36).

Values

A value is a cluster of emotions and beliefs concerning an object or individual. A value forms the affective/cognitive part of an attitude which leads to consequent action. Professional

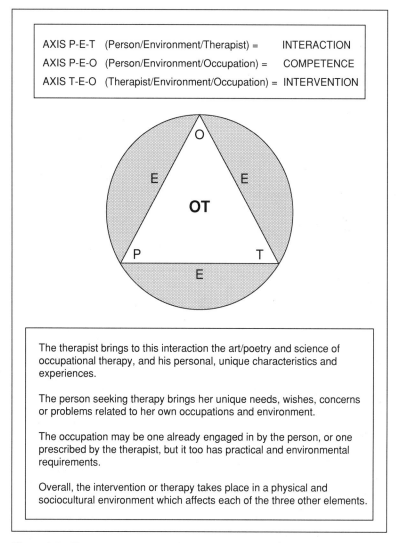

AXIS P-E-T (Person/Environment/Therapist) = INTERACTION
AXIS P-E-O (Person/Environment/Occupation) = COMPETENCE
AXIS T-E-O (Therapist/Environment/Occupation) = INTERVENTION

The therapist brings to this interaction the art/poetry and science of occupational therapy, and his personal, unique characteristics and experiences.

The person seeking therapy brings her unique needs, wishes, concerns or problems related to her own occupations and environment.

The occupation may be one already engaged in by the person, or one prescribed by the therapist, but it too has practical and environmental requirements.

Overall, the intervention or therapy takes place in a physical and sociocultural environment which affects each of the three other elements.

Figure 3.7 The core components of occupational therapy: the central triad.

values form 'the deeply held convictions of the discipline which pertain to the rights of those served and the obligations of the practitioner. They define what ought to be done in practice' (Kielhofner 1992). Values, like attitudes, may be positive or negative, but the emphasis tends to be on those which are positive. A value often has a moral, ethical or philosophical basis, concerning what is considered right, good, just or desirable. Once formed, a value-expressive attitude is slow to change.

Over the past decade, since the production of Yerxa's list of values (1980), there has been an active attempt to produce a code of values which the whole profession can use. Values are discussed by, e.g. Yerxa (1983), Kielhofner (1992), Polatajko (1992) and Turner (1992). All texts on the philosophy and theory of occupational therapy make value statements, either implicitly or explicitly.

Values are viewed as a means of unifying the profession, providing a unique professional identity, and promoting coherent practice. Our values have a fundamental effect on what we do as therapists, leading us to select or reject theories, assumptions, and actions. Values influence clinical reasoning. (Fondillar et al 1990, Fleming 1993).

Box 3.2 summarizes some of the main values listed or discussed in recent literature in relation to the three segments of the core.

Values concerning people, occupations and environments relate to culture. The therapist must therefore reinterpret these when occupational therapy is practised in a particular culture, or is related to a person of a different culture than the one in which the therapist practises. The skill of the therapist lies in the

---

Box 3.2 Values of occupational therapists

Segment P-E-T (person/environment/therapist)
Occupational therapists value:
1. The uniqueness of each person.
2. The intrinsic dignity and worth of each person.
3. The individual's right to autonomy and all other human rights.
4. Respect for each person's ethnic, social, cultural and religious background and beliefs.
5. The subjective perspective of the individual.
6. Life experiences which have meaning for the individual.
7. Life which offers both quality and quantity of experience to everyone including those who are handicapped or otherwise disadvantaged.
8. Each person's need for satisfying personal and social relationships.
9. A therapeutic relationship of active partnership and mutual cooperation – working with the client to identify the need for, and goals of, therapy or intervention.
10. The potential of each individual, and her adaptive capacity for change.
11. The person's capacity for choice, self-direction and responsibility.
12. A view of the person which takes full account of physical, emotional, cognitive, social and environmental factors.
13. Each person's right to the maintenance and enhancement of health.
14. The person as an active agent in promoting her recovery from or adaptation to illness, trauma, disability, handicap, dysfunction or other disadvantage.

Segment P-E-D (person/environment/occupation)
Occupational therapists value:
1. Occupations, activities and roles as essential components of human life.
2. The differing contributions which work, leisure, play, self-care and rest make to a person's life.
3. The capacity of a person to acquire skills, abilities and competencies, and the contribution which occupations, activities and environments make to this process.
4. The capacity of a person to take control of her life by means of occupations and activities.
5. The experience of meaning in life and of personal identity provided by engagement in occupations or activities.

6. Personal capacity for productive creativity through the use of mind and hands.
7. The ways in which individuals can act to shape and control their environment, rather than being controlled by it.
8. The role of the environment in providing a person with opportunities.
9. The role of the environment in enhancing quality of life.

Segment T-E-D (therapist/environment/occupation)
Occupational therapists value:
1. Employing their personal traits, abilities and competencies in service to the client.
2. The use of their accumulated experience and clinical judgement in partnership with the client.
3. The provision of high quality service, meeting professional standards and producing consumer satisfaction.
4. Having the necessary time and resources to provide a quality service.
5. Having, maintaining, and seeking to increase professional knowledge and methodology.
6. The maintenance of professional ethics and standards of behaviour including adherence to moral and legal principles, objectivity, honesty, integrity and confidentiality.
7. The ability to exercise self-discipline and sound judgement in action.
8. A dedicated, responsible attitude to the welfare of others.
9. The ability to act as advisor to and advocate for the client.
10. Positive supportive relationships with colleagues.
11. Positive action to seek personal support and supervision.
12. The potential of occupation/activity to enable, enhance and empower the life of the client.
13. The potential of the environment to enable or enhance performance.
14. The unique contribution which occupational and environmental adaptation can make to the life of the client.
15. A positive expectation of the outcomes of intervention.
16. Evaluation, reflection and research as aids to the development of practice.

ability to undertake such interpretation for/with a client, rather than imposing upon her some predetermined cultural norm. This is one of the factors which renders a tightly defined paradigm inappropriate for occupational therapy, for a paradigm permits of no interpretation (Mocellin 1992).

Assumptions

An assumption is a statement which is accepted as being true for the purpose of argument or action (COD). There may be scientific evidence for this, or the assumption may be based on a theory or hypothesis which is acted upon, tested and modified. Much of the practice of occupational therapy is based on assumptions about the nature of people, occupations and environments and the practice of occupational therapy. Values and assumptions are closely linked and help to shape each other.

There is no agreed list of the central assumptions of occupational therapy. Some authors (e.g. Reed & Sanderson 1983, Mosey 1986, Cynkin & Robinson 1990, Turner 1992) have described their personal view of assumptions, but these inevitably become coloured by the writer's model or frame of reference.

American texts frequently quote Reilly's central assumption 'that man, through the use of his hands as they are energized by mind and will can influence the state of his own health' (Reilly 1962). There are, however, many differing assumptions concerning how this may take place. For this reason, assumptions concerning the four core components are discussed and summarized in the following chapters.

Knowledge

Knowledge encompasses the theoretical and practical understanding on which practice is based. It includes facts, information, explanations and theories, in other words, knowing *about* things.

Epistemologists (those who study the nature of knowledge) make a precise distinction between various levels and types of knowledge. To incor-

porate these in a simple model of the core would only confuse; however, knowledge in the sense of 'knowing about' needs to be distinguished from methodology, which is 'knowing what should be done and how to organize it', and procedural knowledge which is 'knowing how to do it'.

In a practice-based profession such as occupational therapy, 'knowing what and knowing how' are related to our understanding of the processes of therapy, or of various approaches or models of practice. This type of understanding forms the outer ring of the core, and is augmented by the content of the theoretical belt.

The form of knowledge which exists in the inner layer of the core is 'knowing about'. This concerns the basic study of people, occupations and environments. An unnecessary amount of anxiety has been caused over the fact that this knowledge base is not unique to occupational therapy. What may prove to be unique, (once the content of the core is properly defined) is the precise combination of the elements of knowledge and the conclusions which the profession draws from this amalgam. This is a case where the whole is certain to be different from the sum of its parts.

One difficulty encountered in defining this knowledge lies in distinguishing between what should be inside the core, and what is outside, either within the theoretical belt, or excluded completely. Knowledge from many frames of reference has been incorporated into the core (e.g. humanistic psychology, cognitive psychology, developmental theories, physiology), yet these same theories are also presented as options located outside the core as frames of reference in the theoretical belt.

Knowledge has a habit of being added frequently to the core, while subtraction is far rarer. Some of the knowledge base of the profession therefore is internally inconsistent or inconsistent with values and assumptions.

It would be an impractical task, in our current state of understanding of the core content to attempt to make a firm distinction between included and excluded knowledge. In general, core knowledge is related to an organismic, phenomenological, positive relativistic view of reality, but it is too simplistic to use this as a touchstone for rejecting all views which are based on determinism, scientific realism or logical empiricism.

Knowledge is focused on understanding and explaining the associated facts and phenomena. There is no single view of these things, although a consensus may be developing. The literature contains a variety of perspectives – retrospective, current and prospective. By exploring these in relation to the core components of person, therapist, occupation and environment, some of the underlying knowledge base of the profession becomes more explicit.

Summary of core principles

To conclude the discussion of this layer of the core, it seems that it is now possible to make a generally acceptable, though still not universally agreed, list of professional values. This is a considerable step forwards, for it provides the benchmark for the critical evaluation of other principles.

Despite considerable discussion, assumptions and knowledge cannot yet be stated with certainty. Further academic work is needed to achieve a defined statement of these essential core principles, and to confirm the content which should, or should not, reside in the core. It is likely that central assumptions will be agreed in time. Agreement on core knowledge, however, may prove more difficult.

It is possible that, if we wish to retain a knowledge base derived from multiple frames of reference and their associated assumptions, these would be better placed in the theoretical belt, leaving only the philosophy and values of practice within the core. Alternatively, the most applicable frames of reference may move into the core, leaving a smaller theoretical belt containing other optional frames of reference and alternative models of practice.

The fact that there is such uncertainty helps to explain why therapists find it difficult to explain the principles of their profession, and why the core is still vulnerable to invasion by inappropriate assumptions or knowledge.

CORE PURPOSES

No meaningful action can take place without a purpose. Purposes are cognitive constructs which define the intentions and consequent objectives which are to be translated into action; they concern 'what one means to do' and 'why one means to do it'. Purposeless action is merely random and unproductive use of energy. Purposes focus action to use the available energy economically to achieve a desired result.

Occupational therapy has three purposes: enabling, enhancing and empowering.

1. To enable means to improve or extend ability. This may be a new ability, or one which the person had, but has now lost. The person may be enabled by her own skills and endeavours, or by alterations, to remove barriers to the performance of activities or the use of the environment.

2. To enhance means to heighten or intensify. Skills may, through practice, be enhanced. The content of environment may be altered and intensified to provide interest or enjoyment. Perceptions of objects, people or experiences may be heightened by appropriate intervention. Quality of life may be enhanced through pleasurable experiences, relationships and activities. A person's self-concept may be enhanced through engagement in meaningful activity.

3. To empower means to provide a person with the means to become autonomous, to claim her rights, and to exercise active control of her own life in a responsive and responsible relationship with others.

These purposes form the third layer (Fig. 3.8). They serve to coordinate action which is carried out through the processes in the outer ring. They are compatible, and may simultaneously inform and direct action. These are the purposes of occupational therapy, and thus, of the therapist. They must also be related to the purposes of the patient/client, who, although she may not choose to use such language, seeks help from the therapist in order to become more able to do things, more in control of his life, or more fulfilled by personal activity and environment.

These purposes imply the need for action: if the client does not share the perception of this

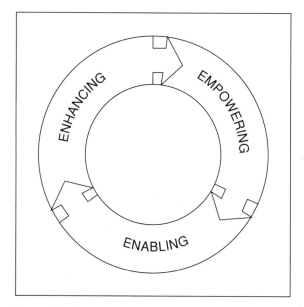

Figure 3.8 Core purposes.

need, therapy or intervention cannot take place. It is not uncommon for the first stage of an intervention to be directed towards enabling a person to accept the purposes of therapy as related to her own life.

This section concerning a conceptual model of the core of occupational therapy was written in 1993, before publication of the position statement of the College of Occupational Therapists (COT). It is interesting to compare it with the COT document which states the philosophy of occupational therapy and the framework for practice as follows:

Philosophy of occupational therapy

Occupational therapy promotes and restores health and well-being of people of all ages through using purposeful occupation, as the process or as the ultimate goal.

In this context occupation is the meaningful use of activities, occupations, skills and life roles which enable people to function purposefully in their daily life.

Framework for practice

The central values and beliefs of occupational therapy are that people with disabilities are valued as people

with physical, emotional intellectual social and spiritual needs.

Occupational therapists use their core skills to enable and empower people to make choices and to achieve a personally acceptable lifestyle, with the goal of maximising health and function.

(College of Occupational Therapists 1994)
The similarity in views and terminology provides further evidence of a developing consensus concerning the core philosophy, principles and practice of the profession.

CORE PROCESSES

In most occupational therapy texts the terms 'occupational therapy process' or 'treatment planning process' are used to describe a process which I prefer to call 'case management'. My rejection of a widely-used term needs justification. First, I believe that occupational therapy has several core processes, and it is therefore inaccurate to refer to case management as *the* occupational therapy process, implying that there is only one.

Secondly, and more fundamentally, it is not a unique *occupational therapy* process, since it is based primarily on problem-solving/analysis, which is adopted by other health-related professions in very similar formats. The 'treatment planning process' (Trombley 1989) is a more accurate description, but treatment planning is only part of the process, which is usually conceptualized as including information gathering, planning, implementation and evaluation. I will therefore use the term 'case management'.

Case management, which includes clinical reasoning and problem analysis forms the inner layer of the fourth ring of the core. The remaining processes form the final, outer layer (Fig. 3.9). These six processes are related to the three segments of the core, however they, like the rest of the core, interact in a manner too complex to be indicated on a simple two-dimensional figure.

The case management process is the central, organizational process whereby a client or patient is accepted for intervention or therapy, decisions are taken about what is to be done, the

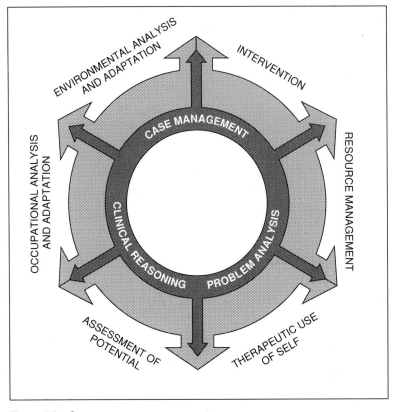

Figure 3.9 Core processes.

other core processes are integrated and employed, and the selected intervention proceeds until it is considered to have been completed. This may be viewed as a linear process or as a circular one.

The process provides both a sequence for action and a framework for problem analysis and clinical reasoning, which are inseparable parts of case management. Clinical reasoning occurs at each stage in the process and is the means whereby, through the knowledge, judgement, skills and experience of the therapist, the generic core of the profession becomes applicable to the unique situation and needs of an individual.

A crucial point in the case management process is the selection of a suitable model or frame of reference. All subsequent action and conceptualization depends on this. The effects of taking this decision at different points in time have fundamental consequences, and exploration of these differences can illuminate the complex

relationship between core concepts and the theoretical belt, which will be described shortly.

The process of case management serves to integrate and organize the other core processes of occupational therapy. These are processes which are either unique to the profession, or which the profession employs in a particular manner which is determined by the principles, purposes and practice of occupational therapy.

The core processes of occupational therapy are illustrated in Box 3.3.

These processes are discussed and described in Part 2. A central proposition in this view of the core processes is that they are fundamentally generic, involving the acquisition of core skills, knowledge and attitudes. This raises the question of whether there is a difference between core skills and core processes.

The list of 'core skills' (COT 1994) defines the unique core skills of occupational therapy as

---

Box 3.3   Core processes

- Case management including problem analysis and clinical reasoning
- Assessment and evaluation of individual potential
- Occupational analysis and adaptation
- Environmental analysis and adaptation
- Therapeutic use of self
- Implementation of therapy/intervention
- Resource management.

---

occupational and environment adaptation and analysis. These have been included as processes in Box 3.3. Further core skills for practice are listed, related to these unique skills, including enabling, prophylaxis, education, therapeutic intervention, advocacy, support for carers, adaptation, partnership with other care providers, and the ability to influence social policy and legislation.

The COT's definition of skill is 'expert knowledge. A craft or accomplishment; to make a difference'. However, the definition continues: 'Related to the paradigm of occupational therapy the core skills are the expert knowledge at the heart of the profession' (COT 1994), which resembles my concept of process. Indeed, the practice skills described are necessarily generic, and more like statements of processes or parameters for service provision.

In this text the use of the term 'skill' has been rejected because at this level of description I believe we are dealing with a more complex level of performance. The process describes what happens; the skill describes a particular instance of the applied use of knowledge, skill and attitudes.

Core skills certainly exist, but at a lower level of analysis. For example, occupational analysis is a process, but breaking down an activity into tasks is an activity which requires core skills – some of very many such skills which the therapist will acquire during his professional education.

In view of the difficulty of making a comprehensive list at this level, it may be questioned whether it is practical to enumerate core skills, and the associated competencies, except in the context of educational documents – and even

here there is a divergence of opinion over the usefulness of such listing. However, with our current state of knowledge, it seems that the use of either term is legitimate provided that the subject matter is the same in each case.

Whatever the semantic quibbles, a consensus does now appear to be emerging over the unique processes/skills of the profession. It is also clear that practice must remain true to the core, for if, in applying a theoretical structure, the therapist loses sight of the core philosophy, principles and purposes he is in risk of moving away from the practice of occupational therapy. It is precisely this loss of focus which has caused the 'wobbles' to which I referred earlier.

THE CORE OF OCCUPATIONAL THERAPY

It is now possible to present a conceptual model of the whole core, which indicates how the central components influence what is both known and believed by therapists, and also how the purposes and processes of therapy, as integrated by the process of case management, are related to these components (Fig. 3.10).

The central 'nucleus' contains the four components: person, occupation, environment and therapist. This is the philosophical core which gives rise to three segments in each of which occurs a differing combination of the core elements. These segments concern competent action, interaction and the provision of therapy/ intervention.

The first ring beyond the 'nucleus' contains the values, assumptions and knowledge of the profession – the core principles on which practice is based.

The second ring contains the central purposes of occupational therapy: enabling, enhancing and empowering.

The third ring contains the organizing process of case management and the processes of clinical reasoning and problem analysis through which the intervention or therapy is applied to a specific client or patient. The outer ring contains the remaining processes of therapy.

There are many more interconnections than

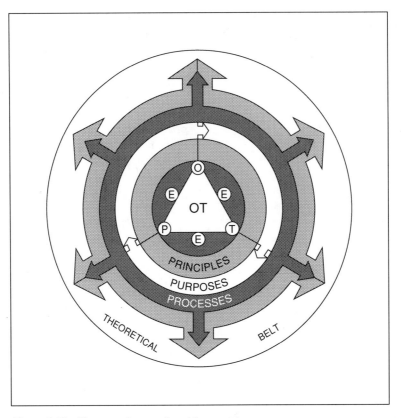

Figure 3.10 The core of occupational therapy.

can be shown here, but Figure 3.10 illustrates those which are most significant.

The theoretical belt is the layer beyond this core.

THE THEORETICAL BELT

The theoretical belt surrounds the core and contains the additional theories and methods which therapists have borrowed, synthesized or found useful. The core contains theory, as does the belt. The problem is that we have at present only a hazy definition of which theories are inside and which are outside the core. This problem is compounded by the fact that some theories – those derived from the humanistic frame of reference are good examples – seem to be both within the core *and* available as options within the belt.

The theories within the belt, although closely related to the core, are separate from it because, unlike the core content which is axiomatic and pervasive, the content of the belt represents options which may be selected by the therapist to fit a particular situation or to provide a specific focus for therapy.

The therapist's knowledge of the core theory forms his identity and action as a practising therapist. He then selects from the belt the theory which fits the problem of the client or is appropriate to his interests, expertise, or practice location. So, for example, he will be continually aware of the humanistic, client-centred nature of therapy and perception of the individual, which is an integral part of the profession. In addition, he will be aware that, if he encounters a patient who needs it, he may draw upon the humanistic frame of reference to provide a more overtly client-centred approach, or techniques of teaching, counselling or psychotherapy.

Although the belt is called 'theoretical' for the sake of convenience, it has two layers: theoretical and practical (Fig. 3.11). The inner, theoretical layer contains the conceptual structures – models and frames of reference – which provide the cognitive and organizational framework for therapy guiding the interpretation of data, analysis of data and synthesis of therapy. The outer, practical layer contains the means of application – approaches which provide assessments, techniques, methods, a style of relationship, relevant media and all the practicalities required to conduct therapy or intervention.

A simplified version of the total model of the core and belt is shown in Figure 3.12.

THEORETICAL STRUCTURES

The discussion of theory is yet another area that is bedevilled by semantics. Is there or is there

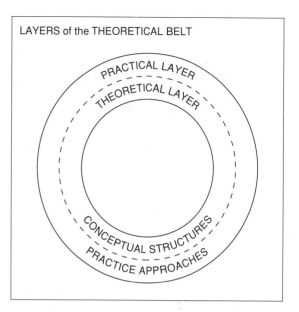

Figure 3.11   Layers of the theoretical belt.

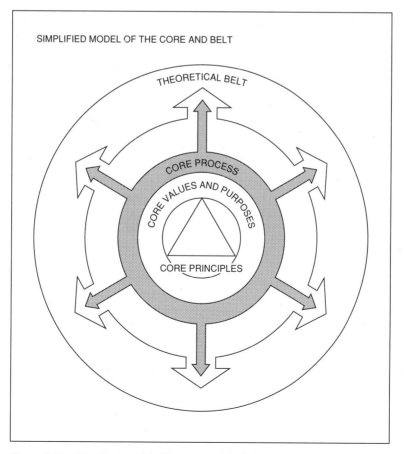

Figure 3.12   Simplified model of the core and the belt.

not any difference between models, frames of reference and approaches? Although everyone is agreed that there is a definable theoretical basis for the profession, there seem to be almost as many opinions over the ways in which this should be described or structured as there are theoreticians.

Again, the debate over terminology obscures the understanding of the basic issues, rather than illuminating them; yet words do need to be defined in order to avoid confusions.

Of the three terms defined below, 'approach' seems to be least controversial. The difficulty lies in deciding if there is a difference between models and frames of reference, and if so, which theories should fit into which category.

Frame of reference

A system of theories serving to orient or give particular meaning to a set of circumstances, which provides a coherent conceptual basis for therapy.

Frames of reference are derived from knowledge which is *external* to occupational therapy, and typically provide an explanation of a single view of human identity, psychology, or action, e.g. physiological, behavioural, psychodynamic or cognitive, developmental and humanistic.

The confusion between these and models arises because therapists then interpret this basic theory in the context of occupational therapy, and create applied frames of reference, or approaches, which give details of how treatment should be provided, including relevant assessments and techniques, in relation to a specific theory or set of concepts about therapy or the individual in a defined clinical setting.

Approach

Ways and means of putting theory into practice.

An approach is derived from a frame of reference, but may be used in isolation, or within the organizing context of a model. Selection of an approach leads the therapist to use particular assessments, treatment techniques or style of relationship appropriate to the needs of the patient/client (e.g. biomechanical approach, client-centred approach).

Model

A simplified representation of the structure and content of a phenomenon or system that describes or explains the complex relationships between concepts within the system and integrates elements of theory and practice.

This is perhaps the most controversial term. Mosey (1981) avoids the use of 'model', and writes of 'frames of reference'. Reed (1984), on the other hand, avoids the use of the term 'frame of reference' and describes numerous models under the headings metamodels, supermodels, health and rehabilitation models, occupational therapy models – generic, descriptive, parameter. As she states, models do appear to cluster in related areas, but how should these clusters be defined? However hard one tries to provide a taxonomy something fails to fit, or classifications proliferate to an unmanageable degree.

My view is that there is a fine, but useful, distinction to be made between models and frames of reference. A frame of reference provides the cognitive 'conceptual lens' which focuses on the patient and enables the therapist subsequently to put into practice an approach consisting of appropriate and compatible techniques. It might equally be described as providing 'blinkers' or 'tunnel vision', for it also limits greatly the scope of view.

A model is a more comprehensive entity, the essential function of which is the integration of a 'basket' of different ideas about people and their occupations, within a concept of occupational therapy, It is this integrative nature of models which is the chief means of distinguishing them from frames of reference. A model usually tries to explain 'life, the universe, and everything' in one coherent whole, whereas a frame of reference gives a unified but narrow view of a particular aspect of human function.

There are two types of models.

Integrative occupational therapy models give explanations of humans as occupational beings in relation to their environment, and of the therapeutic benefits of occupation. Such a model typically coordinates philosophy and theory to provide a coherent and comprehensive description of the individual, a concept of function and dysfunction, and an indication of how the model may be used in practice (Creek 1992). It suggests, implicitly or explicitly, compatible interventions or treatment approaches. It therefore provides both conceptualization and an organizing framework for action.

A model of this type is generic and should be equally applicable to all age groups and to a wide spectrum of conditions. It does not necessarily explain how the therapist should intervene in a case, but it will provide a conceptual structure by means of which clinical reasoning may take place.

Problem-based models explain the differing origins of, and consequent management of, problems in social and occupational performance. Once the nature of the problem is understood an appropriate treatment approach or intervention can be selected.

Admittedly, all of this is academic, bewildering, and may be seen as irrelevant to practice. The important issue is not what these theories are called, or how they may be classified, but how they are used by therapists and how they affect therapy.

To avoid repetition of confusing terminology the theoretical bases of the profession will be referred to in the next section by the generic 'theoretical structures' or 'structures'.

There are numerous models and frames of reference, discussion of which is rendered more complex and confusing by the variation in names and concepts. Box 3.4 provides only one, partial, version.

These structures have now been described in detail by a number of authors (e.g. Reed 1984,

---

Box 3.4 Theoretical structures

Physiological	Biomechanical
	Neurodevelopmental
	Sensory integration
Cognitive	Cognitive–perceptual
	Cognitive–behavioural
	Cognitive development and
	disability (Allen 1985)
Behavioural	Behavioural
Psychodynamic	Analytical
	Interactive
Humanistic	Client-centred

Integrative occupational therapy models
(include associated approaches)
Model of human occupation (Kielhofner 1985)
Adaptation through occupation
(Reed & Sanderson 1983)
Activities health (Cynkin & Robinson 1990)
Ontogenesis and adaptive skills (Mosey)
Occupational performance (DNHW, CAOT)

Problem-based models and associated approaches

Rehabilitation	Physical and social rehabilitation
	Various approaches, e.g.
	biomechanical, interactive,
	cognitive-perceptual,
	cognitive–behavioural
Education	Various approaches, e.g.student-
	centred, teacher-centred,
	cognitive, problem-based,
	experiential
Development	Various approaches, e.g.
	neurodevelopmental, sensory,
	integrative, interactive, cognitive
Adaptation	Various approaches, e.g.
	environmental, biomechanical,
	social, humanistic, analytical

Allen 1985, Bruce & Borg 1987, Kielhofner 1992, Hagedorn 1992) and repetition of this material here seems unnecessary.

These theories have variously been described as having the function of 'tools', 'spectacles' (Finlay 1988, Hagedorn 1992) and more elegantly, 'conceptual lenses' (Kielhofner 1992). Such descriptions provide metaphors which illustrate the idea of selecting a structure as a tool for a specific purpose to achieve a therapeutic goal, or of using a theoretical concept to 'colour' or bring into focus, and thereby explain or define a view of the patient or the means of therapy. As will be explained, there is a considerable difference between the views of a theoretical structure as a conceptual lens and as a tool.

TWO PATTERNS FOR IMPLEMENTING THERAPY

One of the most interesting features of this multilayer model of the core and the belt is the relationship between the various parts of the core and that between the core and the belt.

It has already been explained that the core contains theories and provides a view of a person as engaging in occupations within the environment. Each therapist will, in the course of training and subsequent practice, define his own view of this generic core – his understanding of 'what occupational therapy is all about'. Once attained, this perception becomes integral to practice and cannot be shed.

When a therapist begins to deal with the needs of a new patient or client it will be as an occupational therapist, not as a nurse, physiotherapist, psychotherapist or other professional, even if some of the differences are subtle.

However, the core is a large entity. How does the therapist select, interpret and define a particular case in order to take appropriate action? How are the specialized frames of reference, or integrative models in the theoretical belt, used to aid clinical reasoning, to conduct the process of naming and framing the situation, and to decide what to do?

The way in which a therapist selects an appropriate conceptual structure from the belt can only be a matter of hypothesis. I propose that there are currently two distinct patterns whereby therapists use the available core principles, purposes and processes in relation to the theoretical belt.

The existence of these differing patterns has caused confusion and misunderstanding, because the fundamental cognitive schemata, although apparently similar, are conceptually quite distinct. I will refer to these patterns as theory-driven and process-driven.

The crucial difference between these patterns is the point at which the decision is taken to adopt a theoretical structure (model, frame of reference or approach) to direct subsequent therapy or intervention.

In the theory-driven pattern the decision is taken at or before the start of intervention. A model or frame of reference is selected from the theoretical belt to use as a conceptual lens which alters and colours all subsequent clinical reasoning and therapeutic actions – resulting in therapy being theory-driven, even though the fundamental case management process remains problem-based. The 'problem', and indeed the person, is interpreted by means of the theory.

In the process-driven pattern the decision about the selection of an approach is postponed until sufficient information has been gathered and evaluated in the case management process to enable a decision to be made about the nature of the problem, the intervention required and the selection of a suitable treatment method and medium. An approach that is appropriate to a specific problem is selected on a 'tool from a rack' principle.

There is, clearly, a basic conceptual difference between these patterns, which makes it difficult for therapists who are accustomed to working in a process-driven manner to adopt a theory-based approach; they tend to regard each of these structures as 'another tool' to be added to the rack, not as a conceptual lens which alters total perception before one begins to deal with an individual case. On the other hand, theory-driven therapists may criticise the process-driven model as overly eclectic and inconsistent.

A further cause of confusion is that, when it comes to implementation, all practice is based on a version of the problem-solving process (the process of case management) which I have already placed as the central, integrative process of occupational therapy. This may make the process of therapy using a theoretically-based model chosen at the start of therapy look similar superficially to that employed when using the process-driven, problem-orientated model where the decision is delayed.

Neither of these patterns is 'right' or 'wrong',

they merely differ. Each has its place, but they cannot be merged. These ideas will be discussed and expanded in the following pages. It may be helpful to bear in mind that the difference is not so much one of action, but one of cognition.

THE THEORY-DRIVEN PATTERN

This pattern is illustrated by Creek's presentation of the process (1990) (Fig. 3.13).

It has also been presented explicitly by Pedretti & Zoltan (1990), and implicitly in the model of human occupation (Kielhofner 1985), Sanderson & Reed's adaptation through occupation (1983), Allen's cognitive development model (1985) and Cynkin & Robinson's model of activities health (1990) all of which require the user to adopt the model and *then* treat the patient.

It seems to me that this process takes place in two stages. In the first, the therapist moves from the core into the inner ring of the belt to select a theoretical structure. This provides the conceptual lens or pair of spectacles through which she then views both the core and the available approaches and techniques. This filter acts to enhance some features and eliminates others.

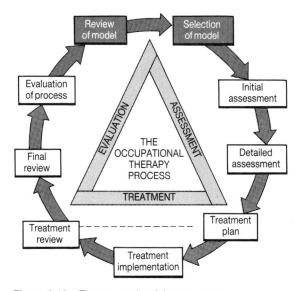

Figure 3.13 The occupational therapy process. (Reproduced from Creek 1990 Occupational therapy and mental health, with permission.)

The therapist then investigates the situation and needs of the patient/client *through the filter of the conceptual lens* in order to understand and describe her situation and the need for intervention.

In the second stage, still 'wearing' the selected filter the therapist chooses a suitable approach by which the theory can be translated into practice.

Selection of a frame of reference at the start of therapy

The therapist begins by adopting a frame of reference by means of which the remainder of his actions and judgements will be focused and organized.

The reasons for early selection may be situational – the therapist works in a unit or a specialty which always uses that frame of reference; or conceptual – the therapist believes that it is 'right' and uses no other, although such a purist view of occupational therapy is very rare.

The therapist in a stroke unit, e.g. adopt a neurodevelopmental frame of reference. This will lead him to use a neurodevelopmental approach in which particular interpretations of data, methods of assessment, manner of handling the patient, style of writing objectives and language for recording will be used. In a psychotherapeutic unit, on the otherhand, he will adopt a psychological approach.

The chosen frame of reference provides an explanation of human behaviour, function and dysfunction which alters the view of the patient. Using this conceptual lens, perceptions of the core are filtered, exaggerating some aspects and modifying or eliminating others. In the inner ring alternative models or frames of reference are rejected. In the outer ring the relevant approach is highlighted, excluding the others. Thus the conceptual filter colours views of core, belt and patient (Fig. 13.14).

Early selection produces clear advantages in coherence of approach and economy of action, provided that the occupational focus of the core is retained. It simplifies clinical reasoning by narrowing the range of potential interventions, and may well accelerate the pace of therapy. It

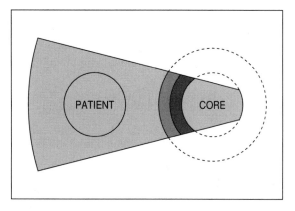

Figure 3.14   The exclusion effect of selecting a frame of reference.

allows the therapist to become an expert within a defined and limited field.

Many of the frames of reference are specialty-biased, and are more appropriate to work in structured clinical settings. They do not, therefore, lend themselves comfortably to work in other settings such as the community, where a generalist approach is needed.

There is also an inevitable narrowing of vision which may result in a reductive attitude, excluding facts, interpretations or actions which do not fit the frame of reference but might have been beneficial. The degree to which the therapist remains flexible and in touch with the core will determine the degree to which he is able to 'see past the theory' and to switch to another if it seems to constrain therapy. However, circumstances within the working environment – time, resources, policies, attitudes of colleagues – may prevent him from moving away from the dominant theory.

Selection of an integrative model at the start of therapy

As explained earlier, an integrative model of occupational therapy usually provides a definition of the occupational nature of the individual, and the consequences of this for the processes of therapy. Once the model is integrated into practice the therapist will assess and treat the patient

within the language, concepts and forms of the model. Consequently all, or most, of the core is likely to be viewed through the conceptual filter, as are the approaches which are compatible with the model. Fewer of the potential approaches will be excluded, although some may be incompatible. The unselected models and incompatible frames of reference will be rejected, as before (Fig. 3.15).

These models do not explicitly 'tell the therapist what to do'; they tell her 'how to think' about people, occupations and therapy.

A well-designed, comprehensive, integrative model can be successfully used only as a total package; the model cannot simply be added to the list of tools; it must change fundamentally the view of both core and client. Partial use is less likely to be successful and may give rise to inconsistencies.

Being widely based there are fewer disadvantages in using a model of occupational therapy from an early stage, and considerable advantages in compatibility and coherence, provided that the therapist remains versatile, well-acquainted with the various approaches and capable of understanding when to apply them.

Characteristic of such models are sophisticated, often complex and elaborate concepts, frequently expressed in a language evolved by and specific to the model, and generating a body of literature communicating in a specific style. This can make

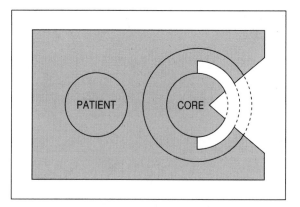

Figure 3.15   The integration effect of selecting an occupational therapy model.

the use of the model somewhat impenetrable to those unfamiliar with it. Although a sophisticated model may impress, it may also make communication with other professionals or clients more difficult since the model must be 'translated'.

It might be argued that the ultimate goal of the theorists who construct integrative occupational therapy models is to find a model so comprehensive that the distinction between core and conceptual belt is submerged within a coherent, organized whole. The ejected material could then be regarded as permanently irrelevant to practice. However, it would take a brave theorist to claim that he or she had achieved this goal, even if it was thought to be desirable or achievable.

THE PROCESS-DRIVEN PATTERN

The primary choice here is the adoption not of a *theory* but of a *process*. In fact, this pattern relies on the integrative function of the problem-based case management process as a means of directing therapy.

This process has been described by Foster (1992), Trombley (1989) and Hagedorn (1992). The necessity for therapists to retain flexibility and use several frames of reference has been stressed by Mosey (1986) and Mocellin (1992a,b).

The basic problem-based case management process is illustrated in Figure 3.16A. I believe that in British practice this is used in relation to four primary problem-based models: development, education, rehabilitation and adaptation. The first three of these models, like frames of reference, are derived from sources external to occupational therapy, but have become an integral part of practice, being reinterpreted within the context of occupational performance. The model of adaptation has been generated largely by the practice of occupational therapy itself.

Although the problem-based process is well-understood it has not previously been presented in this way, and will therefore be explained at this stage. The following description should be read with reference to Figure 3.16B.

Selection of the process-driven pattern eliminates from the theoretical belt all but the four problem-based models and their associated approaches.

The remaining theories are placed to one side; they will be used only if all the problem-based models and approaches prove insufficient for the needs of a particular case.

The therapist begins by drawing the client into the case management process and assembling data on her physical, social and psychological situation, her occupations, activities and roles, her physical and psychosocial environment and her personal needs, wishes, goals and aspirations. The aim of this is to 'frame' (identify and understand) the problem or problems.

The process is as much a matter of elimination as selection: as data is gathered it becomes clearer which of the problem-based explanations of dysfunction will be most relevant and which parts of the occupational therapy core are applicable. Hypotheses are constructed and pointers towards particular approaches are noted, while those obviously inappropriate are discarded. When sufficient data has been gathered the relevance of the four problem-based models can be ascertained. The distinctions are simple but significant (Box 3.5).

Each model provides an explanation of the origin and nature of the problem and a set of approaches with which suitable intervention or therapy can be carried out.

It is important to maintain a general view of the patient and also of other human and non-human factors affecting his situation. One of the strengths of this pattern is that it is possible to recognize that the problem may lie not with the patient, but with others, or with the environment, or even in the mind of the referring agent. If the problem is seen as unsuitable for occupational therapy intervention, for any well-justified reason, an alternative intervention (or no intervention) may be recommended. Alternatively, the education or adaptation models can be used to address a problem *external* to the patient.

The flow from core to problem-based model to approach is separated by periods of problem definition. Indeed problems or priorities may be redefined, and new approaches selected, several times in the course of an intervention. Once an approach is selected further assessments, treatment techniques and methods will be chosen.

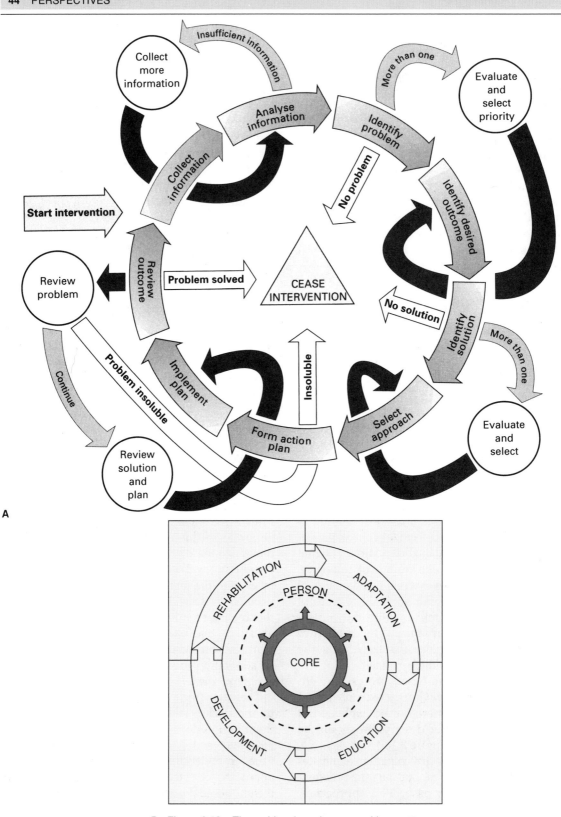

A

B Figure 3.16 The problem-based, process-driven pattern.

Box 3.5	The four problem-based models

Basis of problem	Indicated model
The person has potential to acquire a skill or ability, but is not yet developmentally ready to do so. Foundation skills must be gained before she can become competent.	Development
The person is able to become competent but lacks the knowledge, information, practice or experience which are needed. She must learn how to become competent or how to recognize her competence.	Education
The person has had an ability but has lost it, and requires therapy to restore the lost function and competence.	Rehabilitation
The person is faced with barriers or problems in the social or physical environment, or within her own body, personality or cognitive processes, which need to be changed, or to which she must adapt.	Adaptation

The four models are entirely compatible with each other and it is possible to use one, or all, simultaneously or sequentially in a treatment programme. All provide means whereby the central purposes of enabling, enhancing and empowering may be translated into action.

Development

Development refers to the process of maturation through which the infant finally reaches adulthood and attains a repertoire of adult skills (Fig. 3.17). This process is determined by a complex inter-action of genetic inheritance, environmental conditions and opportunities. Llorens (1976) describes how aspects of development occur over time, both simultaneously and horizontally, and longi-tudinally and chronologically. Thus skills are developed both in related clusters at around the same time (horizontally and simultaneously),

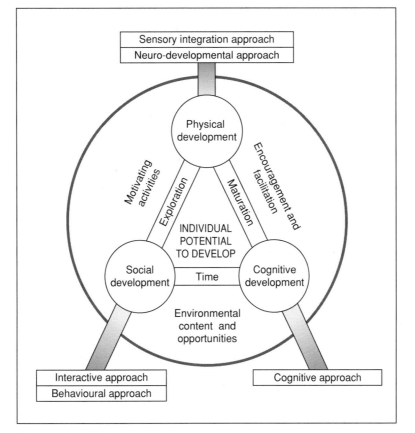

Figure 3.17 Development.

and incrementally over the period of maturation (longitudinally and chronologically) from birth to around the age of 21 years.

Occupationally the developmental model refers to the proto-occupational stage (see Ch. 5) where skill components are assembled into skills, skills into the ability to perform task segments, task stages and tasks until finally tasks are assembled into activities.

There are a number of developmentally-referenced approaches relevant to sensorimotor, perceptual, social, affective and cognitive development. Some of these deal with 'normal' development, and others with the need to redevelop following damage. The occupational therapist tends to be concerned with the former where development is delayed for some reason, and with the latter as the preliminary stage in a process of rehabilitation, e.g. neurodevelopmental

approaches such as Proprioceptive Neuromuscular Facilitation (PNF) or Bobath, sensory integration (Ayres 1972) Trombly 1989 and recapitulation of ontogenesis (Mosey.)

There is obviously a very close link between development and education; however they are not the same. Development is concerned with turning potential into usable ability, in creating the building blocks of skills which can be used and established as part of the person's repertoire. Education is directed towards extending and improving the use of skill and establishing competence in a range of tasks, activities and occupations.

Education

Education is concerned with the person as learner (Fig. 3.18). Skill must be practised, refined and

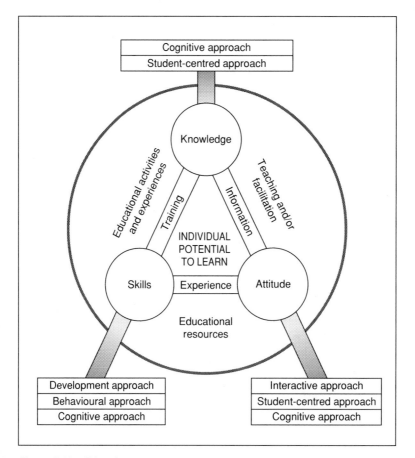

Figure 3.18 Education.

extended for competent performance. The person must acquire knowledge of her world – social, physical, and spiritual – and must become functional within it. This process takes most of childhood and extends on a continuum throughout adult life.

The therapist integrates education into much of his practice; skill development and education in use of skills go hand-in-hand. Sometimes education takes precedence especially when new learning – of activities, information, use of resources – is required.

There are numerous educational approaches; those most commonly used by therapists include the behavioural approach, used at the proto-occupational level, and various teacher-led, student-centred or cognitive approaches used at higher occupational levels.

Rehabilitation

Rehabilitation becomes relevant when damage has occurred to remove an ability and reduce competence in occupational performance (Fig. 3.19). Rehabilitation may be preceded by development, and may include education. (Indeed it is sometimes referred to as re-education).

The aim of rehabilitation is to regain the previous level of function (not necessarily maximum function, for the patient may not previously have used maximum function, or may not require it for the purposes of her own roles and occupations).

Rehabilitation approaches are derived from various frames of reference and are chosen for their application to a specific problem, e.g. a motor problem involving joints or muscles may be treated biomechanically, a problem in the central

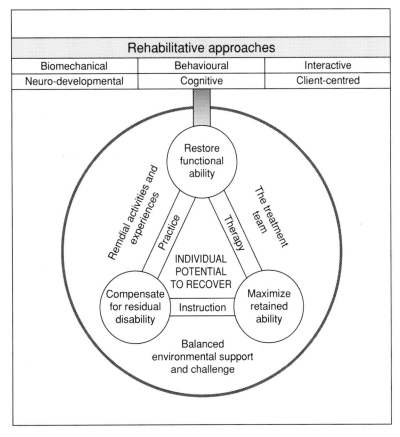

Figure 3.19   Rehabilitation.

nervous system neurodevelopmentally and a perceptual or cognitive problem cognitively. However, rehabilitation ought to retain a holistic perspective, since the various areas of function are so closely interdependent as to be inseparable. When rehabilitation is consciously used as one model within the four-part structure it is easier to avoid the reductionism with which it is sometimes associated.

Once rehabilitation has reached its conclusion, i.e. when no further recovery can be attained, it may be necessary to proceed into the model of adaptation, in order to assist the person to compensate for residual disability, and to rebuild and reshape her occupations and interactions.

Adaptation

This involves adaptation of the environment, including other people, to meet the needs of an individual, adaptation of roles, occupations and activities and adaptation of some aspects of the individual's functioning in order to cope with the demands of the environment and occupations (Fig. 3.20).

Adaptation is a very important process in which the complex individual patterns of occupations and roles become highly significant, as does the basic potential of the person to adapt.

Sometimes the therapist must return to the developmental model in order to develop the ability to adapt before adaptation can begin.

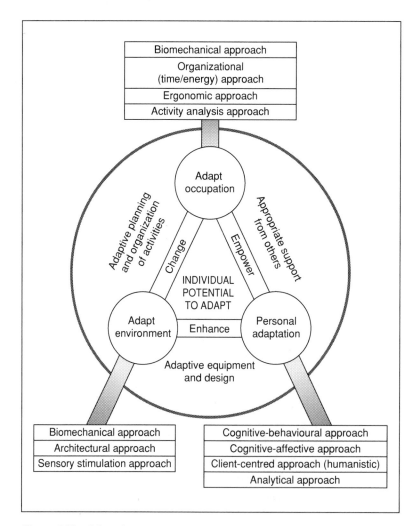

Figure 3.20 Adaptation.

Adaptive approaches are focused on the environment (mechanical, architectural, aesthetic), on other people who must in some way change their own behaviour, occupations or roles in relation to the individual, or on the individual herself. The individual may adapt physically, usually through biomechanical means such as splints or prostheses, or cognitively, affectively and socially, by means of interactive, psychotherapeutic, humanistic and other approaches.

The adaptation model recognizes that some situations are either insoluable, or liable to deteriorate, but that something may usually be done to minimize the adverse effects of such circumstances, provided that the individual is prepared and able to change, or that it is possible to change elements of the environment, or reactions or behaviours of others.

Approaches to the patient within the process-driven pattern

In therapy, three possible approaches to the client can be identified along a continuum:

Therapist-directed → partnership → client-directed

In the directive approach the therapist states 'you give me the facts, and I will tell you the nature of your problem and the solution'. In the client-directed approach the therapist asks the client 'tell me the nature of your problem and your solution'. There are disadvantages to both these approaches, the former being prescriptive and the latter expecting the client to perform an exercise which, if she were able to do so, would render intervention unnecessary. It is therefore the 'partnership' approach which is most effective in the problem-based process model.

Advantages and disadvantages of the process-driven pattern

Advantages of this pattern are that nothing is excluded too soon, options are left open and automatic assumptions and preconceptions are avoided. The case is evaluated thoroughly and the final choice should therefore be reasoned,

justified and appropriate. Flexibility is retained; as further information is gathered the option of changing to a different, more appropriate approach is left open.

On the other hand, initial information gathering and assessment may be slower; it takes time to sift the relevant from the irrelevant. This requires highly developed clinical reasoning, and having all options open can lead to a bewildering proliferation of explanations and potential courses of action, resulting in confusion rather than clarification. It also requires a versatile therapist who has a sound understanding of the professional core and who is equally skilled in, and comfortable with, a variety of approaches, media and techniques.

It may be argued that it is impossible for a therapist to approach the core without a conceptual filter of some kind, but if it is accepted that the filter in this case is provided by the process rather than a theory, and that the relevant knowledge and assumptions for the preliminary stages of intervention are contained within the generic core, this becomes less problematic.

PATTERN SELECTION IN PRACTICE

In everyday practice the majority of therapists will probably take only occasionally the primary decision about whether their practice is to be theory-driven or process-driven. They may may well do so at an almost subliminal level. The decision is taken during training, or when moving into a new job, when choosing an area in which to specialize, on being impressed by a new theory, or simply as a result of accumulating experience by means of which the therapist evolves a personal style or expertise derived, consciously or otherwise, from one of these patterns.

The chosen pattern becomes integrated into practice. Decisions from that point are related primarily to selecting an approach. In the case of a specific frame of reference, even that decision may be unnecessary since only one approach is available.

An occupational therapy model can provide a clear basis for practice with well-described explanations of dysfunction and justifications for therapy. It may, however, cause the therapist to 'squeeze' the patient to fit the parameters of the model. It is still possible, however, during the process of intervention, to select appropriate assessments and techniques based on compatible approaches.

When working within the problem-based models, decision-taking should, ideally, be a more conscious, reasoned, and frequent occurence. Although the problem-solving process remains the consistent factor, the choices between the four available models, and several approaches, need to be made each time an individual is referred, and must be justified, individually implemented, and modified when required.

The reader may by now have deduced that, while accepting the theory-driven pattern as an alternative, my preference is the process-driven pattern.

CONCLUSION

A number of propositions have been made concerning the philosophical and theoretical basis of the profession and its relationship with practice. These are summarized in Box 3.6.

Box 3.6 Propositions

1. The debate concerning an occupational therapy paradigm continues, but there is an emerging consensus that it is possible to distinguish between a relatively stable central core, defining the profession's philosophy, principles, purposes and processes, and a changeable theoretical belt, containing optional frames of reference, models and approaches.
2. Both central core and belt are as yet imperfectly described, and the relationship between elements within and between them are complex.
3. It is suggested that the core components of occupational therapy are a triad consisting of the person seeking therapy, the therapist and the occupational element. This triad operates within a physical and sociocultural environment. Occupational therapy can exist as an entity only when the triad remains unbroken within a suitable environment. The values, assumptions and knowledge of the profession are related to and derived from this core content.
4. The process of case management (the occupational therapy process) is the central, organizing process of occupational therapy which coordinates the use of other processes, including: problem analysis and clinical reasoning, therapeutic use of self, assessment and evaluation, occupational analysis and adaptation, environmental analysis and adaptation, resource management.
5. A crucial point in the process of case management is the selection of a theoretical structure for practice which will direct subsequent intervention or therapy.
6. There are two patterns for this decision. In the theory-driven pattern, the choice is made before the start of intervention, and results in the selection of either a specific frame of reference, or an integrative occupational therapy model which affects perceptions of core and patient/client. In the process-driven pattern, selection of a problem-based model follows preliminary data gathering assessment and problem identification. Subsequently an appropriate approach (or a selection of compatible approaches) is chosen, by means of which therapy or intervention is conducted.

4

The person

HUMANITY

What does it mean to be human? The explanations are as diverse and contradictory as humanity itself. Are we amoral and aggressive naked apes with a thin veneer of socialization? Are we intrinsically moral and altruistic, with free will, adaptively seeking personal growth and wisdom? Are we nothing but a well-mixed potion of basic chemicals animated by a weak electric current, programmed by genetic inheritance and chance contact with the environment, or do we possess souls and potential for higher life?

We cannot at present prove which, if any, of these and numerous other explanations is most true. Whether we ever will is yet another matter of philosophical and scientific debate. It is not the answer, but the fact that humankind asks the question at all which is deeply significant; as far as we know we are the only life form on this planet which is capable of doing so; the capacity for introspection and abstract thought, for the examination of the past and the imaginary construction of the future is one of the features which defines humanity.

The other, and most basic, distinguishing feature is the ability to make and use tools for wide-ranging, adaptive, creative and unstereotyped performance. The crucial change signalling a development from the earliest hominids towards *homo sapiens* was the making and use of primitive flint tools by *homo habilis*, 'skilful man', some 2 000 000 years ago.

Even allowing for the recent evidence that

mankind may be genetically nearer to the apes than was previously thought, there is a very wide gap between the simple use of tools and social communication of the primates and the elaborate complexities of human skills and cognition.

Equally significant in defining humanity was the production, perhaps some 40 000 years ago, of objects such as cave paintings or etched carvings, which had symbolic, not utilitarian, purposes. Humans are uniquely capable of manipulating imaginary ideas and using symbols, creating not only images of the real world, but also conceiving of worlds or creatures which do not, or cannot exist.

Buckminster-Fuller (1969) has described humans as 'artists–scientists–inventors'. The primary focus of occupational therapy was, and remains, the two unique characteristics of humanity: the ability to choose, think, solve problems, invent and plan, and the skilful, creative ability to perform occupational tasks and roles. The therapist is therefore dealing with the fundamental components of human existence.

Wilcock (1992) explores the three-way link between survival, health and occupation from early human history. She describes the ways in which human occupations have shaped cultures as well as individuals. She concludes:

Occupational therapists should be willing to reconsider approaches so that they cover more adequately the complexities and values of occupations to humans, and recognize a much broader role in shaping individual lives, societies and cultures in the future.

It may be appropriate to adapt. Descartes' famous dictum 'Cogito, ergo sum' (I think, therefore I am) to 'Cogito *et facto*, ergo sum' (I think and I make, therefore I am). Certainly this view of humanity forms a fundamental assumption of occupational therapy.

THE UNIQUE INDIVIDUAL

The sole reason for the existence of occupational therapy is the person referred for the therapist's services. This person is unique. He is also, inescapably, a member of the human species and therefore 'Like all others, like some others and like no other' (Rogers 1986).

The therapist may relate to the individual in different ways, depending on the approach used and the therapy environment. Views of the nature of humanity and the explanations of human behaviour are diverse and conflicting, stemming from philosophy, psychology, science, and theology.

In general they derive from one or other of the 'metamodels' (Reed 1984), the reductionist or organismic views of the world and humanity. The reductionist view sees the person as a machine, running within systems which have set parameters and which are capable of objective study and reduction to component parts with consequent description of established facts. This is the logical–positive–realist view of science, medicine and of some psychologists and educationalists.

The organismic view sees the person as an interactive, adaptive system which has to be studied as a whole, considering both objective and subjective factors within the context of the environment, and accepting the phenomenological, existential view that personal experience and perceptions are legitimate and of prime significance to the individual. This is the view of the sociologist, anthropologist, human ecologist and some psychologists and educationalists.

Related to these two perspectives are the still unresolved fundamental philosophical arguments of at least 2000 years' standing over the degree to which a person is a 'free agent' in his actions.

The determinist sees human behaviour as responses to a set of external influences (a deity, astrological predestination, conditioned responses) or internal imperatives (subconscious drives and mechanisms, biological necessities, genetic inheritance). The opposing view, which may stem from a religious or cultural basis, or from philosophical ideas loosely termed humanistic or existential, sees the person as having free will and the ability to steer his own course of actions to achieve personal growth and eventual wisdom.

In the face of such deep and abiding dissention

on the nature of humanity and the dynamics of individual human behaviour, discussion can become heated and unproductive.

For the therapist the uncertainties are likely to be resolved by the personal values, beliefs and attitudes directing the therapeutic relationship. However, she should beware of inflicting her own ideals and ideas on others, and especially on her patients.

Is there then any constant focus on the individual which can be grasped by the occupational therapist among intense metaphysical speculation? Whatever the context of therapy and the frame of reference, the core concerns of the therapist should focus on the individual as a participant in roles and occupations. This leaves room for interpretation and debate, but is at least a comprehensible concept.

THE AUTONOMOUS PERSON

Most highly evolved societies struggle to balance the basic paradox of protecting the rights of the individual to do as he wishes, while imposing upon him constraints and responsibilities. Some of the rules are implicit; others are explicit, in the form of laws, rituals and customs. If an individual fails to confirm, penalties, either social or legal, are likely to be imposed.

In Britain, where much behaviour is implicit and dependent on history, custom and practice, the citizen is expected to fulfil a duty of care to himself and to any dependents (e.g. by keeping himself and them clean, fed, warm, housed, clothed, to his neighbour (by being ethical, honest, considerate, helpful, careful and unobtrusive) and to the State (by contributing active labour and paying taxes). In return his neighbour is expected to offer the same duty of care, and the State is expected to maintain a basic infrastructure for healthy, safe, daily life and to provide for the individual and his dependents if he is, through no fault of his own, unable to care for himself.

This is, of course, a simplistic view of a highly complex 'contract' which evolves and changes,

and is subject to frequent stresses and strains. Today, for example, the rights of the individual seem to be expressed more often than the reciprocal duties. Nonetheless, the fundamental expectations in any culture of what an autonomous individual should do, and what the State or society should provide, colour the provision of health care and need to be understood.

It is surprising, in view of the importance of the role of the 'autonomous person', that there is no single, generic title in common use to indicate such an individual. 'Citizen' implies social duty rather than the duty of self-care, while 'voter' implies a political role.

People tend to be classified into subgroups with implicit rights and duties; e.g. *consumer* (duty to spend money, right to receive high quality services and products), *worker* (duty to provide personal effort, right not to be exploited by employer) and *pensioner* (duty to be frugal and if possible useful, right to state pension).

Autonomy cannot be viewed simply as the ability to survive on one's own, for humans are essentially interdependent social animals and true self-sufficiency is a myth. In this sense no-one is autonomous; nor is autonomy a stable concept, for expectations vary according to an individual's age, sex, culture, role and responsibilities.

Therapists tend to speak of a person as 'autonomous' when in fact they mean 'capable of exercising choices and control over one's personal life', and as 'independent' when they mean 'able to do what is required to remain healthy, without needing someone else to help'. Occupational competence seems to imply the ability to cope adequately with the three 'duties of care', to self, neighbour and State, while occupational dysfunction implies a breakdown in one or more of these areas.

The concepts of independence and autonomy and the criteria whereby their absence or presence are judged, therefore, need careful examination, and must take close account of complex cultural and social expectations.

Autonomy carries with it implicit assumptions about individual choice. It has already been noted that occupational therapists tend to take the view that a person does posses some degree of free will and is capable of making choices and decisions which direct his life. The constraints of environment or ability are acknowledged, but the person is able essentially to make positive decisions, through his choices, even in unfavourable circumstances.

Sartre wrote that man is 'condemned to choose'. Choice is both a burden and a blessing, for we can never be certain that we have made the best decision, nor that the alternative would not have been preferable. This burdens us with guilt and regret.

Therapists accept that an individual does not always make the right decision, but insist that the ability to choose is, on the whole, positive. In therapeutic contexts people can choose to change, to adapt, to learn, and to embark on the threatening and uncertain road to personal growth or achievement. The therapist can facilitate, or perhaps guide, the process of choice but the decision rests ultimately with the individual.

HOW ARE CHOICES MADE?

On what basis do humans make their choices? A baby starts to choose from the moment he reaches to grasp a red toy instead of a blue one, or spits out the pudding he dislikes. The ability to choose seems to be innate, yet must be affected by environment and experience. Once again we are faced with a multitude of explanations, relating to past learning, opportunities, likes, dislikes, attitudes, values, culture, other people, emotions, unconscious mechanisms and conscious or symbolic meanings.

Many of the effects of institutionalization result from the restricted choices available to people who, deprived of autonomy, eventually become incapable of choice. However, Allen (1985) points out that rational and planned decision-taking requires also a high level of cognitive function, which may be absent due to basic organic inadequacy, damage or illness, rather than simply to inappropriate environment.

Facilitating choice is a delicate art. Freedom to choose is dependent on realistic opportunities and alternatives, and on the possibility of risk-taking and poor decision-making. We know that the best choices are made when the person feels safe and unrestricted, understands the issues, and can see relevance and personal meaning in the thing chosen. Poorer choices are the result of control, coersion, insecurity, anxiety, stress, lack of information, lack of opportunity and lack of relevance to personal wishes or experience.

THE IMPORTANCE OF MEANING

People tend to choose to do those things which they find meaningful, and to avoid things which are meaningless. It is important therefore that the occupational choices offered are meaningful to the individual.

The importance of meaning in relation to occupations or activities is stated often. Kielhofner (1985) writes that 'An individual's experience and participation in the environment result in the building up of certain images about various activities or occupations which are very personal and evoke strong emotions.' He defines meaningfulness as 'An individual's disposition to find importance, security, worthiness and purpose in particular occupations.' The sources of personal meanings are various, but he concludes that 'Developing occupations which can have personal meaning and incorporating them into one's lifestyle is critical since a lack of meaning in life produces anxiety and depression.'

Cynkin & Robinson (1990) also stress the importance of meaning and add 'It is of critical importance that activities be examined ... to determine their meaning and relevance to the individual as a member of a sociocultural group.' They point out that meanings are contextual and unstable – the same basic activity may assume different meanings in different environments and social contexts.

The meaning attributed to a specific activity by an individual is clearly an acquired attribute; however, familiarity and past meaningfulness may be no guarantee that the person will continue to find an activity pleasurable, relevant or meaningful, especially if a change in circumstances has affected his ability to engage in it at the previous level of competence. In this case, negative meaning may rapidly supersede positive meaning, as the person's sense of incompetence is reinforced by his failure to experience his former level of success and pleasure.

THE PERSON AS A PARTICIPANT IN ROLES AND OCCUPATIONS

PERSONAL SURVIVAL

As a biological organism the person needs to provide himself with the necessities of life in order to maintain homeostasis and health. He must therefore be able to meet these needs by his own endeavours, or by the cooperative endeavours of the society in which he lives. If he cannot meet these needs, for reasons of age, disability or pathology, then someone else must provide them, if he is to remain healthy and to survive.

Maslow's hierarchy of needs (1970) suggests that, when poverty or hostile environment causes a person's existence to focus solely on survival, the higher occupational goals of personal meaning, self-actualization and creativity become irrelevant; there is simply no surplus energy to direct into such activity. This is observable in extreme circumstances such as famine where the victims sit listlessly in their camps, too exhausted to do more than cling to existence until the next supply of food is issued.

It may, however, be simplistic to assume that Maslow's hierarchy operates rigidly in less extreme circumstances. Sustaining personal meaning and cultural affirmation may actually become an important means of survival in adverse circumstances, even though the basic necessities of physical survival are in short supply. For example, in the besieged, bombarded city of Sarajevo, undernourished actors have rehearsed Samuel Beckett's play 'Waiting for Godot' and musicians have practised the classics, in a deliberate and symbolic rejection of the potential descent of daily life into dehumanizing barbarism. Spiritual and cultural sustenance may be needed to make the continuing struggle for the basic necessities seem worthwhile.

In western culture the concept of personal survival is imbued with a plethora of attitudes, based on moral, social, and religious values. Survival is both a right and a duty; a person must act to preserve another's life at all costs, and must not contribute to ending it, even if the other person wants to die.

A person has a duty to do his utmost to survive, for the benefit of himself and his species, and should not take any action which will end his life. However, personal autonomy dictates that a person may take risks if he is considered mentally competent to do so, and paradoxically, self-sacrifice in the service of others is regarded as heroic. In terms of medical ethics this is a moral minefield.

The conflict between personal survival and personal meaning is highly relevant in occupational therapy. Is a life which lacks any occupational quality or personal meaning worth sustaining? If a person has a very limited supply of energy, should this energy be directed solely towards basic survival, leaving no capacity for pleasurable or meaningful occupation, or should some other person be asked to help the limited individual with basic survival, thus freeing his energy for more rewarding occupation?

THE PERSON AS A WORKER

Work provides a person with personal identity, social status, and economic independence and security. This is not a new concept; since the days when early humans began to develop more skills than one person could master, divisions of labour have resulted in complex attitudes and hierarchies.

In the remote past, status was given to people whose expertise promoted survival and prosperity, e.g. the skilled smith, dyer, hunter or farmer. Expertise led to mystique; those who could not grasp the complexities of a skill shrouded it with magic.

The complexity of specialization is now far beyond the comprehension of the averagely educated person. We live in a world full of things which we use but do not understand – perhaps that has always been true to some extent, but now technological advances have widened the gap between understanding how to use something and comprehending how it is made and how it works.

The changing patterns of employment in Britain and the rest of the 'developed' world in the 20th century have provided much material for sociologists, economists and politicians. People work shorter, more flexible hours, in a greater diversity of occupations which require, in general, more varied skills. More women work, both part-time and full-time. Changes in work have altered family structures and roles, as well as changing standards of living.

Education and training have had to adapt in order to provide suitable, employable workers to sustain the economic and productive viability of the State and the ever-increasing complexities of the global economy.

Work remains a major component of most people's adult life, but constant employment between the ages of 16 and 65 is already faltering and may one day be a thing of the past. Retirement comes earlier; people may no longer maintain the same job throughout their working life. Even well-qualified people may find themselves without work for a period or faced with the prospect of re-training.

Technology has made many jobs, especially manual ones, obsolete, and comparatively fewer new occupations have been created. Developments have tended to have affected most adversely those who are already disadvantaged by poor skills, poor education and abilities which, although perfectly adequate for the multitude of less skilled jobs available in the past, cannot cope with the stressful complexities of the modern workplace. Advanced technology results in dysfunction being re-defined.

The need to find a means of paying benefits to an increasing number of people when they are not working, when fewer workers are paying taxes to sustain these payments, is a socio-economic nightmare.

Occupational therapy was born at the close of an era when work was regarded as both a right and a duty, employment was relatively plentiful, and only the rich and aristocratic or the feckless or sick did not work. Social values and attitudes are notoriously slow to change; society is still grappling painfully with the realization of the enormity of the socioeconomic changes which have already occurred and which will hit harder in the next century when work may become even less readily available. Have therapists caught up with the changes? Does the notion of a required balance between work, rest and leisure hold good when that balance is no longer stable, and when patterns become so variable?

The boundaries are already blurred. Complex technology enables increasing numbers of people to work from home rather than in an office. Work does not always have to mean paid employment, e.g. voluntary work for a charity, education, work for a pet project or hobby, working for oneself (described by Pahl (1984) as 'domestic self-provisioning'), e.g. DIY and housework, are all forms of work, yet the participants may or may not recognize them as such.

Occupational therapists are potentially well-placed to help people to develop new and adaptive patterns of occupation to replace those inherited from the 19th century. However, many of the profession's own concepts and assumptions concerning work are still rooted in the past and will need considerable revision if therapists are to cope with providing occupational meaning and purpose for people for whom paid employment is a minor, or missing, component of their lives. Perhaps this is an area where occupational therapists can intervene to change a culture, rather than to perpetuate it.

THE PERSON AT LEISURE

Leisure, a concept developed and refined in the 20th century, is of relevance chiefly to young people and working adults in western-style societies. It means little to children, who play, rest, learn and explore in an unbroken continuum, and has little relevance to the very old who also tend to ignore artificial divisions of activity. For the very rich it ceases to exist because leisure becomes a total way of life, sometimes elevated to an art form; for the very poor it also disappears, for the struggle to survive leaves little space for it.

An absence of work does not constitute leisure, although it is often spoken of in that way. For people who desire, but do not have work, an occupationless limbo is created in which time not working is not leisure time, for leisure implies the use of discretionary time and money. Many unemployed or retired people have too much time and too few resources to exercise the limited choices which they do have.

People who are unemployed are not usually envied for possessing leisure but ironically people who have retired from work may be envied, although they are, in fact, in a similar situation to that of the jobless person – having an unlimited supply of unstructured time, and finding this an uncomfortable experience.

In both cases it may well be the lack of structure which is the problem; people brought up in western cultures generally seem to need to design structures and patterns for use of time if these are missing, but not everyone has the skills to do this effectively.

The more externally structured a pattern of occupations has been the harder the pensioner or unemployed person is likely to find the creation of a meaningful and purposeful structure for himself. Time becomes filled with routines, with stereotyped behaviours and with aimless pursuits such as habitual walks, long periods of watching television, or reading the papers; life become sterile and low in engagement or meaning.

Despite the inequalities of opportunity, leisure, once the prerogative of an advantaged few, is now a profitable and marketable product for many. To the adult worker, leisure may be seen as an antidote to, or an escape from, work, as complementary to it or as a separate 'compartment' of life. Personal perceptions of work may be idiosyncratic, but to a lesser degree than the individuality of perceptions concerning leisure. The only common denominator in leisure occupations and activities is the element of choice.

When free time is available people choose how to spend it – having fun, being creative, being sociable, or simply sitting in the sun may all be regarded as leisure, as may altruistic use of time to help others, or working for oneself. Perceptions of leisure are essentially subjective.

It has become accepted in occupational therapy texts to view leisure as a means of creative self-actualization. This may be the case for some people, but self-actualization is in danger of being a middle-class hobby, or rather, the routes towards it tend to be viewed as middle-class.

Occupational therapists should be well-placed to give people an understanding of how to use personal time effectively and meaningfully; education for healthy living should, ideally, include such instruction as a matter of course, and from an early age.

THE PERSON AS AN OWNER OF ROLES

Occupational roles identify the person as a 'doer' of particular jobs, arts, crafts or techniques. Social roles identify relationships.

Internalized self-concepts often involve recognition of one's occupational and social roles; 'I' may be an amalgam of worker, friend, relative, child, driver, club member, churchgoer, gardener and many more. The 'I' present at a particular time in one role may be, in subtle or even quite marked ways, different from the 'I' presented and experienced in other roles. Loss of role or failure to cope with an important role such as parent or spouse can have profound effects on self-concept and identity.

Roles imply required actions, knowledge, skills, attitudes, duties or responsibilities, and may exclude the role-holder from other, incompatible activities. Competence is often linked to the ability to handle many roles well and adaptably; people who are dysfunctional typically have difficulty in sustaining roles, and, reciprocally, role conflict can produce dysfunction.

The ways in which roles are acquired, retained, changed, exchanged, owned or rejected are important to the therapist because of the ensuing effects on the occupations and activities engaged in by the person. Role acquisition is a 'chicken and egg' affair; occupations bring with them roles, and roles lead to occupations or activities. The would-be artist may purchase paint, brushes and canvas and equip a studio in order to act out the chosen role; the active and competent business person is elected to a local committee and becames Chair; the single child unwillingly becomes the carer of an aged parent.

The most valued and rewarding roles are those leading to close interpersonal relationships in which the people involved can experience the positive emotions which Maslow regards as essential human needs to be met before any others can be satisfied: love, safety and belonging. These relationships engage the strongest of human emotions and in consequence are also potentially the most volatile, challenging, dangerous and threatening.

A few basic basic skills can be taught, but ultimately every person is on his own when it comes to building close relationships. To the therapist trying to help a person with difficulties in this enormously important, intensely personal area of life, it can feel like walking across quicksand on a spider's web bridge. Perhaps we need also to remind ourselves at times that there are areas of human life where, as occupational therapists, we ought not to venture too far.

THE PERSON AS A MEMBER OF A CULTURAL GROUP

The need to belong is powerful and can be met through cultural affiliation and affirmation. This may include attachment to country, state, town, locality, ethnic group, religion, society, club ar any group of like-minded people. Culture is learned, and often produces strongly held, if imperfectly articulated, concepts, beliefs and attitudes – some positive, some negative.

Culture permeates every aspect of daily life, and can alter fundamentally the way in which the individual perceives his world. Some cultures have strict rituals, customs or taboos; all have 'rules', explicit or implicit, by which the members of the group must abide. Most cultures also evolve celebrations – feasts, festivals, rituals, holy days, marches, parades – and use art, dance, drama and music as a means of cultural affirmation.

Sensitivity to, and understanding of, such needs, especially when dealing with a culture different from her own, is essential for the therapist.

OCCUPATIONAL COMPETENCE

The concept of the person as a competent performer of occupations, roles and activities is central to occupational therapy, even though the precise definition of 'occupational competence' may vary. A strong proponent of the importance of this concept is Mocellin. He states that the driving force of occupational therapy is based on the concept of competence: 'the core, the fundamental assumption, the philosophical basis of occupational therapy is, and always has been, based on the concept of competence' (Mocellin 1992). More controversially, he continues:

Thus, it is not occupation, in whatever way this may be defined or conceptualized, that is therapeutic but the experience of efficacy, control and of self-determination . . . referred to as competence . . . which may be achieved through occupation but also through many non-occupational activities.

Since the therapist is concerned with identifying whether or not the person is a 'competent performer' (Kielhofner) or a 'competent actor' (Cynkin & Robinson 1990) there needs to be a concept of 'competence', an understanding of the elements of which competence is composed and how it may be identified. This is not simple. Competence means skilled performance of purposeful actions with the implication of an acceptable but not necessarily perfect, level of achievement.

At first sight it seems possible to define competence objectively. Given defined purposes and standards the therapist may observe performance of actions or interactions and define how far the objectives and standards were met by the performer.

However, even this supposedly objective evaluation is liable to become subjective, for it requires highly accurate observation and recording, the process of observation itself may alter the outcome, and who sets the criteria? Are the purposes and standards those of the individual, those of the therapist, or those of some external agency such as social norms, or the requirements of an employer? Competent performance may mean different things to different people.

In assessing performance two approaches can be used: 'criterion-referenced', which means using a defined set of standards relevant to an individual on a specific occasion; or 'norm-referenced', which means judging performance against a notion of the average which may be expected from, or have been achieved by, a group of people.

In general therapists use a form of criterion-referenced assessment, measuring the person's abilities against standards which are appropriate to, and set in conjunction with, that individual.

Being competent is not, however, simply a matter of performing ably the action or inter-action on one occasion. Performance must be consistent, replicable and generalizable from one situation to another with appropriate flexibility and judgement. It is of no practical value if a person can act competently within a protected environment, such as an occupational therapy daily living area, but becomes incompetent when faced with the stressful demands of the 'real world'.

Competence is situational and can be unstable. Most of us have experienced incompetence when faced with emotional stress, illness, sudden change, lack of accustomed resources or excessive environmental novelty or challenge. It may also be possible to be quite competent in some areas of life, and incompetent in others; the communicator who is fluent on paper may be paralysed if faced with public speaking. This may not matter to an author, but would matter very much to a person who wished to become a lecturer. A level of competence which may be quite sufficient for one individual to cope with the requirements of his life may be inadequate for another whose requirements are more exacting.

Competence also implies subjective recognition by the participant of satisfaction, comfort, completion of purpose, efficacy and efficiency. It is usually of little use simply to reassure someone who views his performance as unsatisfactory that he is, in fact, managing adequately.

For Mocellin this central concept of competence implies that the role of the therapist is as a teacher: 'the "therapy" in occupational therapy

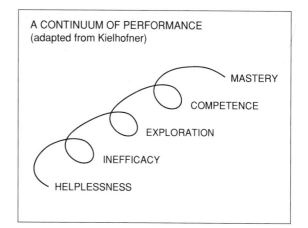

A CONTINUUM OF PERFORMANCE
(adapted from Kielhofner)

MASTERY
COMPETENCE
EXPLORATION
INEFFICACY
HELPLESSNESS

Figure 4.1

is about teaching patients functional skills so as to make them as competent as possible.'

The concept of competence has become linked to the concepts of function and dysfunction. Kielhofner (1985) has suggested a continuum of performance from helplessness via inefficacy to exploration, competence and mastery. He defines competence as 'The quality of being able or having the capacity to respond effectively to the demands of one or a range of situations.'

OCCUPATIONAL DYSFUNCTION

The use of the term 'dysfunction' throughout this text requires some justification. It is selected as a useful shorthand for a complex concept. Kielhofner (1992) uses the term 'occupational dysfunction', and explains its multifarious nature as follows:

Occupational dysfunctions result from the interplay of biological, psychological and ecological factors. For example a limitation of physical capacity may not be a sufficient condition for occupational dysfunction. A dysfunction in occupational performance, however, is likely when the individual with limited capacity lacks confidence, does not know how to problem-solve effectively to compensate for limitations, and encounters physical and social barriers.

Words such as 'disability', 'handicap' and 'impairment' tend to be unduly influenced by the medical model, and are also view primarily in physical terms. It is perfectly possible to be disabled, yet highly competent. It is equally possible to have no disability, but to be dysfunctional.

The word 'dysfunction' is used therefore to indicate a temporary or chronic inability to cope with and engage in the roles, relationships and occupations expected of a person of similar age and culture. The causes of such inability may include physical, social, psychological or environmental factors.

It is easy to recognize severe dysfunction because the person is observably, and catastrophically, unable to perform. It is much harder to recognize, prevent or treat the impending onset of dysfunction or performance deficits which, although not resulting in total inability, are nevertheless subtly and cumulatively damaging to the life of the individual.

As functional competence is more than the simple ability 'to do', so dysfunction is more than simple inability. As noted, many people are disabled, e.g. lacking movement, sight or hearing, but are *not* dysfunctional. They manage to lead perfectly competent lives, albeit with some restrictions. Dysfunction implies a much wider inability to cope in the view either of the individual or of society.

As described by Kielhofner and by Reed (1983, 1984), dysfunction feeds on itself, spiralling the individual down the continuum. Dysfunction not only disenables, it disempowers as well. If the individual recognizes this state, and is able to seek and use help to change it, the problem of identifying the need for intervention is lessened. However, dysfunction produces the paradox that those most likely to need assistance are also those least likely to be able to seek and make use of it.

In view of this, it is particularly unfortunate when societies and cultures are intolerant and judgemental concerning dysfunction, and treat the dysfunctional individual as a scapegoat. They react not so much to the inability to perform as to a perception that the dysfunctional person is 'different' (and therefore unacceptable or threatening), unable to cope, and also, apparently lacking the desire to do anything about this (thus not only neglecting his own social obligations, but also imposing duties of care upon others).

Because perceptions of dysfunction are culturally loaded it can be difficult to draw the line between people who are genuinely dysfunctional and those whom society labels as 'odd' or 'deviant' because they do not conform to the social norms of the majority. Travelling people (gypsies or new age travellers) are an example of people who attract such labels.

The fact that it may be society itself, or elements in the environment, which have produced and maintain the dysfunctional state, rather than some basic inadequacy in the person himself, is now more generally acknowledged by health care professions.

The belief in the ability of people to learn, change, adapt and find identity, even in challenging circumstances, is the foundation of occupational therapy, which provides the occupational and environmental interventions to enable and enhance this process.

Explanations for dysfunction are as far-reaching as explanations for human learning and behaviour, and stem from the same frames of reference (Table 4.1).

We should beware of using too freely labels associated with dysfunction: using Kielhofner's continuum, we are dealing more often with inefficacy; much of the therapist's occupational intervention or therapy is geared towards *preventing* incipient dysfunction, and if successful, the label is unnecessary. People who are genuinely dysfunctional typically face a multiplicity of organic, motivational or environmental problems, the unravelling and remediation of which challenge all the therapist's skills and ingenuity.

THE PERSON AS A SKILLED PERFORMER

Competence implies the effective use of skills – but what is meant by skill? The word can be

Table 4.1 Explanations for dysfunction

Frame of reference	Explanation of dysfunction
Medical	Person is suffering from organic or functional disease, deficit or injury which renders him unable.
Environmental	Person is affected by social and/or environmental barriers, deprivation or hostile, stressful past or present circumstances.
Educational	There is a deficit in learning affecting knowledge, skills or attitudes which consequently affects social or productive performance.
Occupational	Person has an insufficient, or inappropriate, repertoire of necessary occupations and roles, lacks skills or shows occupational imbalance.
Developmental	Person lacks developmental potential and/or has not experienced suitable environmental opportunities to promote development of functional ability.
Biomechanical	Strength, range of movement or coordination of movement has been affected with consequent limitation of normal function.
Neurodevelopmental	Person shows congenital developmental delay, or delay or regression due to acquired damage to the sensory and nervous systems.
Cognitive	Problems are due to faulty perception and processing of information, memory, rational thinking, planning, organizing or problem-solving.
Analytical	A deficit in, or lack of integration of, the personality resulting from unconscious causes derived from childhood experiences or relationships leading to disturbances of thought, emotion, action or relationships.

used to indicate both innate potentials and the transference of those potentials into effective practice; it may also be used as a synonym for an activity or task, but this is confusing and best avoided.

Lovell (an educationalist) for example, uses skill in the sense of abilities or competencies (1987):

All skills, whether they are industrial skills or the skills of day to day life, whether they involve physical activity or are predominantly mental, have a number of characteristics in common. All are learned, all involve the building up of organised and co-ordinated activities in relation to some specific object or event, and all involve the ordering or co-ordination of a number of different processes or actions in a temporal sequence. They are serial in nature, that is to say one activity follows another.

Behaviourists are concerned solely with observable skill, by which they generally mean a component of performance. Other theorists tend to agree that skilled performance requires the integration of three elements, knowledge, skill and attitude, and that learning of each element takes place in subtly differing ways, and therefore requires differing methods of instruction. Gagné (1977) is particularly clear on this distinction.

Various educationalists, psychologists and occupational therapists have proposed differing ways of classifying and defining skills. Gagné describes five human performance skills. The first three relate to types of knowledge, the fourth to motor skill and the fifth to attitude:

1. Intellectual skills, including using symbols and rules, forming concepts, making discriminations and using procedures.
2. Cognitive strategies – effective ways of learning and remembering.
3. Verbal information – use of language, verbal concepts and 'labels'.
4. Motor skills – the ability smoothly to chain and engage gross or fine motor skills in intended actions.
5. Attitudes – feelings which influence choice of action and so direct behaviour.

The view of skills as the learned 'building blocks' for performance of activities is probably the most commonly held view in occupational therapy.

SKILL COMPONENTS

A person is born with potentials for performance, not with skills. Potentials are derived largely from genetic inheritance. Recent developments in genetics suggest that, in addition to personality traits, factors such as dispositions to be interested in, or skilful at, various pursuits may also have a genetic basis. The exact balance between genetic influence and the effects of environment remains unclear, but there must be suitable opportunities and experiences before a potential can be developed into a skill.

Human performance is so highly integrated that even the smallest performance unit, a task segment, requires the use of many skill components. The process of skill acquisition can be conceptualized as a spiral – skill development leads to performance which becomes established and integrated into the repertoire, and this in turn enables the individual to move towards the next level of competence and performance complexity.

The list of skill components in Box 4.1 is derived from the AOTA *Uniform terminology*, second edition (Hopkins & Smith 1993). Some modifications have been made to the list to take account of British terminology and practice, and to include some terminology used by others, including Mosey (1986), Reed (1983), and Gagné (1977).

Young & Quinn (1992) point out that 'humans master an astonishing array of skills ... many are culturally-specific, but all cultures require skills of some sort from their members and these change as cultures evolve.' They continue: 'Occupational therapists teach two broad classes of skills, motor (or perceptual motor) and social/communicative skills.'

Reed & Sanderson (1983) stress the role of the therapist in developing skills, and list motor, sensory, cognitive, intrapersonal (internal psychological mechanisms relating to concepts of self and reality) and interpersonal (roles and communication) components.

Kielhofner (1985) proposes that the performance subsystem in the model of human occupation consists of three types of skill, communication/interaction, process, and perceptual motor, each of which has symbolic, neurological and musculoskeletal constituents.

It is useful to separate the consideration of skill – the learnt, coordinated application of skill components to achieve a task or activity – from the evaluation of potential. In the case of skill, the question is 'how well can he do it?', i.e. has the task been learnt and mastered and has

---

Box 4.1 Skill components

Sensorimotor components

Those required for the execution of movement and for the appreciation of position, and the reception of input from the environment. These include:

Sensory integration	Integration of sensory input, motor output and sensory feedback, by means of sensory awareness, sensory processing and perceptual skills.
Neuromuscular skills	Those required to produce, control and utilize movement, including reflex integration, postural control, range of movement, strength and endurance.
Motor skills	Those required to produce coordinated, purposeful movement, including gross motor coordination, fine motor coordination, praxis, unilateral movement, bilateral movement and visual–motor coordination.

Cognitive components

Those involved in learning and the application of knowledge. These include:

Cognitive strategies.	Skills which enhance learning, including attention, memory, storage and retrieval of information.
Process skills	Those concerned with the application and integration of knowledge, including generalization, integration and synthesis of learning, sequencing, time management and problem solving.
Intellectual skills	Logical thinking, reasoning and deciding; internal manipulation of spatial relationships, concepts, time, language and number.

Psychosocial components

Those required for communication and interaction with others, including awareness of self in relation to others. These include:

Interpersonal skills	Social conduct, communication, self-expression, social cooperation, dyadic interaction and group interaction.
Intrapersonal skills	Those related to the development and maintenance of self-concept, identity and integrity, including self-control and coping skills.

effective performance been produced. In the case of potential, the question is 'has he the capacity to learn to do it?', i.e. does the person possess the basic physical or intellectual requirements to reach a suitable level of ability.

Education is as subject to the influence of frames of reference, models, theories and fashions as is occupational therapy. Indeed, many of the debates are identical, since both professions are concerned with the nature of learning (epistemology – the study of the nature of knowledge and methods of obtaining it) and with methods of promoting learning (theories and practice of teaching).

There are numerous educational textbooks and other texts on occupational therapy which deal with the nature of learning, to which the reader is referred for a detailed study; a summary of some of the main ideas will follow.

INFLUENTIAL THEORIES ABOUT THE NATURE OF LEARNING

Each theory tends to develop its own definitions of learning, but a useful, reasonably generic definition is given by Lovell (1987): 'The relatively permanent changes in potential for performance that result from past interactions with the environment'.

As Mocellin (1992b) points out: 'The ideology which equates occupation with health does not need complex explanatory models since healthy people are, on the whole, optimally occupied.' Cynkin & Robinson (1990) define *activities health* as 'a state of well-being in which the individual is able to carry out the activities of everyday living with satisfaction and comfort, in patterns and configurations that reflect sociocultural norms and idiosyncratic variation in number, variety, balance and context of activities.' Both these views imply that the individual must achieve and maintain competence in a great variety of learnt roles, occupations and activities. The individual as a learner is therefore of great interest to the therapist, but what is meant by learning, and on what does learning depend?

The chief debates concerning the person as a learner are those relating to the nature of motivation (mechanistic/deterministic versus organismic/free will conflicts) and to the nature of learning – the same conflicts with the addition of the 'nature versus nurture' debate.

These educational debates may be summarized in terms of the following questions:

- what is the nature of learning?
- what role does genetic predisposition play in learning?
- what role does environment play in learning?
- what motivates the person to learn?
- what role should the teacher play?
- how can learning best be promoted and encouraged?

It is clearly important for a therapist to have accurate methods for evaluation of potential and for identification of skill levels or deficits, since competent performance rests on the use of skill, and therapy is directed frequently towards skill improvement or acquisition.

THE PERSON AS A LEARNER

For many decades the debate has waxed and waned over whether 'nature' or 'nurture' decides human behaviour. It is now generally accepted that both contribute, but there is still much discussion about the balance between the two. In the 1980s the environmentalists and developmentalists were at the forefront; recent research has suggested that genetic inheritance may be more significant than was previously thought, at least in predisposing the individual to certain traits or abilities.

However this debate is eventually resolved it is clear that only a very small portion of human behaviour is totally instinctive and innate. All concepts, roles, relationships, styles of communication and occupational behaviours are learned. Each person is born with potential, great or small, to develop knowledge, skills or attitudes. The degree to which he does so will determine the degree to which he is able to be healthy and successful in occupational terms.

BEHAVIOURISM

Behaviourism is derived from the principles of classical conditioning as modified by later theorists into behavioural theories of learning. The behavioural definition of learning is 'an observable change in behaviour'. Behaviour is a conditioned response to the environment, therefore 'A person does not act upon the world, the world acts upon him' (Skinner 1938). Learning is thus a comparatively passive process which 'happens to' the learner without the necessity of active choice.

The chief contribution to teaching practice has been the use of backward or forward chaining to break into small stages – the behaviours to be learnt stimulus-response chains, each step of which can be taught by means of practice and appropriate shaping, cueing, prompting and reinforcement; these steps are gradually chained together until a complete behaviour has been achieved. 'Unwanted' behaviours can be removed by a similar process. In order to teach using this method very precise behavioural objectives must be set, and the teacher must control all elements of the learning situation.

Some educational theorists straddle the behavioural–cognitive divide. Bandura (1977) extended behavioural theory to include the concept of social learning – that people do not learn only by direct personal experience, but also by observing the rewards and sanctions obtained by other learners, whose rewarded behaviour can then be imitated. This allows for some personal thought, choice and insight, thus Bandura was able to write that 'People are at least in part the architects of their own destinies.'

Gagné (1977) proposes a cognitive–behavioural hierarchical structure for learning, and a system of instruction which is particularly applicable to occupational therapy, since it deals with skill acquisition.

COGNITIVISM

Cognitivists are prepared to accept that humans view the world 'from inside looking out'. Introspection is not only valid but important. They consider that the learner gradually constructs a model of reality (hence the term 'constructivism'). These ideas are concerned with the internal mechanisms of learning, and explore the ways in which learning may be inferred to take place (inferred because no-one may directly observe them), the physiological processes involved, and the data processing, perceptions and connections which occur in the 'internal space' of the learner. Learning is 'the discovery of meaning'.

The teacher's role is to identify the student's perceptions and to present material in the way most likely to promote learning; learning will not occur in the absence of motivation, for motivation precedes attention, the first stage of memory. Some cognitive researchers have studied the styles and strategies which people employ when learning.

RATIONALISM

Rationalists propose that individual learning involves the unfolding and discovery of innate understanding and knowledge which need simply to be 'brought out' of the learner, perhaps by a question and answer method known as 'Socratic dialogue'. If the learner is asked the right questions he can be conducted towards discovering the 'right' answers.

DEVELOPMENTALISM

As some theorists straddle cognitive–behavioural ideas, so others are cognitive–developmentalists. Bruner is quoted frequently in occupational therapy literature, having written extensively about the processes of learning, and the way in which the person constructs models of reality. Bruner suggests three modes of representation: enactive – being able to remember and enact appropriate motor responses; iconic – the internal, perceptually organized, imagery of the mind; and symbolic – the use of language in thought (Bigge 1987).

His ideas suggest ways in which material should be presented and organized to engage these representational modes, and advocate particularly experiential and problem-based styles of learning. Like Gagné, he is interested in the implicit and explicit 'rules of behaviour' and the ways in which these are learned.

Other developmentalists have been concerned with charting the stages of learning, e.g. Piaget (1952, Piaget & Inhelder 1969), who explains the developmental sequence in the child, or Perry (1970), who describes the 'nine positions of adult learning'.

Knowles (1978) has a developmental–humanistic perspective and has concentrated on exploring the ways in which adults learn, coining the term 'andragogy' to indicate adult learning. He too stresses the importance of personal perceptions of meaning, relevance and relationship with experience in motivating adults to learn.

Developmentalists view learning as a continuous and lifelong process, and acknowledge the importance experiential person–environment reactions. Impoverished or inappropriate environments which limit the scope for exploration and experiment severely constrain the learning process.

PERSON-CENTRED LEARNING

With the exception of the behaviourists, who maintain control and direction and do not consider subjective aspects of motivation or the processes of cognition, each of the schools of thought views the learner as an active and motivated participant in learning, and the teacher as instrumental in structuring relevant learning experiences, and providing information or instruction.

The person-centred theory of learning places the responsibility for learning squarely with the learner, and sees the role of the teacher as a facilitator of the learning process. This theory derives chiefly from the work of Rogers (1983), and therefore relates closely to his ideas concerning therapy which developed from his experience as an educationalist.

Rogers' statement about the person as learner: 'Man is subjectively free: his personal choice and responsibility account for the shape of his life; he is in fact the architect of himself', is, possibly deliberately, the antithesis of the views of Skinner and Bandura.

Rogers states even that it is impossible for one person to teach another anything. The 'teacher' can only help to facilitate learning; the learner must set his own goals and evaluate his own progress.

The goal of education if we are to survive is the facilitation of change and learning ... (which) rests upon certain attitudinal qualities which exist in the personal relationship between the facilitator and the learner.

These attitudinal qualities are precisely those which Rogers advocates in the therapeutic relationship, e.g. authenticity, openness, prizing, acceptance, positive regard and trust.

REASONS FOR INEFFECTIVE LEARNING

Unfortunately, learning is a complex entity which relates to organic, motivational and environmental factors. It may be difficult to untangle these strands in the life of an individual and typically there is more than one reason for failure to learn. Some examples are given in Box 4.2.

PSYCHOLOGICAL PERSPECTIVES

Psychology, like education, has a variety of models of the description of the person (indeed, many educational models are derived from studies of the psychology of learning). Occupational therapy has borrowed from most of these in its history; physiological, behavioural, analytical, cognitive, social, developmental and humanistic theories have each been influential in their turn. The fact that these frequently provide contradictory explanations of the human condition has not in the least deterred the therapist, who is happy to accept these as alternative explanations which may, in different situations and for different clients, provide helpful explanations.

This seems to be another example of the acquisitive therapist wishing to use these alternative frames of reference as tools, rather than selecting one to provide a total 'world view'.

Box 4.2 Reasons for failure to learn

Organic reasons
- Damage to the person's physical capacity to learn. The person is unable to perceive, store or recall information, as a result of neurological or sensory damage or deficit.
- Damage to the person's ability to perform. The person may be able to learn how to do something, but cannot execute the required actions due to damage to or deficit in the sensorimotor functions of the body.

Motivational reasons
- The benefits of learning – intrinsic or extrinsic rewards – are viewed as insufficient or inappropriate by the learner.
- The person perceives no need for learning. Material to be learned is viewed as irrelevant, useless, meaningless or culturally inappropriate.
- The person is inhibited from learning by feelings of anxiety or insecurity, by negative perceptions of the thing to be learnt or by previous unsuccessful experiences of learning.
- The person is suffering from a disorder affecting motivation and the ability to initiate the action required to learn.

Cognitive reasons
- There are deficits in the internal environment which affect readiness to learn, e.g. lack of foundation skills (cognitive, perceptual, sensorimotor, interactive), foundation concepts, rules or discriminations required for learning.
- The learner's perceptions of his environment exclude, for some reason, perception of, or attention to, things to be learned.

Environmental reasons
- Past environments have limited learning opportunities so severely that the basis for new learning has not been established.
- There are deficits in the learning environment so that the external conditions of learning – opportunities, conditions, tools, materials, suitable model or teacher – are not available.
- Sociocultural values, customs and attitudes inhibit or prohibit learning.
- There is a failure of communication between the teacher and the learner.

There has been, however, in the last 15 years or so, a noticeable trend way from deterministic explanations, towards organismic and phenomenological explanations. These ideas have filtered into the core, being related by some theorists to the early philosophy of the profession, suggesting that in some ways our founders were ahead of the field in promoting this phenomenological perspective of the person.

Although this may be true to some extent, it has to be remembered that these founders did not, some 90 years ago, have access to the research evidence or evolved conceptualization currently available. Our ways of thinking may be similar to theirs, but they cannot be the same – reinterpretation is a continual occurrence.

SOCIOLOGICAL PERSPECTIVES

THE PERSON AS A MEMBER OF SOCIETY

Historically, the focus of occupational therapy has been on the individual rather than on society. Sociology has long been ignored, while the profession has drawn its scientific background from psychology, physiology, medicine, psychiatry and other disciplines which are concerned primarily with the individual in isolation or in only immediate relation to others.

Social psychology is now included in the curriculum, but sociology as such remains largely excluded. A scan through the references drawn by therapists from academic sources will confirm rapidly that sociologists are seldom quoted. This is puzzling, as occupational therapy is itself a type of social science, being concerned, as discussed in the preceding pages, with cultures, attitudes, beliefs, the study of work and leisure, and the effects of the sociopolitical environment on health and social adaptation. All of these concerns are in the domain of sociology, at least insofar as it deals with the analysis of the individual in relation to small groups, rather than to large groups or cultures.

There are clear parallels between some of the statements in academic writing about the theory of occupational therapy and some of the more significant sociological theories of the past 30 years. This is noticeable particularly in American texts, and it is surely no coincidence that many of the prominent sociological theorists of the past 50 years were American. It is debatable whether this a case of the parallel development of ideas within two different professions, or whether sociological theory has filtered into occupational therapy thinking without recognition or acknowledgement of the source; it may be that both mechanisms have contributed. The following models are worth summarizing in view of their relevance to occupational therapy.

FUNCTIONALISM

Although functionalism has largely been replaced by other theories, its influence lingers. Haralambos (1985) described the functionalist view of society as organic; social institutions such as the family or religion are understood with reference to the contribution they make to the system as a whole. This has some similarity with the occupational therapy view of the 'functional' individual, in which the totality of actions contributes to the well-being of the individual.

Functionalists have tried to identify 'functional prerequisites' which any society must have if it is to be maintained and developed. Talcott Parsons (O'Donnell 1992) is a functionalist to whose work occupational therapists may relate. He believes that only a commitment to common values provides a basis for order in society and that value consensus forms the fundamental integrating principle in society. Common goals are derived from shared values.

Roles provide the means whereby values and goals are translated into action . . . The content of roles is structured in terms of norms which define the rights and obligations applicable to each role.

Haralambos states that:

Parsons views society as a system. He argues that any social system has four basic functional pre-requisites – adaptation; goal attainment; integration and pattern maintenance. These can be seen as problems which we must solve if we are to survive. . . . Adaptation refers to the relationship between the social system and its environment.

While it is plain that Parsons, being a sociologist, is referring to *society*, these ideas echo closely some therapists' views of the *individual* as an adaptive, purposeful, integrative system; the model of human occupation with its organic system basis and concern with values seems to relate to this perspective. It is also interesting to note the efforts of therapists in the USA to provide a coherent scheme of values as a unifying force for the 'occupational therapy society'.

Functionalism has been criticized heavily on the basis that it is overly deterministic and that it is very difficult to prove the kind of consensus of values in a society which Parsons suggests.

SYMBOLIC INTERACTIONISM

The American philosopher George Herbert Mead is a principal contributer to this theory. Interactionism takes a phenomenological view of human thought, experience and behaviour as essentially social. The most important aspect of the theory is, as its name suggests, that people interact in terms of symbols which impose particular meanings on objects and events. The development of language promotes this symbolic view of the world.

Human society relies on shared meanings; through these we are able to understand the actions of others and make our own actions compatible with theirs. We respond not only to overt behaviour, but also to our own implicit intentions, and those of the others in the same situation. Role play and role-taking are important in helping a person to build an identity and to understand others.

Symbolic interactionism is too complex to be described in this text, but six basic propositions are quoted in Murphy (1984):

1. Human beings are different from animals in that we assign symbolic meanings to stimuli and interact on the basis of these meanings.
2. What characterises human action is the fact that it has both overt and covert aspects.
3. The starting point for socialization is the fact that the infant is born into and participates in a world of meanings.
4. The child develops a self through interaction with other people.
5. Socialization both enmeshes the individual in a social world and makes it possible for the individual to transform, oppose or counter-define his/her social world.

6. Socialization is never finally and absolutely complete.

Again, the relevance to occupational therapy is clear: there is increasing emphasis on the importance of personal meanings and symbols and of how the situational aspects of any activity or interaction change the reactions and roles of particpants.

SOCIAL ACTION THEORY

This is a development from structuralist theory originated by Max Weber who set out to analyse the individual person in sociological terms. O'Donnell (1992) categorizes Weber's views on social action into four types, motivated by reason, values, emotion or tradition, as follows:

Instrumentally rational action (geared to 'the statement of the actors' own rationally pursued and calculated ends').

Value-rational action ('determined by a conscious belief in a value for its own sake . . . independently of its prospects of success').

Affectual action ('determined by the actors' specific affects and feeling states').

Traditional action ('determined by ingrained habituation').

This again has similarities with those occupational therapy theorists who view motivation from a cognitive–behavioural perspective.

PHENOMENOLOGY AND ETHNOMETHODOLOGY

Phenomenologists reject the notion of a fixed objective reality in favour of the idea that each individual makes his own version of reality through interpretation of personal perceptions and experiences. Therapists have taken a firm hold of this view, maintaining that the individual's personal perspectives must be discovered, respected, and taken account of in therapy. Objective reality (or rather the version of reality as perceived by the therapist or others) is less significant than the reality which the patient is currently experiencing.

However, from a sociological perspective, meanings are developed not just by the individual, but also by individuals in a group who develop shared perceptions of reality and shared cultural interpretations which become so deeply integrated into their lives, that the individuals are unaware of the subjective nature of their views.

Ethnomethodology (founded by Harold Garfinkle in the early 1960s) was a deliberate attempt to apply the phenomenological perspective to sociological research. Ethnomethodologists rely on observation to document actions in a situational context with reference to the meanings that the actors ascribe to them. Meaning and event are interrelated and interdependent (indexicality and reflexivity). Any attempt to interpret or structure these meanings or to generalize them beyond the given situation is strictly avoided. Life appears orderly or patterned because people see it, describe it and explain it as such, but they tend to impose structure where none exists. Ethnomethodology seeks to understand how people set about this task of making sense out of the world.

Because these methods are qualitative and descriptive rather than quantitative, and because they eschew artificial and external interpretation of actions within situations, they offer possibilities for research into occupational therapy in areas where scientific, hypothesis-based methods are inappropriate.

THE HEALTHY PERSON

Social perspectives on health and illness

Medical sociology has also had a considerable effect on the core assumptions of occupational therapy. There is nothing very new in the idea of ill-health being associated with causes such as poverty, deprivation, working conditions, stress or cultural practices, and the effects of health and social policy on health care – in other words, with social, rather than purely organic or physical, factors.

Throughout the 1980s there has been an

increased awareness of the significance of these factors.

Not only are diseases now more identified with multiple causal factors which are distant in terms of time from the end result, but, more importantly, this shift in ideas about disease processes suggests that health care provision ought to be directed more towards intervention in the state of affairs prior to the ultimate manifestation of the disease.
(Patrick & Scambler 1986.)

The 'new' ideas concern a phenomenological view of health and illness. O'Donnell (1992) describes three 'cultural paradigms of health'. He lists the magical and religious view, the modern scientific medicine view and the humanistic view of holistic medicine. Illness, with its causes, meanings and effects, is constructed in the mind of the individual and in the collective perceptions of society. Even the data collected to give statistics about ill-health has been shown by ethnomethodologists to be subject to our selectively organizing and patterning perceptions and interpretations.

The therapist needs to be as, or more, concerned with how the patient feels and thinks about his own health, how significant others perceive this, and how the social and physical environment affects health, as with what is wrong with him. Cynkin & Robinson (1990) state that 'health (and its practical correlate function) is manifested in the ability of the individual to participate in socio-culturally regulated activities with satisfaction and comfort.'

The holistic view has been strongly influential in occupational therapy, although in practice the concept may be honoured more by words than by action since there is a tension between this view of individual health and that proposed by the medical model. This dichotomy between the medical and social models of wellness and illness has been discussed by Reed (1984).

Occupational therapy, being a medically prescribed therapy, has absorbed much of the medical view of the ill person as having a condition to be diagnosed, for which treatment is prescribed, and a 'cure', or at least improvement, sought. The majority of therapists continue to work in medically dominated settings and must communicate with doctors 'in their own language'. However, the occupational therapy view of the ill or disabled person is fundamentally closer to the social model than to the medical one.

The whole purpose of therapy is to concentrate on wellness; to enable and empower the individual (both sociological words) through his own actions, to take charge of his own life, to improve his own health and to deal with the effects of his condition or disability. The therapist seeks to facilitate this by removing the physical, psychological, social and environmental barriers which prevent the person taking action on his own behalf or becoming integrated into society.

This is easier said than done. It requires a considerable shift in perspective from both the therapist and society as a whole. The emphasis must shift from providing a group for the person to attend to allowing people to set up and run their own group, from finding a job for a disabled person to making all jobs available to as wide a range of people as possible, from adapting housing or public transport to ensuring that as much as possible is designed so as not to require adaptation. It is the difference between the provision of a 'health service' and an 'illness service', between quantity and quality of life.

CONCLUSION

Many of the perspectives discussed in this chapter seem to have a sociological dimension. Insofar as sociology deals with individual actions in relation to small numbers of others, it offers interesting insights concerning the person who occupational therapists have, perhaps unwittingly, begun to assimilate into their assumptions. A more conscious and knowledgeable use of this theory might be profitable, not least in providing new perspectives to enlarge our understanding of the basis on which we provide schemata and interpretions for the actions, roles and interactions of others.

Social views of health and illness have informed occupational therapy practice, which continues to move away from the medical model. Awareness of societal factors which contribute to health or illness can lead therapists to develop prophylactic occupational or environmental interventions and to work for appropriate changes in health and social policy.

A summary of occupational therapy assumptions is given in Box 4.3.

Box 4.3   Occupational therapy assumptions concerning the person

1. Humans' abilities to think, imagine, plan, make, create and problem-solve are defining attributes of humanity.
2. Each person is a unique individual, genetically, by the nature of personal experience, in the content of his physical and sociocultural environment, and in his precise pattern of roles, relationships, occupations and activities.
3. A person is innately capable of choice concerning roles, relationships, occupations and activities. A person is able, through his choices, to take positive actions or to make decisions concerning his life.
4. Choices may be constrained by the interplay of many complex factors affecting an individual including disability, illness, injury, dysfunction, beliefs, values, environmental or social barriers, lack of knowledge or skill, or economic disadvantage.
5. Active participation in a varied repertoire of occupations, activities, roles and relationships is the essential means whereby a person interacts with the environment for the purposes of personal survival, social survival, cultural affirmation, and the achievement of personal purposes and satisfactions.
6. A person requires the ability to perform competently a variety of occupational and social roles which change throughout life and must be appropriate to his age, sex, social status and culture.
7. A person needs to express and affirm his cultural values and affiliations, and the therapist must take account of such needs in any intervention or therapy.
8. Occupational competence occurs when an individual is able, consistently, and to the satisfaction of personal and cultural standards, to cope with the majority of his personal occupations, activities, roles and relationships.
9. Occupational dysfunction renders a person unable to meet the requirements of his life, and additionally tends to render the person ineffective in efforts to alter this condition.
10. A person requires a repertoire of skills, e.g. sensorimotor, cognitive–perceptual, interactive, process, to be developed in order to produce competent performance. Skill development depends on the opportunities for learning the provision of a suitable environment.
11. Competent participation in, and performance of, roles, occupations and activities, engaging the maximum potential of the individual, depends on effective learning.
12. As competent performance depends on learning it becomes important to identify the reasons for the failure of learning. If the reasons can be found, remedial action may be possible.
13. The person's subjective view of reality and the way in which he makes sense of and interprets his own life and actions should be respected and understood.

5

Occupation

The difficulties of defining occupations and occupational therapy have been discussed in Chapter 2. Occupations, activities and roles have meaning only in the context of human performance, and some aspects have already been explored in Chapter 3. In this Chapter, I shall be less concerned with these broader aspects of occupation, and more with the technicalities of defining and understanding occupations for use in therapy.

DESCRIPTION OF PERFORMANCE

The purpose of having words such as *occupation*, *activity* and *task*, is to describe areas of human performance with precision and, from the point of view of the therapist, to enable analysis of human performance to be carried out for therapeutic reasons. Current general usage in the UK is summarized in Box 5.1.

The levels of performance described in Box 5.1 – if they *are* levels, for this is not generally agreed – seem to overlap. Any therapist who has conducted analytical exercises, using even one of the better-constructed systems of analysis, will encounter difficulties when the available terminology runs out and the threads become too entangled to separate.

Given the amazingly complex, adaptive and diverse nature of human behaviour, it should be no surprise that occupations are not simple to explain or define. It is a matter of concern, however, that with a few exceptions relating to

---

Box 5.1 Usage of terms

Occupation
- A generic title, used in the name of the profession and whenever it is necessary to speak of the total span of human action. An 'umbrella' term.
- Commonly used interchangeably with 'activity' to indicate something purposeful which is done. Occupations are described variously as work/productivity; play/leisure; self-care/self-maintenance/activities of daily living.

Activity Used both as a verb to describe the action of being active and as a noun to indicate a specific instance of being active. Activities are generally seen as divisible into tasks.

Tasks Sometimes used as a synonym for activity, but most usually seen as components of activity.

Skills Performance components required for task completion, variously classified.

---

specific models, our profession still seems rather vague in its terminology concerning, and methods used in, the core processes employed in the analysis and description of occupations. Considerable research and refinement are required if more generally accepted taxonomies and methods are to be evolved.

There appears to be a tension between the desire, on the one hand to view occupations as gestalts, retaining the richness of meanings and inter-relationships and avoiding any mechanistic reductionism, and on the other hand recognizing the need to *be* reductive and analytical when it comes to specific application. Both views seem legitimate in context. Are they necessarily incompatible? I suggest that they are not, but also that the current vocabulary is insufficient and too imprecise to be a useful tool.

This imprecison also leads to difficulties in terms of producing taxonomies for the classification and analysis of occupations; here again, authors vary.

DIFFERING VIEWS OF OCCUPATIONAL TAXONOMIES AND OCCUPATIONAL ANALYSIS

If occupations are conceptualized as gestalts, the reductionist process of analysis into some form of structure or taxonomy has to be accepted as artificial. It is, nonetheless, essential as a therapeutic tool.

Reed (1984) proposes one taxonomy related to her model of adaptation through occupation. She states that:

1. Occupation can be divided into three subcategories: self-maintenance, productivity and leisure, which in turn can be subdivided.
2. Occupation can be divided into component tasks:
   a. Orientation – includes the three dimensions of space, the individual, family or community and three dimensions of time, clock, circadian and psychologic.
   b. Order – includes patterns forward and backward, sideways, up and down, circular, spiral, fixed or flexible.
   c. Activation – includes the ability to move all or part of the body in certain prescribed ways as well as the thinking or rehearsal of movement in order to do an occupation.
3. Occupations can be divided into five performance areas: motor, sensory, cognitive, intrapersonal and interpersonal, which can be subdivided.

Kielhofner (1985) classifies occupations as work, leisure/play and daily living tasks. He uses 'task' to denote 'any occupational activity' within these areas. Tasks have five dimensions:

- complexity
- temporal boundaries
- rules
- seriousness/playfulness
- social.

Task performance requires skill. Skills are 'The symbolic images or rules and biological structures and functions organized into gestalts'. Skills can be divided into communication/interaction, process and perceptual/motor, each of which has symbolic, neurological and musculoskeletal components.

Cynkin & Robinson (1990) offer a very thorough discussion of activities from a number of perspectives, including patterns and configurations, and spatial or locational features. They criticize the standard 'work, leisure' classification of activities (occupations) and propose two approaches to classification: sociobiological (survival needs) and sociocultural (historical, social and cultural factors).

Young & Quinn (1992) give a format for process-based activity analysis rather than a taxonomy. They suggest that:

'Activity may be analysed in terms of:
1. Permanent and unchanging requirements intrinsic to the activity itself.
2. Other requirements, such as those of space, equipment and materials which are always present and need consideration, but which change.
3. Social and cultural perceptions of both the activity and the outcome of the activity.'

Johnson (1992) also describes activity analysis as a process of division into tasks and subtasks: 'an activity is a step-by-step process involving a potentially large number of operations in which sequencing is vital.'

Both Pedretti (1985) and Trombley (1983) give methods of activity analysis based on bio-mechanical and neurodevelopmental approaches.

All these approaches provide information about occupations, activities or tasks, but the proposed structures tend to emphasize a particular area or aspect; they do not distinguish between differing purposes or levels of analysis, and it is difficult to find one which enables the therapist to analyse an occupation through all its levels in sufficient detail.

One form of occupational analysis is the socio-cultural classification of occupations which comprises:

- **Work** (productivity)
- **Leisure** (play)
- **Self-care** (self-maintenance; activities of daily living).

A balance between these aspects of life is often advocated. The apparent simplicity of this classification is deceptive, for there are many anomalies. The significance of these areas of life to an individual has already been discussed in Chapter 4, but it is worth exploring these further as a means of understanding the nature of occupations and activities and their differences.

SOCIOCULTURAL CLASSIFICATION OF OCCUPATIONS AND ACTIVITIES

There are three perspectives on sociocultural classification:

1. The link between occupation and an occupational role title for the participant, and the way possession of such a role may influence the person's position in society.

2. The view of the occupation, and its significance to society as observed by others.

3. The subjective perceptions of the participant concerning his roles and the nature and significance of his occupations which, although individual, are strongly influenced by the culture in which she lives.

Occupational titles and social role titles

Humans are 'labellers' – they like to find names for things and people, and titles to designate roles and relationships. A role is a social designation which has implications of expected responsibilities and actions. There are two forms of role titles, occupational and social. How does a role relate to an occupation?

It should seem a straightforward matter that an occupation (in the sense of employment) has a title, e.g. carpentry, computing, medicine, law, dressmaking, cooking, engineering. The participant's role title when engaged in the occupation is usually derived from, or closely associated with this occupational name: carpenter, computer operator, doctor, lawyer, dressmaker, cook, engineer. There are sometimes also linked verbs, such as to to cook.

Jobs may further be given sociocultural descriptions such as managerial, professional, white-collar or blue-collar. The type of work undertaken may be described further using socio-historic terms such as crafts, trades or techniques. The main performance features of a job may be recognized, leading to descriptions such as sedentary work, clerical work, assembly work, manual work, with associated stereotypes concerning the sex, status or intelligence of workers.

We often ask a new acquaintance 'what do you do?', usually meaning in terms of work, or main role. When we have a reply we are likely to respond to that person according to the above preconceptions. Incorrect attributions of role and status, leading to an inappropriate social response, are embarrassing to both parties.

However, even in British culture such designations, although slow to change, are not fixed. With changing patterns of work and leisure blurring the boundaries, and the opportunity for some people to move more fluidly between occupations, the expression of personal identity by a single occupational role for the majority of life, while still the dominant pattern, is not the only one. It remains unclear what will replace it. In other cultures occupational titles may be even more significant in terms of status or social acceptability than they are in the UK.

The question of role titles in relation to occupations has another interesting feature. Basic activities which are related to personal health and survival do not generally have associated occupational role titles. We do speak of bakers, artists, authors, but we do not talk about 'dressers', 'washers' or 'eaters', and a social role description such as 'independent person' would not be widely understood. It is surely significant that such activities as washing and dressing are customarily referred to by therapists as 'personal *activities* of daily living' (PADL). It does not seem appropriate to refer to these activities as occupations.

Activities of daily living (ADL) become incorporated into occupations as a kind of supportive infrastructure; these activities are antecedant to the main occupation. If we cannot get ourselves out of bed in the morning, wash, dress, and have breakfast, we cannot get to work. 'Getting ready for work' is a preliminary process for working, as is 'travelling to work'. At other times ADL supports social roles such as parent or student.

However, occupational titles need not indicate a worker, but may relate to someone engaged in leisure or self-care. Despite the fact that 'the cook' is cooking for pleasure rather than for payment, the therapist will generally recognize the nature of such engagement as 'occupational'.

A similar nominal distinction applies to casual and intermittent leisure pursuits. People who occasionally swim, ride, play football or paint for fun do not usually introduce themselves as swimmers, riders, footballers or artists unless such an activity forms a highly important area of their lives. Many leisure activities are experiential rather than productive, e.g. watching television, listening to music, sunbathing. These also bring role titles only when the participant spends much time engaged in them.

It can be seen, therefore, that the designation of 'occupation' is related to two linked factors: an extended period of participation, and acceptance by the participant of an associated role title to identify such participation as a separate and significant part of life.

What about social role titles such as parent, child, housewife, grandfather? Are these related to occupations? There are two forms of social role titles: those which describe a relationship, e.g. mother, father, husband, wife, partner, niece, aunt, grandmother; and those which indicate something about what the person does, e.g. student, schoolgirl, housewife, worshipper, volunteer.

The role titles designating relationships imply, at least in western cultures, diverse spheres of action which are not easily defined by a generic noun or verb. A builder is engaged in the occupation of building, he builds things. Law is practised by a lawyer. A sister is not described as having the occupation of 'sistering' nor does she 'sister' or 'practise as a sister'. On the whole, such roles do not have a product in the same sense as does an occupation.

One possible exception is the role of parent. One does speak of fatherhood and motherhood, and there are verbs 'to mother' and 'to father'. There is now also the generic 'parenthood' and 'parenting'. Perhaps this linguistic clue indicates a recognition that parenthood is an occupation?

Social roles which imply some aspect of 'doing', such as housewife, holidaymaker, student, however, do seem more like occupations, for it is possible to define some of the general purposes, products and processes of such a role.

One view would be that these social role titles define important relationships and consequent responsibilities and sociocultural expectations. Another view would be to regard these as occupational roles, albeit of a rather atypical nature, having an organizational function in coordinating complex, individualized patterns of occupations and activities, the analysis of which would be extremely lengthy.

Whether or not they are related to occupations or activities, social roles organize and direct a substantial part of an individual's actions and relationships, and cannot be disregarded. A view of an individual which included only elements having clear 'occupational' titles would be incomplete. I am therefore inclined to place social roles at the top of the taxonomy of occupations which will be presented later in this chapter on the assumption that they have a function in organizing occupations.

Work, leisure and self-care

The classification of occupations into the above categories (or synonyms for these) has become general within occupational therapy. Several integrative models – adaptation through occupation (Reed & Sanderson), model of human occupation (Kielhofner), occupational performance (CAOT) – use this division as an essential part of the model.

The Canadian occupational performance measure gives the following examples of performance areas (Law et al 1990):

- Self-care: Personal care: dressing, bathing, feeding
  Functional mobility: stairs, bed, cars
  Community management: transportation, finances, services
- Productivity: Paid/unpaid work: finding and/or keeping a job
  Household management: cleaning, laundry, cooking
  Play/school: play skills, school performance, homework
- Leisure: Quiet recreation: hobbies, crafts, reading, cards
  Active recreation: sports, outings, travel
  Socialization: visiting, phone calls, parties, correspondence.

Although I agree that this form of classifi-

cation is pragmatic and useful, I believe that it should not be accepted without question. The fundamental problem is that such classifications are sociocultural, contextual and situational, and not, for the most part, inherent characteristics of each occupation or activity.

Although some cultures have reached an agreement on what is generally accepted to fall into each of these classifications, in terms of personal participation, such designation often depends on the context of performance and the perceptions of the participants.

Many occupations and activities fall into two or more of these classifications: one may cook as a job, cook for pleasure or cook for survival – it all depends on the circumstances. To complicate matters further, it is possible to perform different activities simultaneously, e.g. planning an outing while ironing, or in an interwoven manner where performance of each element utilizes short bursts of attention and engagement, e.g. a secretary writing a letter, answering the telephone, replying to queries, reminding the boss of an appointment and deciding where to have lunch, all in the space of 15 minutes.

As already noted, the concept of a division between work, leisure and self-care is culturally biased. While this is recognized by the industrialized western world, a different view is taken by other cultures, especially in developing countries where these boundaries blur and disappear.

Even in the UK boundaries are unclear. Young & Quinn (1992) quote Parker (1971) as identifying differing views of leisure, as an extension of work, the opposite of it, or complementary to it. They add that:

There is no clear dividing line between leisure occupations and work . . . leisure cannot adequately be defined in terms of an inverse relation to work.

They also point out that not everyone is able, wishes, or has the opportunity to define a part of their lives in this way. Cynkin & Robinson (1990) make a similar criticism of the standard definitions.

Age also has a marked effect on the relevance of these classifications. Children play and go to school; it does not seem appropriate to regard these occupations or activities as leisure or work, although they are in preparation for both. Retired people do not 'work' in a formal sense, but may work hard as volunteers.

People who have no job may nonetheless engage in many activities which satisfy the needs otherwise met by work – how should such activities be described? Are the essential, unpaid, chores of daily life work? Probably many people would view them in this way; they certainly contribute to personal and social survival, yet I have known people who regard at least some aspects as leisure.

There are other grey areas. Kielhofner views these classifications as applying to occupations rather than to activities. He therefore excludes sexual, social and religious activities from the work, leisure and self-care categories, and speaks of these as activities. Yet sex can be work in some circumstances (prostitution is certainly an occupation) and it might well be regarded in different situations as either leisure or self-care.

The occupations of priest or rabbi are generally accepted as vocational callings – work – but what about the worshipper? Is the devout Jew, Catholic or Muslim who participates in religious observances which may take up a substantial part of her time, engaged in leisure, or perhaps self-care? Neither is a comfortable description. If such observances are 'spiritual activities' and not occupations, are they excluded from the

---

Box 5.2 Features of work, leisure and self-care

Work
- Has a product or result of value to society, culture, or the individual, but typically is an aspect of a cooperative division of labour which enables the individual to survive as a member of society, and promotes the survival or society as a whole.
- At the occupational level work defines a major life role and provides identity for the participant, specified by an occupational title.
- Work may contribute to self-esteem and self-concept.
- Work performance is normally related to standards, e.g. of quality, quantity, completion, set by an employer or other person, or by an individual worker.
- There is usually a defined reward, but this is not always financial – it may be social approval, an expression of altruism, or something done or made which is of value to the worker.
- There are usually implications of some kind of obligation or commitment, e.g. to provide a needed service or goods, to be a productive member of society, to fulfil a 'breadwinner' role, to provide care for another, to meet a deadline.
- Work is typically structured, perhaps only loosely, in patterns of activity, responsibility and use of time. These patterns may be imposed by someone other than the worker.

Leisure
- Is self-selected and has value and meaning to the participant.
- May satisfy personal needs for self-expression, self-actualization, self-directed learning.
- The standards, goals and duration of participation are set by the participant.

- Leisure provides outlets for playfulness, creativity, fantasy, exploration, adaptation, spontaneity, emotional expression.
- May meet personal needs for affiliation and social interaction, e.g. through membership of group with shared goals or ideals.
- May promote cultural identity.
- May involve elements of rest, reflection and relaxation, as well as productive activity.

Self-care (activities of daily living)
- Promotes physical health and safety, and satisfies basic survival needs which would have to be met by someone else if the individual could not satisfy them herself.
- Promotes the social well-being of the individual, and enables her to maintain social roles and relationships.
- Enables the individual to remain a productive, independent, contributor to society.
- Enables the individual to care for significant others.
- Enables the individual to participate in work or leisure.
- Carries implied expectations of competence related to age, sex and culture.

ADL may be subdivided into:
Personal activities of daily living: those associated with personal survival, maintenance and well-being, e.g. washing, eating, toileting, mobility, communication.
Domestic activities of daily living (also known as instrumental activities): those required to provide and maintain a dwelling, or to maintain dependent or associated others. These activities are sometimes categorized as work.

attention of the therapist? Clearly, to disregard such meaningful or symbolic elements of daily life because they are not easily classified would make no sense, nor does it seem helpful to restrict these designations to 'occupations' when it is clear that 'activities' may also be classified in this way.

These anomalies and ambiguities are as much a reflection of the rich diversity of human occupation and activity, which obstinately refuses to be neatly categorized, as they are arguments for the extension of occupational classification. We must beware of trying to force all human activity into distinct 'pigeonholes'.

In general terms, however, the categories of work, leisure and self-care can be distinguished from each other by a number of features which relate to the purposes and motivation of the participant and the circumstances in which the occupation or activity is performed. Box. 5.2 summarized the main features.

For the purposes of therapeutic analysis an occupation or activity may be placed in a category if it is seen to possess most of the significant features of that category. Apart from practical considerations, the concepts, values and meanings attached to each category may change significantly the individual's motivation to participate in an activity.

However, as noted, some of these categories are restrictive, and some aspects of human interest and endeavour are excluded. If such classification is to be useful, an extended taxonomy might be helpful. Table 5.1 is provisional, and illustrates the disadvantage of proliferating classifications – however much one includes, more seems to be left out.

Summary of classifications

To summarize this discussion so far; an occupational role affects other people's perceptions of, and attitudes towards, the owner. The claiming or rejection of an occupational role is an important affirmation of personal identity. These features help to explain why the loss of a valued

Table 5.1   Classification of occupations and activities

Work	Employment	Having a paid job
	Training for work	Preparing for paid employment
	Education	Work substitute for a child or student
	Domestic work	Necessary chores and DIY jobs
Leisure	Hobby	A continuing leisure interest
	Recreation	An activity engaged in for fun
	Play	Imaginative, experimental fun
	Sport	Including ball games and sports
	Social activity	Involving interaction with others
	Cultural activity	Art, drama, music, festival, parade, etc
	Relaxation	In which the mind and/or body are relatively passive
Citizenship	Voluntary work	Contributing time and effort without payment
	Political activity	Supporting or representing a political cause
	Social responsibility	Being involved in maintaining society
Ritual observances	Religious activities	With others or alone
	Rituals and rites	Cultural, social or religious
	Festive activities	Celebrations shaped by custom
	Cultural affirmation	Activities which promote sense of belonging
Personal activities of daily living (ADL)	Personal care	Activities needed for personal survival/health
	Communication	Activities which express needs to others
	Mobility	Being able to move freely as required
	Sexual behaviour	Participating in a sexual act/fantasy
Domestic activities of daily living (DADL)	Domestic activities	Housework, etc
	Family care	Care of child, partner or dependent others
	Provisioning	Obtaining the necessities/luxuries of life

occupational title (due to unemployment, retirement or illness, for example) is so damaging to the individual, unless a new and satisfactory occupation can rapidly be found.

A social role title has an equally important effect on the perceptions of an individual's identity by herself, and by others, and plays a major part in directing participation in activities or occupations, but such roles are variable and very complex to define.

An activity seems to be something more self-contained, a 'one-off' episode occurring at a particular time and place, and for a particular reason. It may be performed in connection with an occupational role, or as part of a social role, but it may equally have no associated role title. Many activities of daily living and leisure activities seem to be of this nature.

Therefore, until the links and relativities can be made clearer, I shall, for the sake of simplicity, consider people who do not have a specific occupational title in the context of what they are doing to be performing at the level of activity, not occupation.

It is clear that more research is needed on the definition of occupation and activity and the link between role titles and occupations or activities. To return to the questions posed earlier, does this discussion assist in deciding whether there is a difference between occupations and activities, and in deciding whether either, or both, are legitimate areas of concern for the therapist?

There are certainly many ambiguities, but my personal conclusions are as follows:

- The term 'occupation' is a useful generic title for the totality of productive, purposeful human action. It is used in this way in the professional title.
- Occupations and activities are different. Activities may form part of an occupation, or be non-occupational. Both are essential parts of human life. Personal activities of daily living provide an essential infrastructure to enable the performance of occupations and other activities, but they are not themselves occupations.
- It is difficult, therefore, to restrict the occu-

pational therapist's attention only to occupations; activities, tasks and roles must also be included.
- Classifications such as work, leisure and self-care are situational and culturally-biased, and the classification system is incomplete.

Occupational balance

A theory associated with the idea of occupational classification is that of the necessity of a balance between work, leisure and ADL (and, some add, rest) in an individual's life, and the proposal that lack of balance results in dysfunction.

This is an interesting concept, but it is one which should not be accepted without some thought. If, for the reasons described, it is difficult to slot the occupations and activities of an individual neatly into categories, then it becomes difficult to discuss the concept of balance. Balance of what? Should anyone at any age engage in a pattern of occupations which can be classified as work, leisure or self-care? And how can we judge whether a particular pattern – unless obviously extreme – is, or is not balanced?

Most therapists would accept it as significant if a person has no ability to engage in an important area of life. A person who is involuntarily jobless is deprived of a considerable range of expected and desired processes and activities; a person who is deprived of the ability to undertake DADL or PADL for herself has a damaging deficit in her range of performance which is likely to affect her well-being.

One must, however, beware of assuming that such a person is automatically dysfunctional, or disadvantaged. This depends on the individual. Some react well to a major occupational deficit and are able to compensate by the development and enrichment of other areas: facilitating such adjustment, if necessary, is a role for the occupational therapist. It may be more significant if the individual is generally impoverished or shows dysfunction across a range of occupations, activities and roles.

There is also the issue of 'who makes the

judgement'. Is it the therapist's own views, or those of society or of the individual which indicate lack of occupational balance? If the patient is clearly unhappy and concerned about some missing aspect of occupational performance the situation is straightforward, but what if the patient does not see that there is a problem, even though one is perceived by other members of society, or by the therapist?

Objective data on actual engagement can be useful and analysis of patterns of activity can be highly relevant if conducted thoroughly, and with a focus on the needs and circumstances of the individual. If conducted in a mechanistic fashion such analysis could, however, be open to misinterpretation.

As in all other aspects of humanity, the concept of 'normal' is wide-ranging, and cultural influences are very significant. A 'balanced lifestyle' in one culture may be quite irrelevant in another. We possess very little accurate data concerning the patterns of occupations for the population as a whole, or for subsections of it, and even if we did, such patterns are fluid and normative data would provide only general guidance to the needs of an individual.

I find it more useful to discuss occupational balance in terms of the spread and meaning of occupations for the individual (as opposed to some notional 'norm'). Such a complex analysis must take very close account of personal experience and constructs, the significance these have for the individual and the context of performance. This phenomenological view is undoubtedly revealing, especially in cases of psychosocial dysfunction. If the individual lacks any occupation or activity which provides a sense of meaning to her life, the individual is certain to be in some degree stressed or dysfunctional.

One aspect of balance which must be recognized, amid the hectic pace of life, is the need for rest, and for periods of relaxation and comparative inactivity. Being a 'workaholic' may be just as damaging as being inactive.

Both objective and subjective ratings of patterns of activity in the areas of work, leisure and activities of daily living provide useful data on which to base therapeutic evaluation, provided that this is viewed in the context of an individual and her particular sociocultural environment, and is not judged against some abstract or personal ideal of what is 'normal'.

A NEW PERSPECTIVE ON OCCUPATIONS, ACTIVITIES AND TASKS

Current definitions of occupations, activities and tasks have been explored earlier in this chapter, together with approaches to analysis and classification. This exploration highlights various paradoxes and anomalies and leads me to conclude that occupations, activities and tasks are not the same, that they operate at different levels and that they can be analysed in different ways for different purposes.

Human performance is very complex, and an attempt to untangle it is an artificially reductive process. There are many overlaps and 'grey areas'. To avoid confusion, I shall begin, therefore, with a number of statements which summarize the concepts which are about to be discussed (Box 5.3).

The propositions listed in Box 5.3 will now be explored, although it should be understood at

---

Box 5.3 Propositions

1. Occupations are composed of a hierarchy of endeavour which builds performance in stages to achieve highly complex results. Performance occurs at three levels: developmental (basic skills and tasks), effective (activities) and organizational (processes and occupations).
2. The basic difference between occupations and activities is that a person *possesses* occupations, and owns occupational and social roles, whereas she *performs* activities and tasks.
3. An occupation defines and organizes a particular sphere of action over an extended period of time. An activity is the means whereby a specific purpose is achieved on a particular occasion. A task is a component of an activity.
4. Three forms of analysis can be used to explore occupations and activities for therapeutic purposes: basic analysis, functional analysis and applied analysis. These can operate at each of the three occupational levels.

the outset that the definitions, levels and consequent format for analysis are offered as hypotheses, since at this stage insufficient research has been conducted to validate them. It is hoped that a detailed explanation will provide useful tools for therapists who wish to experiment with a more structured approach to the description and analysis of occupations.

LEVELS OF OCCUPATION

The developmental level: proto-occupational

The levels of occupation are arranged in a developmental sequence. The developmental level contains skill components, the 'building blocks' of performance. A task is accomplished by utilizing and coordinating skills to build performance into increasingly complex sequences, but on its own this does not suffice to complete the purpose or product of the activity, only one stage in an activity. For this reason, this level is described as proto-occupational. A single task is completed in a few minutes.

It is at the developmental level that skills and knowledge are evolved. Tasks tend to be learned separately and then, through experience, chained together. It is frequently a problem with task performance which produces dysfunction. A problem at this level inhibits higher level performance.

The effective level: productive

At the effective level something happens which has an effect or consequence. By means of chaining tasks to form routines or procedures and by linking routines together, an activity can be completed. As a result of the energy expended (or conserved) during an activity a product is achieved. Something is changed: an artefact has been created which did not previously exist; some state of affairs has altered; a new idea has evolved; a total event has been experienced.

An activity takes place within a limited period of time on a specific occasion and for a particular purpose, although it may take part of an hour, or a few hours to complete. A person can live a meaningful and useful life at this level, even if activities are not subsequently organized into more complex processes and occupations.

The organizational level: occupational

At the organizational level a particular occupation can be described by its title and processes. On a specific occasion a sequence of activities will combine to complete a version of one, or a combination of several, processes. The specific occupation coordinates, directs and circumscribes a sphere of endeavour, and operates over a long timeframe, typically extending over months or years.

THE OCCUPATIONAL TAXONOMY

The component parts of the taxonomy will now be described following the developmental sequence from the lowest level upwards.

At the developmental level basic skills are first learned, then chained. Skills evolve and become ever more complex and sophisticated with experience. Higher level performance requires higher level skills. The integrative skills, especially process skills, become increasingly important as performance complexity increases (Allen 1985). At the proto-occupational level it is still possible, although time-consuming, to analyse which skills are required for a task, or a stage in a task. Once performance reaches the effective level, however, it becomes increasingly difficult to untangle the specific skills since performance becomes highly integrated and total competencies are more significant than part skills.

TASK SEGMENTS

By integrating skills, a small part of a task can be performed. This is a task segment, which is the smallest piece of performance which can be identified separately. An apparently simple task such as doing up a button comprises several task segments, each utilizing a combination of discrete skill components; e.g. recognize button, recognize hole, grasp button, grasp fabric near hole, bring button edge into line with hole, push button through hole. These segments involve combinations of sensorimotor, cognitive and perceptual skills, and are performed in sequence by means of process skills.

A person has had to learn these movements, concepts and discriminations and master and chain the task segments at some point in her life. Under normal circumstances such learning can happen rapidly and without conscious analysis of the component parts; but a person who has never undertaken any of the component task segments – who does not recognize a button, for example, or has no schema for 'push through hole' – will have severe difficulty. It is sometimes necessary to begin teaching a task sequence at this very basic level.

Training skill components or performance of task segments in isolation, as splinter skills, may sometimes be necessary, but this is ineffective unless it is ensured that such skills are later generalized and integrated.

TASK STAGES

A task stage is a completed act which forms part of the whole task. Thus, 'put arm through sleeve' is a task stage in the task 'put on a jacket'. Task stages form a chained sequence which typically has a fixed order and structure.

TASKS

A task such as 'putting on a jacket' is a self-contained stage in an activity (which in this case might be 'getting dressed for work', 'getting ready for school' or 'going out to dinner'.

Effective task performance is crucial as it is a necessary stage in learning, but on its own it cannot result in functional performance. A person who can do a single task, but cannot chain it to others, is severely disadvantaged. The ability to learn new tasks and to chain these into highly

evolved and complex activities is acquired over a period of time between childhood and adult life, and can continue indefinitely. Under normal circumstances experience of one task leads into learning another so that learning speeds up as the task repertoire extends and networks of performance are evolved.

Tasks tend to be value-neutral. Any personal reactions to tasks, or attitudes connected with them, are likely to be derived from the situational elements affecting the activity in connection with which the task is being performed. Task completion does, however, generally provide some intrinsic satisfaction, and task failure results in frustration or dissatisfaction. Babies and young children obtain pleasure from tasks associated with satisfying basic physiological or emotional needs, e.g. eating, drinking or seeking affection.

The neutral nature of tasks can be illustrated by considering a task which may at first sight be thought of as symbolic, lighting a candle. The symbolism and meaning of lighting a candle are situational:

- as decoration for a child's birthday cake
- to enhance an intimate supper
- to provide light during a power-cut
- as a devotional act in church
- as an act of solidarity with a cause
- to celebrate a religious festival.

It is clear that the meaning in each case is relevant to the whole activity – having a birthday party or offering prayers in church – not to the basic task. It is possible, however, to generalize meanings concerning a task from one context to another by associations, so that lighting the candle in a power-cut suddenly reminds a woman that her husband used to do this and that she lit a candle in church when he died.

ROUTINES AND PROCEDURES

Routines are chains of tasks with a fixed sequence which becomes automated and habitual. Effective routines help to reduce effort and the need for attention and planning, and contribute to the production of a successful result or product. Some routines are formed because task performance has an obvious sequence; in other cases a person evolves routines which feel comfortable and meet her needs. An overly rigid adherence to routines can be counterproductive and may inhibit creativity or problem-solving. A procedure is a rigidly structured task sequence which must be followed to achieve the desired result.

ACTIVITIES

The crucial feature which distinguishes an activity from an occupation is that an activity is conducted for a specific purpose on a particular occasion, and is identified by a short phrase indicating the primary action and objective.

An activity is different from a task both qualitatively and quantitatively. As already illustrated by the example of lighting a candle, it is at this level that subjective feelings, values, symbolism and personal meanings become significant. A participant will place an activity on a series of continua expressing emotions, relevance, liking and significance. This placement depends on past experience and the situational context of performance.

In addition an activity has some stable, inherent features. Cooking provides a useful example. Baking buns (in USA, muffins) is an activity. It is significant that one does not have to be a chef or a cook to engage in the activity of baking buns. The participant might equally well be a housewife, a student, a child, or someone simply baking for fun. Therefore an activity may or may not bring with it a specific social or occupational role title.

The activity of baking buns requires a certain basic familiarity with the actions required, e.g. mixing, measuring, using an oven. The purpose is to produce buns to be eaten. The product will be a quantity of buns. There is a generally accepted method of making buns; this will normally take place in a kitchen and it is possible to list the essential equipment and ingredients. There are routines for collecting ingredients and preparing equipment, making the buns, cooking them and clearing up afterwards.

This is a utilitarian view which takes no account of individual feelings or perceptions.

This basic understanding of the activity has to be informed and adapted by the precise nature of the activity on a specific occasion with a particular participant, and this is where many subjective, mutable and situational elements play a part.

There is a big difference (not just quantitative) between baking ten dozen buns for a coffee morning and making six for the children. Buns can be made in a variety of flavours, with different additions and decorations. They can involve intricate preparation and decoration, or simply mixing the contents of a packet and placing the result in a microwave. The procedure may be carried out carelessly, creatively, or with care and affection. It may be the first time a person has made buns, or a regular event. The buns may be intended for a lunch-box, or for a post-funeral tea. The permutations are innumerable. There is no such thing as 'just baking buns'. An essential element is personal meaning and situational context; appreciation of the situational elements of an activity is therefore crucial in occupational therapy.

It is only through the cumulative experiences of participation in activities that an occupation acquires personal significance or meaning for an individual, as distinct from any general socio-cultural meaning which may be attached to it.

An activity can therefore be described as having a few, relatively stable, requirements which can be determined objectively, and a larger set of changeable elements, objective and subjective, which are situational, and only relevant to a particular participant on a unique occasion. Both stable and situational elements can be considered under the general headings of participant, purpose, product, procedure, practical requirements and performance demand.

An activity is identified by a short description of action and objective. An activity takes place on a specific occasion, during a finite period, for a particular purpose, and has both stable and situational elements. A completed activity results in a change in the previous state of objective reality or subjective experience.

An activity may be a self-contained event which has little or no implication for what happened before or afterwards. More commonly, activities require antecedent and consequent activities extending backwards and forwards in time (Cynkin & Robinson 1990). Sometimes these chains are quite lengthy, and unavoidable. The activity selected as the point from which the chain can be extended in each direction is the pivotal activity; this may be the most significant activity, but could be one at any point in a given chain. A cluster of closely associated activities performed adjacent in time may be described as contiguous activities.

This has implications for the practicalities of therapy, for only one of the activities in the chain may be therapeutically relevant, or there may be insufficient time for a chain to be completed. The amount of preparation and clearing up required for a pivotal creative activity, or social activity are examples. An activity performed in isolation from a chain may have reduced meaning.

PROCESSES

A process describes the means whereby the purposes of an occupation may be carried out and the products achieved.

Metaprocesses are those which organize a chain of processes, e.g. in describing the sequence of a total manufacturing process or, in occupational therapy, the occupational therapy process (see Ch. 11). Metaprocesses can therefore be described in terms of general purpose, product and component processes. They typically extend over a long timescale.

As a shorthand means of conveying its main features, a process may be described in terms of actions, purpose(s) and product(s), and general requirements. An action is not the same as an activity. The word 'activity' is used freely to mean both the thing done, and the action of doing it, which is confusing. An action is identified by a verb describing a 'type of doing'. It is a generic description of a type of act, not a specific example of an occasion on which something was done (an activity).

There are two kinds of process which serve somewhat differing purposes:

A generic process

This gives a generalized description of a typical kind of performance which is part of the occupation and which comprises various skilled actions; e.g. the process 'cooking meat' is a generic process in cooking. Boiling, baking and frying are typical actions in the process, which has the purpose of 'rendering meat suitable to eat', and the product of 'cooked meat'. The general requirement is a suitably equipped kitchen. A generic process is purely descriptive – one does not actually carry out a generic process, only a version of it, for it must be expressed in terms of one or more activities before one can do so.

An integrative process

This describes the order in which a sequence of activities is performed to achieve a product of the occupation, and draws together activities which may use actions from several generic processes. Some integrative processes involve a fixed sequence of activities, e.g. producing a chassis for a car. An integrative process may be further defined by specifying a particular product instead of a generic one, e.g. instead of 'car chassis', 'car chassis for × make of car'. Other integrative processes are more fluid (Box 5.4).

OCCUPATIONS

An occupation provides longitudinal organization of time and effort in a person's life and provides that person with a role. The definition and description of an occupation is clouded by the problem that it can be viewed from two fundamentally differing perspectives, that of the occupation as an entity having intrinsic, relatively stable characteristics, and that of the occupation as relevant to a particular individual. The therapist is, naturally, concerned primarily with the latter, but this involves recognition of a host of contextual, situational factors which originate with the individual's needs and perceptions, rather than with the occupation itself. There remains a need to understand the inherent nature of the occupation.

Box 5.4	An integrative process
Occupation	Cooking (role title: cook; social role title, e.g. housewife)
Integrative process	Cooking a traditional roast lunch
Pivotal activity	Cooking Sunday roast lunch for relatives
Generic processes	*Antecedent activities*
Entertaining	Invite relatives
Menu planning	Plan menu for next Sunday's lunch
Shopping for food	Shop for provisions for the lunch
	Contiguous activities
Table preparation	Lay table for lunch
Flower arranging	Put flowers on table
Kitchen preparation	Get things ready to cook lunch
	Cook lunch – routines (sequence may vary):
Vegetable preparation	Prepare carrots, peas and potatoes
Pie making	Make pastry
	Cook apples and assemble pie
	Bake pie
Roasting	Roast joint of lamb and potatoes
Vegetable cooking	Cook carrots and peas
Sauce making	Make onion gravy
	Make custard
Serving food	Serve lunch
	Consequent activities
Entertaining	Eat lunch with family and relatives
Maintaining kitchen hygiene	Clear up and do the washing up
Relaxing	Rest, snooze or chat

The inherent nature of an occupation

A sociocultural phenomenon

The occupation has features such as the purposes, values, attitudes and beliefs which are attributed by those who, over an extended period of time, participate in, or benefit from it. An external observer can only deduce and infer such subjective views by questioning others to gain a consensus.

These features are stable within a specific culture, and tend to evolve only slowly, but can vary between cultures. An individual may share these perceptions to a greater or lesser degree. Although these attributes may be generated by factors unconnected with, and external to, the occupation they become integral parts of the occupational gestalt, and are features as inherent and as important as the more observable components. Designations such as work or leisure are sociocultural.

An observable entity

It is possible for an observer to watch the performance of an occupation by many performers, over an extended period of time, and to describe its intrinsic features, e.g. generic or integrative processes, products, tools, materials or the skills which need to be used by participants. These features are also relatively stable, but can change as technology improves, or as new designs or concepts are created. An individual will have a personal approach to performance based on experience, but needs to follow the basic format. Ergonomic analysis of observable features enables improvements to be made to process sequences, productivity or equipment design.

Characteristics of an occupation

It is proposed that occupations can be distinguished from other levels of action by the characteristics described in Box 5.5.

The definition of occupation is, therefore:

An occupation is an organised form of human endeavour, having a name and associated role title. A participant engages in an occupation over an extended period of time. It may be described as a sociocultural phenomenon having attributes including principles, positions, possessions, and purposes, and objectively described and defined by observable attributes including products, processes, patterns, practical requirements and performance demands.

These attributes can be used to form the basis of a structure for basic occupational analysis (macro-analysis) which will be described in chapter 14.

THE NEED FOR AN EXTENDED TAXONOMY OF OCCUPATIONAL LEVELS AND DESCRIPTIVE TERMINOLOGY

There may appear at first sight to be an unnecessary number of stages in the completion of

Box 5.5   Characteristics of an occupation

A name for the occupation and an occupational role title for the participant(s)
Sociocultural attributes: intrinsic and subjective

Principles	Fundamental concepts, assumptions, values
Position(s)	Sociocultural organization and ranking; designation as work and/or leisure
Possessions	The sphere of intellectual and/or practical action and influence which is regarded as owned and controlled by the occupation
Purposes	The objective rationale, practical intentions, socioeconomic or cultural benefits of engagement

Observable attributes: intrinsic and objective

Products	Tangible or intangible outcomes
Processes	Chained actions or activities achieving purposes and products
Patterns	Longitudinal arrangements of time and energy
Practical requirements	Human resources, environment, tools and materials needed to perform the occupation
Performance demands	General attributes – knowledge, skills attitudes – which the participant is required to possess in order to perform the occupation

part of an occupation. A few experiments in practical analysis should, however, prove that these are necessary if the whole range of human performance is to be described as a continuum.

This will be illustrated by a brief analysis using gardening as an example.

The organizational level

Gardening is an occupation. It may be situationally described as work, leisure or domestic ADL. It has many different purposes, e.g. growing flowers, growing vegetables or providing an aesthetic environment. There is a multitude of products, e.g. flowers, fruit, vegetables and a well-maintained garden. The generic processes by means of which these purposes and products are achieved include, e.g. propagation, irrigation, soil cultivation, garden design and pest control.

A integrative process combines actions from various generic processes to achieve a purpose and product. 'Growing bulbs' is a process; different types of bulbs require different treatment, so a process variant might be 'growing spring bulbs', involving the typical actions of planning where to plant (garden design), planting bulbs, staking, deadheading, lifting, dividing (propagation) and storing.

To teach someone 'to be a gardener' would take several years. To teach someone the process of 'growing bulbs', one would need to include all types of bulbs. To teach someone how to 'grow spring bulbs' would be more easily defined and accomplished.

The effective level

An activity which might form part of the process of growing spring bulbs is 'planting daffodils'. This requires antecedent activities, which might occur at some distance from the activity, e.g. 'buying bulbs' and 'deciding where to plant them', as well as several consequent activities once the bulbs have grown, also far removed in time. The activity requires two contiguous activities, one antecedent, 'gathering bulbs and tools', and one consequent, 'clearing up after planting'. Planting bulbs has a relatively simple task sequence, or procedure: 'dig hole, place bulbs right way up, fill hole, repeat as required'. It is not difficult to teach someone how to 'plant daffodils'.

The developmental level

Each of the above tasks will achieve only a small part of the purpose of the activity. It is of no use to dig the hole unless the bulbs are planted. 'Digging the hole' has task stages, e.g. 'dig trowel into earth', 'remove soil', 'place soil in heap beside hole' ('repeat until hole is required width and depth').

'Dig trowel into earth' has several task segments, e.g. 'grasp trowel', 'position trowel', 'push trowel into earth'. The skill analysis of 'grasp trowel' would include evaluation of the sensorimotor and cognitive components required.

OCCUPATIONAL ONTOGENESIS

Babies do not have occupations. A baby is a package of potentials who explores herself and her world developing and then integrates the skills for the performance of task components and then tasks. A small child acquires a repertoire of tasks, and slowly builds these into simple routines and activities. Throughout childhood and the teenage years, education and experience build activities into processes and occupations; social roles also proliferate.

During adult life one or more dominant occupations and roles and many subsidiary occupations and roles are engaged in, and the adult also has a repertoire of activities, some necessary and some recreational.

As time passes some occupations are dropped and new ones are acquired. The elderly person continues to develop occupations and activities, but loses several of the roles, occupations and activities appropriate to the middle years. As old age advances the repertoire of roles, occupations and activities diminishes. In extreme old age, as physical and mental capacities decrease, occupations may once again be replaced by activities, and even finally, by a few remaining tasks.

This developmental profile is not intended to imply anything about the quality of life at each stage, merely to indicate that occupations and social roles are primarily the possessions of the central portion of life. In extreme youth and old age activities and tasks become more relevant.

THE DYNAMICS OF PERFORMANCE

In considering the ways in which a therapist can best analyse and evaluate the performance of an occupation or activity, it can be difficult to disentangle the contribution of each of the core elements – the therapist, the occupation, the person and the environment – since all are involved.

The therapist acts as the observer, trying to describe a dynamic situation in which stable and situational elements combine with objective and subjective points of view in a very complex manner.

Although one speaks of an occupation being 'performed', this is really convenient shorthand, no-one could 'perform' a whole occupation on any one occasion for it is too large an entity. An occupation is engaged in, or perhaps more accurately, 'lived' or 'owned', through a variety of experiences over a period of time. What is performed on any given occasion is one or more of the activities associated with the occupation. It is for this reason that the majority of therapists recognize that therapy occurs at the effective level, by means of participation in activities. One may investigate an individual's patterns of occupation and roles, but one cannot prescribe an occupation, only one of its constituent activities.

The person both performs the activity and experiences participation in it. The nature of such experience spans both past performance and present engagement, and may even look to the future as well. The therapist can observe actual performance, but can only infer, or ask the participant questions about, what it feels like, or what it means.

The activity may or may not be part of an occupation. An activity has some relatively stable characteristics such as the usual tools, materials or outcome, and many more which depend on the particular circumstances at the time. The therapist can predict some of these features, but not all.

The environment will greatly affect performance, both practically in terms of suitability and the availability of resources and, more subtly, as sociocultural influences and expectations assume a role.

All these interlocking aspects make the analysis of occupations and activities a complex matter. This is best illustrated by an example: a piano is meaningless without a pianist; it is merely a redundant piece of furniture of no practical use and little aesethic value. To understand the nature of the occupation 'piano playing' it is necessary to observe pianists.

It is possible to make an objective study of piano playing. The therapist can, by structured observation of a number of pianists, report on the ways in which a piano is used, the environments and conditions which may apply and the skills which are required to play the instrument. In this way a defined concept of some of the inherent characteristics of piano playing can be obtained. The analysis is objective because the therapist reports what he sees people do, where they do it, and the outcomes.

Similarly, observation of a particular pianist will enable the therapist to assess her competence as a player. Such a judgement would, however, require the therapist to have a good understanding of the skills and standards involved; it would be very difficult to carry out such observations if one had no concept of piano playing.

Some aspects of piano playing are not, however, so readily defined. These are contextual, mutable, socioculturally determined or dependent on individual perceptions of meaning. Thus a piano may be played at home for pleasure, or used at home to give piano lessons; pianos may be played at classical concerts, jazz festivals and in pubs; a pianist may accompany children singing in school assembly, or taking part in a musical show. Examination of the sociocultural environment is an important means of placing a particular instance of piano playing in context, classifying it as work or leisure, or gaining an overview of the cultural meaning or social importance of playing the piano.

Individual pianists may have very different attitudes to playing. The expert concert pianist is concerned with technique and interpretation and may practise for many hours; the reluctant child grudgingly practises scales; the elderly person experiences pleasure or nostalgia when playing a familiar, sentimental old tune. Inexpert playing may give one person pleasure and satisfaction and another feelings of disappointment or frustration at not being able to play better. What the participant feels about her playing, the meaning it has for her, or the reactions of others, can only be known if the people involved can describe them, or from indications of such feelings, perceptions and attitudes which the therapist may observe.

Finally, the therapist might be concerned with the therapeutic aspects of piano playing. Does the individual require help to restore lost function and enable her to play the piano again? If so, is playing the piano the best therapy, or should some other activity be selected? Is there some physical barrier to be removed – perhaps the pianist cannot see to read the music or reach to turn the pages? Does playing the piano offer a means of forming a relationship with the patient, or provide her with a means of expression, a sense of being valued, or an experience of exploration, control or competence? Here again, it is necessary to understand piano playing sufficiently to answer these questions.

This implies considerable familiarity and one may question how feasible it is for occupational therapists to gain an understanding of the wide range of occupations with which they may be involved, and whether it is possible to do this at a theoretical level only. Experiencing an activity is the means of understanding it, and the therapist at least needs personally to experience and analyse a range of differing activities in order to develop the skills required to analyse those which are unfamiliar.

OCCUPATIONAL ANALYSIS

From the description of piano playing which has just been given, it is possible to see that there are three forms of analysis involved:

1. Basic analysis: to describe an occupation, activity or task in order to understand its nature and the basis for engagement.

2. Functional analysis: to describe an individual's occupational roles and patterns, her knowledge, skills and attitudes, or her ability to perform a specific activity, with a view to gaining an understanding of abilities, difficulties, needs and appropriate therapy.

3. Applied analysis: to describe and analyse an activity or task in order to use it as therapy, or to identify tasks, sequences and performance skills, to enable the individual to function more effectively.

Analysis takes into account objectively observed features and subjective features such as cultural relevance or personal meaning. It extends the therapist's information concerning the individual, and the individual's knowledge of herself and her skills, and enables the therapist to make appropriate choices of therapeutic media. Linked to occupational analysis is analysis of the environment in which the activity or task is performed.

Occupational analysis is a generic title. In practice the three forms of analysis, basic, functional and applied, operate at different levels and have differing purposes. The following summary outlines this proposed structure for analysis which will be described and explained further in Chapter 14.

BASIC ANALYSIS

Basic analysis is largely 'pure' analysis, undertaken for the purpose of increasing understanding of the inherent nature of occupations, activities and tasks as entities divorced from performance by an individual. Basic analysis can be conducted at three levels (Box 5.6).

FUNCTIONAL ANALYSIS

This form of analysis focuses on the occupational patterns, preferences and performances of the individual. Functional analysis is of three types (Box 5.7).

Box 5.6	Levels of basic analysis
Microanalysis	At the developmental level, analysing tasks, task stages, task segments and basic skills.
Activity analysis	At the effective level, considering stable and situational features in the performance of specific activities and routines, under the headings of participant, purpose, product, procedure, practical requirements, and performance demand.
Macroanalysis	At the organizational level, considering the participant, four sociocultural elements and five practical elements (all 10 beginning with 'P'), and describing an occupation as an entity or gestalt using this '10P analysis' structure.

Box 5.7	Levels of functional analysis
Participation analysis	Describing the individual's past, present and future occupational or social roles and patterns of occupations and activities (engagement).
Performance analysis	Describing how well an individual is able to perform an activity or task (competence).
Existential analysis	Describing how an individual feels and thinks about her roles and activities, and her performance of them (cognitive/affective responses).

Performance analysis, is customarily referred to as 'assessment' rather than analysis, although the process is primarily an analytical one.

APPLIED ANALYSIS

This is conducted for therapeutic purposes and involves detailed analysis of an activity or task in relation to the needs of a specific individual in a particular environment. This is related to specific aims such as enhancing or enabling performance, removing barriers, enhancing quality of life, improving health or empowering an individual to achieve personal goals.

One of the chief objectives of applied analysis is the identification of performance demand, so as either to match an activity to therapeutic needs or to understand the performance requirements of an occupation in which a patient must engage.

A further aim is to identify the unstable and situational elements in an activity since these are features which can be changed to enhance therapeutic potential.

The relationship between types of analysis and levels of performance is charted in Table 5.2.

PERFORMANCE DEMAND

The concept of 'environmental demand' (press) will be discussed in Chapter 6. This is an interesting and useful idea: human/environ-

Table 5.2 The relationship between types of analysis and levels of performance

	Core components			
	Person	Occupation	Therapist	Timeframe
	Functional analysis	Basic analysis	Applied analysis	
Organizational level	Participation analysis	Macroanalysis (occupation)		Extended timeframe (past, present, future)
Effective level	Participation analysis Existential analysis Performance analysis (activity)	Activity analysis	Applied activity analysis	Current timeframe (recent past, near future)
Developmental level	Performance analysis (task)	Microanalysis (task)	Applied task analysis	Current timeframe

mental/occupational interactions are certainly important, but this theory seems to imply that the environment determines the way in which the person performs the activity and the nature of what is performed. This is, however, only part of a complex interaction. The activity also places demands on the performer, and on the environment. I suggest therefore another, complementary, proposition, that of performance demand.

The term 'demand' has been used elsewhere. Johnson (1992) uses it to include the following types of demand: motor/physical, sensory, cognitive, emotional, social, independent, cultural. In the context of the cognitive levels of task performance, Allen (1985) suggests a different interpretation of demands, as 'introduced by the presence of material objects' and states that samples, steps (sensory cues and motor actions), tools, potential errors, length of task, time, supplies, storage and setting contribute to demand.

An activity has a set of stable, inherent characteristics which combine to require the participant to possess particular attributes, knowledge, skills or attitudes, and to use a defined set of performance skills to achieve a successful outcome or product. Some activities have strong demand, which limits the potential for participation; others have low demand and the majority of people may engage in them. The latter acti-vities are those which are most likely to be suitable for therapeutic application.

Demand may be observed and analysed at several levels of complexity. The simplest format places the activity on a series of imaginary continua to provide a general description of its principal characteristics, e.g. physical or cognitive, light or heavy, simple or complex, solitary or social. Alternatively, various shemes of detailed analysis can be used, some generic and some relating to a particular frame of reference.

The concept of performance demand amounts to a statement of the commonsense observation that not everyone can do every activity, because some require very specific abilities. This is best explained by some examples.

Examples

Weightlifting is a sport which has very high demand. In order to engage in an activity such as lifting a weighted bar the participant must be very fit, very strong, young, and highly trained. Casual participation would be injurious. Few people become weightlifters, and only those with potential to acquire a suitable physique and level of fitness would be able to train.

Occupations also have demand. Most professions, because of their high demand for knowledge, skills, experience and expertise, can be engaged in only by people who have had long and rigorous training, and who possess the abilities to obtain a qualification. Again, this limits the number of potential participants.

Many occupations with very specific needs for knowledge, skills or ability can therefore only be performed by a minority. The more expert and complex the occupation the fewer people can perform it. There are very few astronauts, and few nuclear physicists, neurosurgeons or prima ballerinas. A person may dream of becoming one of these specialists, but most people realize that the reality is impossible to attain.

Occupations which consist of a majority of activities with high demand usually have little potential for therapeutic application. The therapist would be involved only if a dysfunctional individual in one of these occupations presented for treatment, and would recognize rapidly the very specific demands of such a job, in which dysfunctions which might be insignificant in other areas could become highly disabling. The top weightlifter, or the fireman, is likely to have substantially different fitness criteria from the office worker.

There are many more occupations which require specific training – indeed, all skilled crafts, trades and jobs are in this group – but which have a lower demand. This means that more people have the potential to engage in them, given the desire and suitable training. Selected activities from such occupations may be appropriate as therapy, provided that the need for training is not too great, but the requirements for tools, equipment, materials and environment often make them impractical.

Finally, there are occupations and activities which either have very low demand, or, and this is the significant attribute for the therapist, have a large number of activities (or tasks) which are adaptable and *can be presented as if they have low demand*, i.e. can be made 'user friendly'.

All activities of daily living, and many social and recreational activities come within this category. Most arts, crafts and creative techniques, although they have high demand at the level of expertise, include some simpler activities which can be structured to have relatively low demand and still be performed quite competently. These, historically, are the activities which therapists have chosen to analyse, adapt and apply for therapeutic purposes.

Summary of performance demand

Performance demand defines the type of skill and level of competence required to participate in an occupation or activity. Analysis of demand enables a therapist to:

- identify the level of demand in a person's job, thereby setting appropriate levels for recovery of function
- exclude activities with very high demand as unsuitable for therapeutic application
- identify activities with low or adaptable demand which may be suitable for therapeutic use
- make adjustments to performance demand to facilitate participation or to provide therapy.

It should perhaps be stressed that demand is based on an *objective* analysis of content (activity analysis), and not on an analysis of any subjective aspects of the activity or occupation, such as personal interest, culture or values (existential analysis). Data from both forms of analysis may need to be combined when undertaking applied analysis, and the personal meaning and relevance may be the final deciding factors in selecting a particular activity for a particular person, rather than a number of other potentially suitable ones.

OCCUPATIONAL SCIENCE

Occupational science is a relatively recent field of study. It has evolved from the work of Yerxa, Clark and others in the USA. Clark & Larson (1993) explain occupational science as:

A new social science which grew out of occupational therapy. Its primary focus is the study of the human being as an occupational being, of how humans realize their sense of life's meaning through purposeful activity.

Occupational science is:

The study of the human as an occupational being including the need for and capacity to engage in and orchestrate daily occupations in the environment over the lifespan. Because of the complexity of occupation, occupational science synthesizes knowledge from an array of disciplines (biological and social sciences) and organizes it into a systems model (USC 1987, quoted by Yerxa et al 1990).

Occupational science seeks to understand the nature, scope and meanings of human occupations. It is envisaged as an aid to occupational therapy, but as distinct from it. Philosophically, it is allied with the central concepts common to models of occupational behaviour/performance, although its proponents are careful to state that it is not a 'model' but an area of scientific enquiry.

This field of study is significant in relation to the earlier discussion of occupations as having intrinsic attributes, and of the need for therapists to understand the nature of occupations in order to identify dysfunction, enable or enhance performance, or identify the therapeutic potential of component activities.

Yerxa et al (1990) state that:

Occupation is a complex phenomenon which is highly individualized and which occurs in an environment in the stream of time. Its building blocks are rules, habits and skills which are learned through the course of development and which enable humans to fulfil their occupational roles and achieve a sense of efficacy. Occupation provides opportunities for individuals to experience flow, make a contribution to themselves and others, and discover sociocultural and spiritual meaning through their own actions. The study of occupations requires the study of the person as the author of his or her work, rest, play, leisure and self-maintenance.

They proceed to declare that:

Occupational science will study the person's experience of engagement in occupation recognizing that observing behaviour is not sufficient for understanding occupation. The organization and balance of occupations in daily life and how these relate to adaptation, life satisfaction and social expectations will be central issues as will timing, planning and anticipation. Occupational science will seek to learn more about intrinsic motivation and the drive for effectance. Finally it will need to be true to its humanistic roots by preserving human complexity, diversity and dignity.

The difficulty of this endeavour should not be underestimated. Our understanding of the place of occupation in human life is still limited and this is a highly complex area of study. The proposals I have made concerning basic analysis and performance demand probably fall within the remit of occupational science, whereas functional and applied analysis relate to occupational therapy.

The evolution of occupational science has led to a debate (e.g. correspondence in American Journal of Occupational Therapy 1991) between those who feel it is a separate field of study, distinct from occupational therapy but contributing to it, those who recognize it as valuable, but really an offshoot of occupational therapy rather than a distinct science, and a third faction who argue that it is not something with which therapists should be concerned since research resources are limited and should be devoted towards applied therapy and the development of frames of reference.

The need for research into occupations as well as into therapy seems well-proven. It is legitimate, however, to question how this should be tackled. It should be recognized that sociologists, anthropologists, environmental, social and occupational psychologists, and ergonomists all lay claim to portions of the 'new' territory. As occupational science is developing rapidly it is too early to comment further.

CONCLUSION

Many statements have been made in this chapter about the nature of occupations and activities. The most important points are recapitulated in Boxes 5.7 and 5.8.

Box 5.7 Occupations, tasks and activities

1. Engagement in roles, occupations and activities is a defining characteristic of humanity.
2. Failure to engage in necessary and meaningful roles, occupations and activities has serious consequences for the well-being and health of an individual.
3. Performance occurs at three levels – developmental, effective and organizational; the components of each level of performance are chained to produce the next level.
4. Occupations, activities and tasks are not interchangeable.
5. The basic difference between occupations and activities is that a person possesses occupations, and owns occupational and social roles, whereas she performs activities and tasks.
6. An occupation has a name and brings with it a descriptive role title for the participant. Social role titles may require the person to engage in occupations, but much action is carried out at the effective level by means of activities.
7. An occupation may be defined as an organized form of human endeavour, having a name and role title, which is engaged in by a participant over an extended period of time. It may be subjectively described as a sociocultural phenomenon having attributes including principles, positions, possessions and purposes, and objectively described and defined by observable attributes including products, processes, patterns, practical requirements and performance demands.
8. An activity is an organized sequence of tasks which takes place on a specific occasion, during a finite period, for a particular purpose, and has both stable and situational elements. A completed activity results in a change in the previous state of objective reality or subjective experience. Personal meanings are attributed to activities by an individual as a result of experience.
9. A task is a self-contained component of an activity which may be further divided into task stages and task segments. These require the integrated use of basic skills: sensorimotor, perceptual, cognitive and interpersonal. Tasks are value-neutral.

Box 5.8 Occupational analysis

1. Occupations may be classified as work or leisure, and activities as work, leisure or self-care. Such classification depends on situational and subjective factors, and sociocultural traditions. These classifications should be used only for general guidance.
2. There are three forms of occupational analysis: basic analysis, functional analysis and applied analysis.
3. Basic analysis can take place at each level: microanalysis (developmental level), activity analysis (effective level) and macroanalysis (organizational level).
4. Functional analysis can take place at each level. It is concerned with the abilities and needs of the individual. There are three types of functional analysis: participation analysis (dealing with patterns of engagement), performance analysis (describing how well an individual can perform), existential analysis (describing how an individual feels and thinks about his roles and activities).
5. Applied analysis enables a therapist to prescribe or adapt an activity or task in relation to the therapeutic goals for an individual. It takes place at the effective and developmental levels only.

6

Environment

OCCUPATIONAL THERAPY AND THE ENVIRONMENT

Views of the environment and of a human being's relationship to it are not quite as diverse as views of the nature of humanity, but must run a close second in provoking passionately held theories. The fundamental question concerns the degree to which a person is influenced by the environment, or influences it. The range of views extends from the behavioural, in which environment is seen as providing the positive and negative reinforcements which produce learned behaviours, through the developmental view of the person exploring and adapting the environment and reciprocally being adapted by it, to the view of the person as the ultimate master and shaper of himself and his surroundings.

Environment is a relatively recent addition to the vocabulary of occupational therapy. In the past, a therapist would speak of adapting the home or the workplace, of altering tools or providing stimulation. Currently, the same actions would be spoken of as 'environmental adaptation'. Although therapists have always recognized the importance of physical environmental factors, awareness of sociocultural environmental influences began to filter into occupational therapy in Britain during the 1970s when sociology was added to the curriculum.

The growing use of the word possibly reflects its currency in the media, but also, and more seriously, the real advances in the understanding of environments and in particular the socio-ecological – developmental view of organisms as interactive and interdependent systems both modifying their environment and being modified by it.

The latter view has virtually monopolized the references to environment in occupational therapy literature over the last decade, which at least simplifies the discussion of the significance of environment to the therapist since the views of various authorities have considerable concurrence.

DEFINITIONS OF ENVIRONMENT

Several definitions of environment have been proposed by American therapists. Mosey (1986) suggests the following:

The environment is defined as the aggregate of phenomena that surrounds the individual and influences his development and existence. It includes physical conditions, things, other individuals, groups and ideas. One of the philosophical assumptions of OT is the belief that the individual can neither be understood nor assisted towards a more adaptive mode of behaviour without consideration of the environment, past, present and future.

Mosey proceeds to describe the environment as consisting of:

- cultural environment
- social environment
- physical environment.

Reed (1984) uses slightly different divisions:

- sociocultural environment – people and their cultures
- biopsychological environment – the individual
- physical environment – the non-human world.

The inclusion of the individual as part of the environment is interesting. It recognizes that a person does not exist in isolation from the environment and that he forms part of it. It may also be a reference to the idea proposed in Lewin's *Cognitive Field Psychology*, in which he suggests that the individual inhabits an ever-changing 'amoeboid' lifespace travelling on a trajectory in time and space, in which the psychological environment is composed of the individual's perceptions of self in relation to the physical, social and cultural environment and the meanings which these have for him at any moment. Because of the individual nature of such perceptions, different people in the same environment may have very different perceptions of and feelings about it.

Kielhofner and Barris (Kielhofner 1985) describe concentric environmental layers with the person at the centre, and divide environmental factors into:

- objects – used by persons when they perform within tasks
- tasks – serious and playful situations for performance
- social groups – natural collections of individuals
- culture – values and technology.

Each of these elements influences performance.

Similarly, Cynkin & Robinson (1990) emphasize the importance of environment in the learning process and considers physical setting, people, objects, implicit and explicit rules, timeframe, behaviour and habitat.

THE CULTURAL ENVIRONMENT

Culture is a set of shared understandings held in common by members of a group. (Mosey 1986)

Such understandings or beliefs relate to the non-material aspects of culture and may be:

Descriptive – agreements about the nature of the universe and its contents.
Procedural – agreements about how things should be done.
Ethnic/aesthetic – agreements about what is desirable, beautiful or good (or the reverse) (Mosey 1986).

Culture consists of the beliefs and perceptions, values and norms, and customs and behaviours that are shared by a group or society and passed from one generation to the next through both formal and informal education. (Reed & Sanderson 1980).

Culture may also be used to describe some material aspects of life such as homes, tools, clothes, foods, religious items – but from the therapist's point of view, these are more usually considered as parts of the physical environment, although methods of use, expectations and personal feelings concerning them are affected by cultural values and attitudes.

Culture is learned, but although in a given culture there is a shared understanding, this does not mean that all members of the culture necessarily share identical perceptions or conform to cultural expectations to the same degree. Cultural values continually evolve and change; if the pace of change becomes too fast people have difficulty in adapting and culture may become disorganized.

Considerations of the impact of culture on the lifestyles and beliefs of ethnic groups is very important; questions of integration, assimilation, isolation, and potential prejudice and discrimination are fundamental to an understanding of any society, particularly when it includes members of several differing cultures.

Each culture produces values, perceptions, concepts, beliefs and practices which relate to the fundamentals of human life, e.g. relationships, sexual habits and roles, religion, work, education, material aspirations, permitted foods and ways of eating, dress, manners and death and bereavement. The therapist, therefore, cannot treat a client effectively without an understanding of the culture in which he lives, and an awareness that the strong emotions engendered by cultural pressures can affect the therapeutic situation both positively and negatively.

Culture may also be used to describe a grouping within a larger group, usually then called a subculture, e.g. a religious sect, criminals, addicts, pop culture or the inhabitants of an isolated village.

THE SOCIAL ENVIRONMENT

The social environment is composed of the people with whom an individual has contact. No-one can escape the pressures and pleasures of living with others, short of choosing to live as a self-sufficient hermit: 'No man is an island, entire of itself, every man is a piece of the continent, a part of the main.' (John Donne 1571–1631.)

Each individual has a network of social relationships within the immediate family structure, sometimes including an extended family, and then including the people in the individual's environment – at work, in religious groups, in leisure occupations or in the community in which he lives. Analysis of the pattern of such relationships, and identification of 'significant others' in a patient's life may help to indicate whether he is functioning adaptively or maladaptively.

The social environment typically provides an individual with a range of possible roles and relationships; it also provides the network of support for his life. In western society we survive only because society has been organized so that needs such as food, shelter, clothing, material goods, health care and social support can be provided by people working cooperatively to meet these needs.

Obviously, culture has profound effects on exactly how the social environment is organized. However, society itself generates other considerations such as availability of work, distribution of wealth, provision of housing, provision of social care programmes or education, which may be culturally influenced, but are also, to an extent, supercultural.

Society becomes stratified typically into classes, the occupants of which usually regard those outside their own, or the desired, class as in some way different/inferior/superior; but whether this stratification is related to wealth and 'social status' as it is in Britain, or to other considerations, such as religious practices, intellectual status or artistic skill as it may be in other countries, is a matter of cultural influence.

Society is also usually organized into a series of overlapping groups, sharing a common role or purpose; these sometimes function hierarchically. The structure of the society in which a person lives will determine which roles he must learn to fulfil, and which groups he joins. These affiliations will change as the individual ages. In British society these roles and patterns of belonging can be highly complex.

An analysis of patterns of roles, group membership and the ways in which these have evolved and changed over time in the life of an individual can be highly significant for the therapist. Although an elaborate analysis is not always necessary, it is not possible to treat a patient unless basic information about his social environment is obtained.

There is clearly considerable overlap between the environmental aspects of culture and society, and it is often simpler to avoid the difficulty of disentangling these and to refer to them under the umbrella of the 'sociocultural environment'.

It is important to recognize, however, that while the therapist may, by detailed observation, be able to obtain a concept of the relevant and 'normal' sociocultural influences in a given place, it is wise to view these as providing hypotheses about the sociocultural values, beliefs and attitudes of an individual, which must be checked and confirmed before being accepted as correct. Inflicting a specific set of cultural 'norms' on an individual must be guarded against, for individuals vary greatly.

THE PHYSICAL ENVIRONMENT

The study of the person in relation to his physical environment is covered by environmental psychology and ergonomics; in both cases the focus is the effect of environment on motivation, effectiveness of work, and reduction of stress or fatigue.

Therapists spend a great deal of time investigating and adapting the physical environment of their clients. They recognize the content of the physical environment to be crucial in motivating action, encouraging or inhibiting learning, providing stimulation and enabling the individual to fulfil – or fail to fulfil – his occupational tasks in all areas of life, work, leisure and self-care.

There is a considerable body of research demonstrating the effects on performance of well-designed and badly-designed environments,

and it is clear that physical environment can have a profound effect on both physical and intellectual performance and, less obviously, but equally importantly, on individual emotions, perceptions, values and attitudes. However, the well-known 'Hawthorne effect' demonstrates clearly that alterations to physical environment alone cannot be relied upon to produce consistent effects on performance.

The physical environment is partly natural and partly manmade. The natural environment, particularly in its more extreme manifestations, has always produced an ambivalent response in humans – on the one hand feelings such as wonder, appreciation of natural beauty and the desire to explore and enjoy; on the other hand, fear, anxiety, awareness of danger and lack of comprehension. These reactions may be viewed as combining to lead man to produce the constructed environment, driven by the desire to control and master the environment in order to ensure the basic biological and emotional needs of warmth, food, water, shelter and safety.

The physical environment comprises all the non-human, inorganic elements which affect and surround us, and also includes the organic, non-human components, such as plants and animals.

The non-human elements may include:

- Natural elements which affect the biological organism and which an individual must have available for survival. These may not be capable of control, but an individual or social grouping usually seeks to optimize and regulate what is available, e.g. breathable air, temperature, humidity, light, availability of food and water.
- Natural elements, which people cannot control, most of which are potentially dangerous, and from which people must seek a means of protection, e.g. sunlight, rainfall, cold, wind, drought, earthquakes.
- Natural resources which may be useful to people: metal ores, fuels, timber, crops, animals, which may be exploited or cultivated.
- The other forms of organic life which inhabit the planet.

The human elements include:

- Human constructs which people inhabit or which significantly change the natural environment, and which enable humans to live safely, and to satisfy their biological and social needs, e.g. buildings, towns, cities, roads, bridges, power stations, irrigation, farmland, forests.
- Artefacts (things which people make and use) to help them to control and master the environment or meet basic biological needs, e.g. tools, containers, furniture, modes of transport, machines, computers.
- Artefacts which are created to satisfy symbolic or non-survival needs and to form an environment which is meaningful or pleasurable to people, or to provide recreation, e.g. musical instruments, colour as decoration, art, sculpture, styles of architecture, gardens, theatres, sports facilities.

From an occupational therapy perspective, investigation of the physical environment is often related to identifying and removing environmental barriers to effective performance at work or in the home. In this context aspects such as noise, temperature, humidity, lighting levels, distractions, heights, steps, floor surfaces, access, design of furniture, tools or machines, space and layout, are important.

In a therapeutic context, the positive physical features which affect psychological well-being or the ability to learn are significant. As well as including the above elements, these may also include the less obvious features of environment which contribute to atmosphere or ambience, convey an emotion or imply values and attitudes. Therapists are not alone in considering these aspects of environment – examination of a restaurant, smart hotel or busy shop will probably show that the astute proprietor has spent time and money on these features.

EXPLORATION AND MASTERY

According to Kielhofner (1985), exploration and mastery of the environment is a basic drive behind human activity. This idea is echoed in various forms by other authors. Children begin to discover, by means of exploration, the difference between 'me' and 'not me' and later between organic and human components of their surroundings, and proceed to develop skills and concepts as a result of continued exploration and discovery. An important part of this process is the development of language to name and describe our surroundings.

In adult life the need to continue to explore and master leads to the development of individualized patterns of occupations and activities. Exploration and mastery are intrinsically motivating and self-rewarding, and can produce enjoyable arousal which has measurable physical electrochemical features. Research has proved that a basic level of arousal is necessary for healthy physical and psychological function and that humans or animals in experimental situation will strive to maintain stimulation at all costs. Deprivation of stimulation leads rapidly to marked behavioural disturbance. Too much stimulation, however, is also damaging, producing anxiety, aggression or withdrawal.

ENVIRONMENTAL DEMAND

The concept of performance demand was introduced in Chapter 4. This relates to the abilities which a participant is required to possess in order to perform an activity or task. This is, however, only one side of a complex equation; for as the performance of an activity affects the environment, so the environment calls for certain types of performance, and influences, facilitates or restricts what is done. The therapist can intervene on either or both sides of this equation, either by improving an individual's ability and/or reducing performance demand, or by altering the environment (Fig. 6.1).

The term 'environmental press' is used by Kielhofner (1985) to describe this attribute of environment. He defines press as follows: 'Press refers to environmental expectations for certain

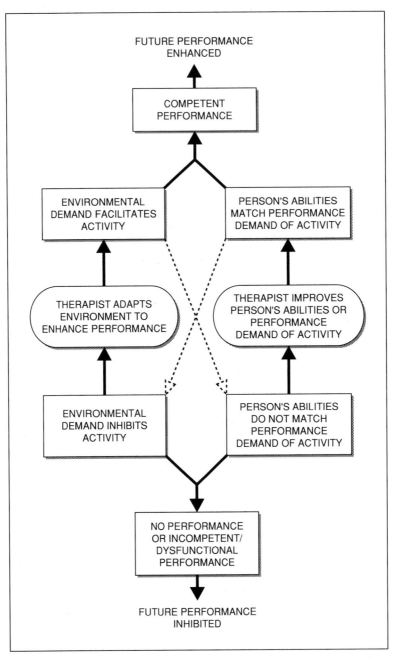

Figure 6.1 The influence of environmental demand and performance demand on the function–dysfunction continuum.

behaviour' (citing Lawton, *Environment and Aging*, as a reference for the term).

A similar concept is expressed by Cynkin & Robinson (1990) as 'field of action', which they state 'encompasses not only physical environ-

ment but also the objects and people in the environment and all the rules that govern the conduct of each activity,' Cynkin & Robinson's view is related to Bruner's concept of 'demand action' which, they explain, means that:

... the field of action creates a behaviour habitat in which expectations of the right kinds of reactions, interactions and transactions are relayed by virtue of the total context in which action takes place. The right kinds of responses are governed by the rules which are not only directives but indicators of expectation for appropriate behaviour.

Environmental content, therefore, affects and alters performance and behaviour. The term 'press' sits somewhat uncomfortably as an explanation for this concept, so I shall adopt the term 'demand', which seems more straightforward, e.g. you expect to cook in a kitchen, to be quiet and respectful in church, to shout encouragement on a football field and to work diligently in the office – each of these environments has a specific demand which helps to create and augment these expectations.

Clearly, the expected response to the demands of a set of environmental conditions must first be learned. Initially, an individual must be motivated to explore an unfamiliar environment and must learn how to do tasks, and use tools, and learn what the expectations of others may be and what are the implicit and explicit 'rules' to be followed.

Social modelling is an important learning mechanism in this context, especially for learning the unspoken, implicit rules of social or cultural behaviour. Individuals who lack 'cue-consciousness' and cannot recognize and respond to demand, and who therefore fail to learn appropriate responses, can become antisocial and dysfunctional.

The individual both acts in response to demand and, by his actions, may change the nature of the demand. People do this automatically in daily life. Given the option, few people spend long in the unstimulating, low-demand environment of a railway waitingroom. Those who must do so take a newspaper. If the children are playing in the kitchen and the radio is turned up to full volume in the middle of cooking supper, the person cooking is liable to evict the children and turn down the noise to reduce the demand to a comfortable level.

On a more important level, the person with a boring job may change it for something more challenging, or may seek an adventurous, high-demand environment during leisure hours. The affluent person may move out of the house which is overcrowded, but not everyone has that choice. In old age, environmental modifications are made gradually to adapt the environmental demands to the changing capacities or interests of the person.

This is an extremely important concept for the therapist, because it suggests that by manipulating an environment to produce relevant demand, or by teaching the individual to recognize and respond to demand, desired performances can be facilitated. Equally, it suggests reasons why desired behaviour may be inhibited, or why inappropriate or dysfunctional behaviour may occur in certain situations, especially when the individual is unable to alter, or is prevented from altering, a stressful level of demand.

Achieving the right level of environmental demand is a very complex matter because it relates to many variables, and these may not obtain the same response from a different individual or group, or even from the same person or group on a different occasion. It is primarily a question of balancing arousal versus lack of arousal. A tension exists between the content of the environment and the desire to interact with it; if there is enough information to be intriguing and interesting, the environment will be explored, choices will be made and participation will be effective; if there is too little, it will not. If there is too much, avoidance reactions, such as anxiety, frustration or withdrawal (flight or fight responses) instead of exploratory ones are likely.

According to Kielhofner (1985), factors which contribute to environmental demand (press) include:

- Physical surroundings and objects – the sensory input which results in perceptions of comfort, safety, colour, sound, presence or absence of distractions.
- People – the number of people involved in relation to the task and their roles within it is crucial; too many people for the job results in poor performance; too few in frustration; in some situations having fewer than might be ideal for the task can actually result in better participation and interaction.

- Tools and materials – having enough for stimulation, but having too good a supply can reduce arousal and lead to less satisfactory performance.
- Culture and expectations of the activities and behaviours to be performed in the environment.
- Tasks which are being performed.

ENVIRONMENTAL ANALYSIS

The importance of occupational analysis has already been explained, and environmental analysis is an equally important, complementary exercise, which also has a number of purposes.

Environmental observation (content analysis) involves noticing and recording the organic and inorganic elements of the physical environment, and the human and sociocultural elements:

- Physical elements (inorganic and organic): e.g. buildings, tools, furniture, artefacts, physical surroundings, plants, animals.
- Human and sociocultural elements: people and things immediately associated with them. Contextual features which guide interactions, cultural significance, emotive associations, ethnic features.

It may be necessary to take measurements or draw plans as part of this exercise.

Analysis of environmental demand and applied analysis involves using these observations for various purposes, e.g.

- to determine environmental demand
- to analyse the effects of an environment on an individual (or group)
- to identify environmental barriers to effective performance or learning
- to analyse the interactions of a person with his home environment thus gaining an insight into the extent to which he is able to adapt, or has been obliged to adapt to, environmental features.
- to adapt an environment for therapeutic purposes.

Environmental analysis can also be related to occupational levels. At the occupational, level a general summary of the main physical and sociocultural features of an environment might be needed.

At the effective level, environmental analysis looks at the ways in which an individual uses or relates to his environment in the course of specific activities. This data can then lead to environmental adaptation to remove performance barriers. Typical interventions of this sort would include evaluation of a disabled person's home to provide suitable alterations.

Applied environmental analysis explores environmental demand and the ways in which this might be used to facilitate performance of an activity or enhance the therapeutic benefit of participation.

At task level, environmental analysis becomes restricted and limited to the area, people and items immediately involved with task performance.

ENVIRONMENTAL ADAPTATION

FUNCTIONAL ADAPTATION

This is aimed at making performance more effective or efficient, less tiring, or more independent.

Adaptation of the physical environment in a person's home or workplace can be a relatively simple matter of either removing problems, e.g. providing a ramp instead of steps or changing the height of a working surface, or adding things which enable or enhance performance, e.g. a different handle, a strategically sited grab-rail. It may equally be a question of designing a total environment with multiple adaptations or computer controlled devices for a person with severe physical disabilities.

Each building and each room or entrance point needs separate evaluation, and the therapist needs to have some basic understanding of building construction and architectural design.

THERAPEUTIC ADAPTATION

Using environment as part of treatment is an integral part of occupational therapy. In physical settings this may amount to making similar adaptations to those just described, e.g. to heights, weights, length and positions, to promote specific movements or to increase or decrease effort. Positioning of tools or materials can also promote cognitive function, choices, problem-solving and decision-taking.

This may mean simply choosing the correct type of chair or table, but it may involve a more controlled use of environment, for example that suggested by Allen (1985) to meet the needs of patients with impaired cognition, which involves very careful selection and placement of tools and materials.

More subtle and interesting is the use of environmental demand to inhibit or enhance interpersonal communication, or carrying out of social roles. Environment can also be structured to create an appropriate milieu for therapy, to permit confidential matters to be discussed, to provide reassurance, or alternatively to challenge or provoke. The calculated positioning of seats and tables, or the presence or absence of carpets and curtains can radically alter the nature of a therapy session.

CONCLUSION

A summary of assumptions concerning the environment is listed in Box 6.1.

Box 6.1 Assumptions

1. The individual may, by means of his activities, effect changes in the physical or sociocultural environment.
2. Physical and sociocultural environmental factors combine to create demands for particular responses from the individual. Appropriate and optimal environmental demand facilitates performance.
3. The individual needs to recognize, and respond adaptively to, environmental demand, in order to perform effectively.
4. By interaction with the environment, the individual is able, through his activities, to alter the nature of the environmental demand.
5. The therapist may intervene to alter environmental demand in order to promote performance or to facilitate subjective responses for the benefit of the individual.

7

The therapist

PROFESSIONALISM

The therapist is also a person. It ought not to be necessary to make such a simple and obvious statement, and yet the fact seems all too frequently forgotten, by employers, by patients, and not least by the therapist trying to fit the mould of the professional stereotype.

The unique element which the therapist brings to the therapeutic interaction is himself. That self has experiences and the combined knowledge, skills and attitudes derived from professional education and practice. That self is human.

The label 'professional' is no easy burden. On the one hand it may bring contingent expectations of omniscience, infallibility and psychological stability which can reach nearly theological proportions. The therapist must have no apparent personal emotions, no prejudices, impeccable ethics, perfect judgement and invariable expertise. The therapist is denied the human luxury of making mistakes.

On the other hand professionalism may provoke negative attitudes and accusations concerning misuse of power, interference, manipulation, arrogance, elitism, 'ivory-tower' intellectualism and protectionist mystique.

These may be the extremes, but some of these expectations and prejudices do filter into everyday situations, and obscure the person behind the metaphorical name-badge, both to the wearer and the viewer. Examples of such attitudes include the checklist for students on placement which, if taken literally, pictures an idealized person, and, in the 'antiprofessional' corner, writers such as Illich (1977) and many examples of the 'de-skilling of professionals' in National Health Service documents of recent years.

Schon's (1983) outline of the professional's perceptions of himself as 'expert' or 'reflective practitioner' is revealing (Box 7.1).

Schon's reflective approach echoes many of the Rogerian principles of honesty, authenticity, acceptance and trust. If living up to the image of 'expert' is difficult and stressful, is it any easier to live up to the ideals of being a totally open, honest and mature individual completely in touch with oneself and one's client? Are both expectations unreal?

It takes 3 or 4 years to convert a person into a therapist. What has happened in that time to ensure that it is safe to let him loose on the public? Does training as a therapist automatically act as a form of psychoanalysis to enable the practitioner not only to gain knowledge and skill but also to internalize all the required attitudes and ethics and to acquire the requisite degree of personal insight? It seems unlikely; it takes most people half a lifetime to achieve some degree of self-knowledge.

Do we select only suitably mature people for training? Perhaps we try – but we know how unreliable selection procedures are. In short, are therapists born or made? I was intrigued to note that, during the First World War, the main characteristic sought by the selectors of girls for training as therapists to work with injured and traumatized soldiers was, simply, 'charm'; yet the efficacy of this nebulous attribute in gaining rapport cannot be denied even in this age of sexual equality. However, the stresses of the late 20th century demand considerably more than charm. The therapist must be both a skilled practitioner and a manager – of resources, people, the client's case, and most of all, of himself.

THE THERAPEUTIC RELATIONSHIP

The special relationship between the person seeking help or healing and the person from whom that help is sought is as old as humanity, and has long been considered both mystical and magical.

Health care professionals, even in western cultures, cannot escape totally from these archetypes, and perhaps they should not try to, for archetypes are powerful entities. The therapist may be uncomfortable with the label 'healer', feeling that it has an unwanted spiritual dimension or that it implies unrealistic expectations of 'cure', yet healing has never been a simple matter, and therapists are healers in the oldest and widest sense.

If intervention is to be successful, the person who seeks help must desire change and be prepared to contribute to it. The first contribution, taking action to obtain help, may be the most crucial, for acceptance of that need requires a definite emotional and cognitive shift.

Box 7.1 Expert or reflective practitioner?

Expert	*Reflective practitioner*
I am presumed to know and must claim to do so, regardless of my own uncertainty.	I am presumed to know, but I am not the only one in the situation to have relevant and important knowledge. My uncertainties may be a source of learning for me and for them.
Keep my distance from the client and hold onto the expert's role. Give the client a sense of my expertise, but convey a sense of warmth and sympathy as a 'sweetener'.	Seek out connections to the client's thoughts and feelings. Allow his respect for my knowledge to emerge from his discovery of it in the situation.
Look for deference and status in the client's response to my professional persona.	Look for the sense of freedom and of real connection to the client as a consequence of no longer needing to maintain a professional facade.

The person enters the relationship with fear, doubt and uncertainty. The healer must transmute this into trust, hope, expectation and openness. The healer must have, or at least seem to have, self-confidence, acceptance of what the person says, understanding of the problem and of the person's needs, knowledge of what can and cannot be done, optimism, and a clear view of possible helpful actions which traditionally are not only done, but seen to be done.

The definition and explanation of health and illness is culturally influenced. Healing clearly does take place in cultures where techniques are very different from our own. It can be proved that western surgery or chemotherapy produces superior results in some conditions, but there are others where the success rate is more debatable, and illness may equally be cured by prayer, ritual, dance, trance, drugs, herbs, homoeopathy or acupuncture. The scientist may explain these results by the fact that many conditions resolve spontaneously in any case, but this applies also to the results of medicine, or indeed occupational therapy!

The 'magical' attitude to medical intervention, in which the doctor represented, and was in touch with, the power of the god or spirit from whom a miraculous gift of healing might come to those who were worthy, is as old as Aesculapius. This attitude has justifiably been criticized when it has led to unnecessary autocracy, mystique and remoteness on the part of the practitioner, and passive credulity from the patient.

THE EFFECT OF VALUES ON THE THERAPEUTIC RELATIONSHIP

The concept and values derived from the principles and philosophy of occupational therapy, influence in turn the quality of the person – therapist relationship, and especially the therapeutic 'balance of power' along a continuum from prescriptive/directive, through partnership to client control. The difficulty lies in using the therapeutic relationship to empower the person

to take control of her own life, and not as a means of the therapist exerting power over the individual and her situation.

In general the therapist is concerned primarily with the needs of the individual patient or client, rather than with those of groups or of society. An optimistic yet practical expectation that improvement is possible, that growth, development or recovery can take place in the life of the individual is fundamental.

The much emphasized (but ill-defined and not always practised) 'holistic' approach seeks to consider the individual and her roles and occupations in the context of a physical and sociocultural environment specific to that individual. In this relationship the therapist seeks to guide or advise, to balance optimism with realism and to be continually sensitive to the needs and wishes of the individual, the two people working in partnership to promote the right to health and quality of life. Occupational therapy cannot be imposed on a patient since active participation is a prerequisite.

THE NATURE OF VALUES

Values are cognitive constructs and emotions with which a person surrounds ideas, objects or people. They are culturally determined and are learnt through primary socialization or, in the case of a profession, through the secondary socialization which occurs during training and practice. The student therapist absorbs, and identifies with, the values of occupational therapy, as demonstrated by the role models with whom she comes into contact during the formative years.

Values, positive or negative, lead to attitudes by means of which these values are translated into action. This is frequently an unconscious process. Therapists, typically, are unaware of their values, positive or negative, unless challenged to define them, yet shared values are a key part of professional identity and can be a powerful method of team-building, especially where these values can be expressed and acknowledged by the whole team. Dissonant values can lead to difficulties in a team, the reasons for which may be hard to unravel until the basic value conflict is exposed and resolved.

Although it is helpful for a therapist to become more aware of positive values which influence his practice, it is necessary also for him to be conscious of negative values which may affect therapeutic relationships or result in prejudices.

It has been shown by Fondiller et al (1990) that values influence both clinical reasoning and the 'helping' relationship. Of the 18 value statements defined by their research several relate to the latter. These include valuing the therapeutic relationship – respect, caring, empathy and the therapists's ability to develop rapport; using effective interpersonal skills; the ability of the therapist to act as teacher, enabling patients to explore new options; and a generally patient-centred approach to therapy.

As may be seen by a review of the statements concerning the aims and nature of occupational therapy guoted in Chapter 2, the therapist also values the individual as an active agent in her own environment – having potential, capable of positive growth and able to make positive decisions and contributions towards her own well-being. Occupational competence is valued as a fundamental attribute of humanity; activities are valued as the means whereby an individual may maintain her well-being in society and achieve her personal goals or social commitments, and as a medium whereby selective participation in activity may be used to promote well-being

Young & Quinn (1992) see these values as part of the core of the profession and quote a list of values codified by Yerxa which covers similar points to those given above, Kielhofner (1992) identifies values as one of three key elements of the central paradigm of the profession. Our values as therapists do seem to be more constant and more easily articulated than some of our purposes and practices.

If we share positive values towards our patients or clients it may be worth considering what we jointly reject: we reject imposing control on others, dislike promoting existence which lacks any meaning or quality of life, refuse to encourage passive and negative attitudes to ill-health or disability, reject constraints imposed by the environment on the individual, and condemn attitudes which accept that an inability to engage in a range of meaningful, purposeful activity is a normal, acceptable outcome of handicap, ageing, or social disadvantage. All of this is ethical, altruistic and commendable, but it is necessary to take a critical look at how far these values are put into practice.

PUTTING VALUES INTO PRACTICE

Once again it is a question of language: there are disturbing paradoxes concerning the terms which therapists use to describe their patients. As shown in the definitions analysed in Chapter 2, therapists regard their clients or patients as 'in need of therapy'. They are variously described as ill, injured, disabled, maladaptive, dysfunctional or incompetent – labels that contradict the values which have just been described.

How do we dare to label an individual in this way? If the individual comes to us in distress, explaining her difficulties and seeking help to resolve them, we may be on safer ground, but what if the person concerned does *not* see the need for help? What if it is society, or the family, or another professional who makes the judgement? Clearly, this is dangerous territory. Ultimately, the patient has the right to refuse to conform to our stereotypes, and may refuse therapy.

Secondly, is it not odd that we, as therapists, 'need' damaged or dysfunctional people in order to earn our daily bread? In this we are no more at fault than other health care professionals whose ultimate goal, in an idealized, healthy world, would be to work themselves out of a job. In his critical, antiprofessional essay 'Professionalized Service and Disabling Help' McKnight offers the following conclusion (Illich et al 1977):

To sum up, professionalized services define need as a deficiency and at the same time individualize and compartmentalize the disabling components. The service systems communicate three propositions to the client:
  You are deficient
  You are the problem
  You have a collection of problems.
In terms of the interest of the service systems and *their* needs the propositions become:

We *need* deficiency
The economic unit we *need* is individuals
The productive economic unit we *need* is an
individual with multiple deficiencies.

This has enough truth in it to make any honest
professional wince in recognition, although it
does, of course, exaggerate and generalize to make
the point. It is nonetheless a timely warning. It is
all too easy for both therapist and client to slip
into these stereotypes and to accept the given
language, without questioning its relevance. At
least the occupational therapist is more aware
than most people that the 'problem' may well
not be 'in' the patient, but due to circumstances
in her environment, or her occupations.

By entering into the therapeutic relationship,
the therapist has entered into a contract with the
patient; this implies a set of expectations on each
side which can easily be mismatched. Schon
(1983), continuing his discussion of reflective
practice, explores the differing attitudes of the
client in both the 'traditional' contract between
client and professional, which can lead to the
type of imbalance of power implicit in McKnight's
criticism, and in a contract derived from a partnership model of 'reflective practice' (Box 7.2).

While many therapists will recognize the
reflective model as the one they might ideally
wish to use, they will also recognize that it is considerably more demanding than the traditional
'professional–client' model, not simply in terms
of the openness and honesty required of the
therapist, but also in the responsibilities placed
on the patient, who must take an active and

intelligent interest in her therapy. Unfortunately,
the nature of dysfunction means that it disenables, disempowers, and demotivates, and it may
be too much to expect this level of insight and
participation from the client. There is security
for *both* parties in the traditional model of
relationship.

It is likely that a therapist wishing to move
towards the partnership model may spend the
first part of the therapeutic intervention simply
in enabling the person to move from the
dependent/compliant/grateful/respectful role
of the traditional 'patient' towards the role of
responsible, active participant and partner in
therapy. This demands not only skill but, more
importantly, time, which is likely often to be in
short supply. Whatever style of relationship is
practised, therefore, it is essential to have a clear
view of the values which guide our practice and
to be sure that we have a secure understanding
of the boundaries of 'normality' for an individual,
the points at which occupational competencies
break down, and the signals for intervention.
Effective management of the therapeutic relationship requires the use of highly developed personal
skills, coupled with honesty and insight.

THERAPEUTIC USE OF SELF

DEFINITIONS

Mosey (1986) coined the term 'conscious use of
self' to describe the involvement of the therapist

Box 7.2 Traditional and reflective contracts (Schon 1983)

Traditional contract	*Reflective contract*
I put myself into the professional's hands, and in doing this I gain a sense of security based on faith.	I join with the professional in making sense of my case, and in doing this I gain a sense of increased involvement and action.
I have the comfort of being in good hands. I need only comply with his advice and all will be well.	I can exercise some control over the situation. I am not wholly dependent on him; he is also dependent on information and action that only I can undertake.
I am pleased to be served by the best person available.	I am pleased to be able to test my judgements about his competence. I enjoy the excitement of discovery about his knowledge, about the phenomena of his practice, and about myself.

in the therapeutic relationship. She defines this as:

A planned interaction with another person in order to alleviate fear or anxiety, provide reassurance, obtain necessary information, provide information, give advice, and assist the other individual to gain more appreciation of, more expression of, and more functional use of his or her latent inner resources. Such a relationship is concerned with promoting growth and development, improving and maintaining function, and fostering a greater ability to cope with the stresses of life.

Mosey is careful to distinguish therapeutic use of self from rapport which is 'a comfortable, unconstrained relationship of mutual confidence'. Conscious use of self involves the person-centred qualities of valuing the whole persona, as she is, and as worthy of respect and affection.

Some therapists have expressed discomfort over the term, suggesting that the premeditated nature of it implies an excessively clinical, 'cold-blooded' attitude which leaves no room for spontaneity or intuition. I do not believe that was what Mosey intended, but, perhaps they have a point.

Schwartzberg (1993) employs the term 'therapeutic use of self', which she defines (following Siegel 1986) as having three essential ingredients: Understanding, empathy and caring. She adds that:

The therapist accepts the patient as he or she is . . . is tolerant and interested in the patient's painful emotions . . . is able to communicate to the patient what the patient expects of the therapist. By remaining neutral but engaged, the therapist encourages the patient to interact.

The term 'therapeutic use of self' will be used in this text.

Whatever words are used to describe it, there can be no doubt that the relationship between the therapist and the patient can be a deeply powerful agent for positive change. When managed well it transforms the nature of therapy. It might be argued that, given expert therapeutic use of self, it ceases to matter what else is done; the use of activity becomes incidental. Yet I reject that hypothesis.

Occupational therapy is not 'talking therapy' it is 'doing therapy'. The use of activity provides the focus and framework for the interactions between therapist and patient, smooths the way, speeds and facilitates natural responses, and allows for awkwardnesses to be rapidly glossed over.

DEMANDS ON THE THERAPIST

Therapeutic use of self requires the therapist to have a finely tuned self-awareness, and the ability to use a repertoire of roles and styles. It demands sensitivity, empathy and even a degree of vulnerability and acceptance of personal change, and yet also the ability to step back from a situation in order to evaluate the most helpful response to it without becoming over-involved. This is a difficult balance to achieve, and is particularly demanding on personal coping strategies, communication skills and intellectual and emotional resources.

It demands also a habit of reflective analysis and a probing self-evaluation which may be described as 'creative dissatisfaction'. This involves asking, in a positive manner, what was done, whether it worked, and how it could be improved upon, learning equally from both successes and failures.

Therapeutic use of self may be likened to walking a tightrope. If the therapist expects too much of himself or of his clients, he may end up frustrated and 'burnt out' from the effort of trying, single-handedly, to 'heal the world'. If the challenge of coping with an open and dynamic therapeutic relationship becomes too great the simple answer may be to retreat behind the professional persona. It is so much more straightforward to be able to 'act the expert' and to disclaim, even to oneself, any feelings aroused by the frustrations, problems and human tragedies with which one may be faced. That too is a route to burn-out.

The techniques of conscious use of self can sound mechanistic or even manipulative: choosing to speak or to listen; tone of voice, eye contact, body language; giving or witholding praise; prompting, reflecting, intervening or withdrawing help; providing a model by acting the fool or the logical planner – part actor, part teacher, part therapist, part salesman. In fact, although some of these decisions may be planned or conscious, during an interaction the therapist is only and can only be himself. Yet it is a self which has learned to understand and accept some part of his own strengths and limitations in relationships, and knows how to use these for therapeutic advantage; a self which has learned to be aware of, and to filter out or to exaggerate if necessary, the normal social signals of voice, posture and expression which we all unconsciously adapt and adjust as we meet different people.

This is why the experienced therapist can change responses in mid-session on the basis of 'gut-reaction', without having to think about it at the time. Afterwards, the student may ask 'Why did you say that at that moment?' or 'why did you stop the session just then?' It may well be difficult to recall; usually it will have been right. However, the wise therapist will spend time reflecting on his own reactions and interactions in order to monitor them; therapists are no more prone to total rationality, and no more immune from assumptions, preconceptions, stereotypes and biases than anyone else.

It may sound unduly pious to say that a therapist needs humility. This is not currently the most fashionable of virtues and must not be confused with being 'humble'. Yeats wrote 'tread softly for you tread on my dreams.' The therapist must often come close to the places where people keep not only their dreams, but also their nightmares and the most vulnerable and insecure parts of their private selves.

It would, of course, be quite wrong to give the impression that all therapeutic interactions are at some deep and delicate interpersonal level. Many remain simple, safe and relatively short transactions, and anything else would be inappropriate, but the therapist must be prepared to dare to enter the dangerous territory, and may sometimes find himself there without warning – a sense of your own powerlessness and your own power is necessary if you are to enable another person to explore safely in such terrain.

Why should therapists be expected to treat all patients with impartial success? We do not relate equally easily to all members of the human race.

Leaving aside the obviously unacceptable influence of racial or other prejudice, there will occasionally be a patient with whom one simply does not 'get on' (or even, with whom one begins to get on far too well). It is far better to acknowledge this and, if possible, to find a colleague who does not share your problem, than to battle on, giving the patient substandard therapy as a result.

Use of self, with or without the tag 'therapeutic', is not limited to interactions with patients; interpersonal skills are of great importance also in dealing with relatives, friends and neighbours, as well as with the plethora of managers and fellow-professionals with whom the therapist must transact.

THE THERAPIST AS AN ETHICAL PRACTITIONER

All therapists are bound by the statements of ethics of their professional association and, in Britain, of the statutory controlling body, The Council for Professions Supplementary to Medicine. The public rightly expects that persons in responsible positions dealing with people who are in some ways vulnerable, must exhibit professional behaviour of a high moral and ethical standard.

Remarkably few practitioners in the annals of the profession in Britain have ever shown less than total probity. Ethical behaviour is not, however, simply a matter of obvious attributes such as personal honesty, integrity, competence and morality. It extends to judgements concerning confidentiality, giving or withholding services, maintaining personal competence and refraining from actions for which one is unqualified.

The therapist is not expected to be perfect. He is expected to use reasoned judgement and to avoid negligence. In the legal maze of modern legislation and litigation the therapist must not only act wisely, but be seen to do so, and be able to prove by suitable records that wise action was taken on the basis of sound evidence.

Ethics are related to values; the values of the profession have already been mentioned. For a therapist who genuinely values his patient as an individual, much of the required ethical behaviour becomes axiomatic. Seedhouse (1988) describes values concerning the individual and concepts of health which are very similar to those espoused by occupational therapists. He states:

Work for health is always designed to remove obstacles that lie in the path of biological, intellectual and creative potentials latent in individuals. . . . there is an ultimate and fundamental link between the idea of health and the idea of morality. . . . Simply, ethics is the key to the new era of health work.

Seedhouse proposes an 'ethical grid' as a tool for directing practitioners towards ethical concerns. He emphasizes that this grid should be used dynamically rather than mechanistically, but it is a very useful presentation of the issues (Fig. 7.1).

The grid consists of four layers. In the centre is the core rationale for health care: respect persons equally, respect autonomy, serve needs before wants, create autonomy. The second layer contains the duties or purposes of the practitioner: promise-keeping, truth-telling, minimize harm, intent to enable. In the third layer are the consequences or intervention: increase of individual good, increase of self-good, increase of the good of a particular group, increase of social good. The final layer contains external factors which affect ethical choices: the responsibility to justify all actions in terms of external evidence, effectiveness and efficiency of action, the risk, codes of practice, the degree of certainty of the evidence on which action is taken, disputed facts, legal rights of others, wishes of others.

The language of this grid is clearly derived

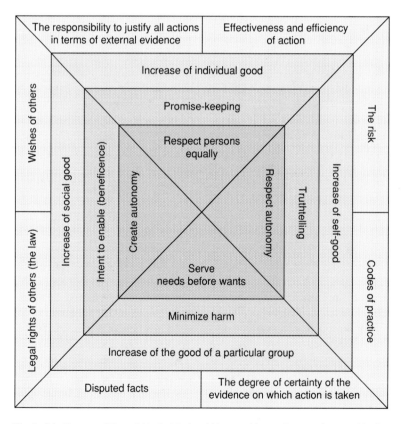

The limit to the use of the grid is that it should be used honestly to seek to enable the enhancing potentials of people.

Figure 7.1 The ethical grid. (Adapted from Seedhouse 1988 Ethics: the heart of health care, with permission.)

from the humanistic frame of reference and is particularly applicable to occupational therapy. The ability to take ethical decisions has been called 'moral reasoning' and is at least as important as clinical reasoning – indeed, the two are interdependent, for the therapist must not only choose to do 'the right things' but also to do them 'for the right reasons'.

The Victorian presumption that a professional person's ethical values must be carried equally into private life was possibly polite fiction, yet the notion lingers and should not be ignored. It is, in any case, questionable whether a therapist demonstrating obvious double standards between public and private life would be totally effective.

PERSONAL SUPPORT AND DEVELOPMENT

'Carers need care' is a slogan that is seen often on therapy office noticeboards. It is true, and the therapist should understand taking appropriate action to acquire the 'care' he needs for himself to be a key part of his professional responsibilities. Everyone who works closely with people in stressful situations needs somewhere to discuss cases in confidence and to seek personal guidance and support. It is not a declaration of a lack of coping skills to seek supervision, rather an affirmation of them.

In a career which may span several decades it is also essential to work at remaining fresh, interested and up-to-date with a continuing sense of personal discovery and adventure within the profession. Managers of therapists have a responsibility to provide resources for self-development; therapists have a responsibility to use them.

THE THERAPIST AS A TEACHER

Since learning is accepted to be the means whereby a person is enabled to become a confident and competent actor in his own world it is not surprising that occupational therapists spend much of their time 'teaching' in one way or another. Indeed, according to Francella (1982) 'above all else the occupational therapist is a teacher'. Mocellin's view of the central importance of teaching as therapy has already been noted. Imparting knowledge and skill to another person is not simply a way of extending performance, but also a means of empowering that person to take more informed control of his own life.

Therapists require a comprehensive understanding of human learning and of various styles of communicating skills, knowledge or attitudes. Although more formal 'teacher-centred' styles of instruction may be required, on the whole therapists tend to prefer indirect, client-centred and experiential styles of facilitating learning. 'Learning by doing' has always been a primary tenet of occupational therapy. In many ways client-centred teaching is simply another form of 'therapeutic use of self'.

Cynkin & Robinson (1990) write: The contract for interaction, whether implicit or explicit, requires that the occupational therapist serves as a competence model with whom the patient/client can interact in activities situations, which by their structure will call forth the will to learn on the part of the patient/client.

Increasingly, writers on occupational therapy speak of the therapeutic process in terms of facilitating learning; not simply developing part-skills, but ensuring that skills and knowledge generalize into meaningful activities and productive occupations.

THE THERAPIST AS AN 'ARTIST–SCIENTIST–INVENTOR'

I am much attracted by this description of humankind, and moreso by the thought that occupational therapy is above all a profession in which these three attributes are employed equally.

The therapist is an artist not only in the use of personal artistic skill and creativity, but also in the 'art' of therapy. Artistry adds heightened awareness and sensitivity to perceptions of people and situations. Therapists also value, and look for, creativity in others.

As a scientist the therapist must have a firm foundation in medical, biological and psychological sciences, with some knowledge also of ergonomics, kinesiology, mechanics and information technology. Fimilarity with scientific research methodology is required as is a knowledge of research methods derived from the social sciences. In particular, the therapist needs to cultivate the scientist's abilities to hypothesize and test, to be an objective and rational observer and recorder and to distinguish objective from subjective elements in a situation.

As an inventor the therapist must design, adapt and problem-solve with a wide range of materials and in diverse situations, being able both to make simple devices and adaptations himself and to communicate effectively with engineers or architects when the need arises.

Invention is the use of creative imagination to project different solutions into a hypothetical future until a desired 'fit' is found between a solution and the desired outcome. Mattingly's view (described in Kielhofner 1992) of the therapist using creative invention to describe and make sense of a patient's life story, script the next chapter and plot the means of reaching a desired end, is another example of therapeutic use of invention.

A more flexible view of the therapist deftly juggling the art, science and inventiveness of therapy might relieve some of the professional anxiety which occurs when we are confronted suddenly by the inevitable tensions which arise when these differing perspectives collide. Perhaps the tensions themselves are valuable parts of the dynamics of our profession.

THE THERAPIST AS A MANAGER

In 1964 MacDonald wrote of the therapist 'She must be a consultant, a teacher, an able organizer and administrator, capable of harnessing her therapy team.' More recently Cynkin & Robinson (1990) described how the therapist acts 'to plan, organize, evaluate progress, serve as an advocate for the patient/client with professional colleagues or agencies, or as counsellor with the family . . .'

Every major basic text on occupational therapy discusses the therapist in the role of manager, but frequently this is interpreted somewhat narrowly in terms of resource management. The therapist is a manager in four different but interrelated areas:

- manager of self
- manager of knowledge
- case manager
- manager of resources.

MANAGER OF SELF

In many ways this is related to therapeutic use of self, but management of self concerns the practicalities of efficient and effective delivery of personal service, e.g. attending meetings or clinics, being on time, using time well, being organized, remembering, prioritizing, sorting out competing demands of a caseload, keeping up-to-date, seeking supervision.

The good self-manager is aware of his role, his place in the structure within which he works, his relationships with other colleagues, which must be developed, fostered and cherished, and his value as both a therapist and a person. He is appropriately confident, and capable of self-control and of appropriate assertion when needed. Self-management has to be acquired and learned.

MANAGER OF KNOWLEDGE

At a simple level, the therapist must be a manager of knowledge in the sense of information. The hundreds of thousands of pieces of information gained during and following professional education, about people, pathology, techniques, media, adaptations, legislation, social provision and services must be mentally filed, cross-indexed and recalled at need. This requires either an impeccable memory or an excellent grasp of information processing and data management systems – and probably both.

Far more interesting and complex is the

management of knowledge in order to apply it to practice. The largest data base is of no use unless the therapist can recognize which of the vast number of pieces of information it contains are relevant, here and now and for *this* patient.

The processes of clinical reasoning, whereby knowledge of why, what and how is converted into knowledge of what to do *now*, in this therapeutic situation, are as yet only partially understood. Research to date has been limited, but indicates substantial differences in cognition and processing between inexperienced, competent and expert practitioners (Slater & Cohn 1991), and suggests that experienced therapists conduct a form of internal narrative as they try 'to make sense of the case' (Mattingly 1991).

Reasoning takes place as an internal dialogue. Fleming (1993) identifies four forms of clinical reasoning: hypothetical reasoning, interactive reasoning, pattern recognition and procedural reasoning. The inner dialogue which comprises these forms of reasoning may not be consciously articulated, and the more expert the practitioner the more subliminal the process becames until correct decisions are apparently arrived at 'intuitively', although they are, in fact, based on rapid processing of previous knowledge and experience.

Schon (1983) makes the interesting suggestion that reflection during and after action is a means by which a practitioner may build into his practice methods for examining the actions he is taking and the reasons for decisions, in order to better understand and develop the processes of clinical reasoning. Schon also makes the link between clinical reasoning and the use of the problem-solving process for the 'naming' (identifying) and 'framing' (deciding what to deal with, and how) of problems.

Selection of an appropriate model or frame of reference is linked also to clinical reasoning in a complex interrelationship: sometimes the selection of a frame of reference actually affects the naming and framing process, by limiting options and perspectives to those within the chosen framework; at other times the naming and framing process provides the information whereby an appropriate frame of reference may be chosen.

Kielhofner (1992) offers a particularly clear account of this process.

It may be argued that if therapists become too introspective concerning the processes of therapy it is possible that they would be totally inhibited by the apparent impossibility of what they are attempting to do; yet they manage to practise. A more in-depth knowledge of how these processes occur must be beneficial, but in an entity as complex as occupational therapy this is clearly going to be difficult to achieve, and an attempt to do so offers the profession one of the greatest challenges of the next decades.

CASE MANAGER

The process of case management begins as soon as a patient or client is referred to a therapist. This has been described in several texts, usually under the heading 'the occupational therapy process', which integrates the other processes of occupational therapy. The foundation of this process is the problem-based approach.

Foster (1992) lists four distinct stages in the process:

• gathering and analysing information
• planning and preparing for intervention
• implementing intervention
• evaluating outcomes.

These four processes are central to practice, and require the coordination of all the therapist's managerial and clinical skills and knowledge to enable a long list of tasks and activities to be performed.

The AOTA standards for entry-level practice include competence in:

• screening
• evaluation
• reassessment
• programme planning
• intervention
• documentation
• discontinuation of intervention
• service management
• research.

MANAGER OF RESOURCES

The personal attributes and training which make a therapist a good therapist also equip him to be a good manager. Indeed, training for management in industry now deals as much with inter-personal skills, communication and counselling as it does with marketing, quality management and financial control. The latter topics are now very much part of occupational therapy management training; the former have existed for decades.

The 'three Es' – efficiency, effectiveness and economy have long been managerial bywords; in the modern health service they are holy writ. Occupational therapists have actually had a headstart, having been involved in resource management since the early days of the profession.

MacDonald (1964) lists the headings buying, selling and purchasing. If 'management' is substituted for 'administration', her introduction to the chapter with the latter heading is still entirely relevant:

Good management is essential to occupational therapy, because of the contribution it makes to the successful treatment of the patient and because it ensures that the treatment service takes its place smoothly among other allied services . . . Management is a means to an end, not an end in itself. It involves foresight, the ability to plan and organize, the ability for sympathetic understanding and leadership, and a knowledge of facts and objectives.

In the 1960s a varied stock of hundreds of craft items had to be ordered and accounted for; now there may be a six-figure budget for adaptive equipment or wheelchairs. Then, the head therapist managed a team of colleagues and support workers; now, as Director of Services, she may manage other professions as well. It involves a change of scale rather than one of content. Occupational therapists remain very competent at managing resources.

THE THERAPIST AS A RESEARCHER

All practitioners have a duty to add to the sum of professional knowledge and skill. This is not an optional extra, although it may be very difficult to convince employers or managers of this fact.

We still know comparatively little about the fundamental dynamics of occupational therapy, about why and how it works, and about the processes which therapists use to achieve results. Research does not have to be thought of with a capital 'R'. Writing up interesting cases, small-scale evaluations, reports of innovation and records of reflection on practice, are all useful, can readily be integrated with everyday practice and should not be dismissed as lacking scientific validation. Admittedly, larger-scale research requires time, resources, understanding of research procedures and active commitment. A primary benefit of a graduate profession ought to be increased attention to research.

Therapists have often been down the track of 'medical model' or 'psychology model' research in the quest for proof of professional validity and measurable outcomes. In a profession which deals primarily with the unique problems of unique individuals this 'control group' approach is of minimal relevance. This does not mean that research is impossible, simply that different methods must be used.

Sociology, anthropology and ecology can all provide models of methodology that have been developed to investigate complex interactions or the outcomes of 'single case' illuminative studies.

SUMMARY OF REQUIREMENTS

Occupational therapists claim to be adaptable and versatile, which seems entirely justified. The person wishing to practise as a therapist must integrate a set of demanding and idealistic values, acquire breadth as well as depth of knowledge, and many practical skills. He must be artist – scientist – inventor, teacher, manager, analyst and researcher, and must have a highly mature, insightful concept of self.

Is it possible to gain so many skills and attributes in 3 years of professional education? On the face of it, this does seem a somewhat unreasonable set of expectations to place on any one person. On the other hand there are many excellent and expert practitioners across the world who do embody the ideals of the profession.

Expertise does not come at once; it must be worked for and consciously developed. The basic values of the profession in relation to people and their occupations are a driving force behind much practice. Ethical and clinical reasoning evolve from the application of these values, together with the knowledge and skills of occupational therapy. Reflective practice informs and advances the process. Research provides validity.

In an increasingly complex and rapidly changing world it may become more important to equip practitioners with a sound understanding of the basic principles of occupational therapy, together with a new set of '3 Rs' – reasoning, reflection and research – than to overwhelm them with quantities of specific information and technical skills which may soon be obsolete.

THE CENTRAL TRIAD: THERAPIST, PERSON, OCCUPATION

I suggested in Chapter 3 that this triad is at the very centre of occupational therapy. It is therefore worth spending some time on analysing how the insertion of occupation into an otherwise dualistic relationship changes the dynamics of the situation, and affects the therapist's use of self.

It may be easiest to do this by reflecting on the nature of situations in which people interact without the medium of an activity. You may come to the conclusion that these are few in comparison to the bulk of human interaction which takes place in the context of 'being somewhere and doing something'.

The situations where little or no activity is involved tend to be of three types: highly intimate, where physical proximity and verbal and non-verbal communication are used to take a relationship to a deep level; somewhat formal, e.g. an interview; or highly superficial, e.g. the trivial remarks about the weather which strangers may exchange when waiting for a bus. None of these situations is therapeutically appropriate; the first is too invasively close, the second is too

remote and possibly threatening and the third lacks impact and is swiftly forgotten.

People react most comfortably with each other in the context of an environment and an activity because these provide the structure for the interaction and the roles and 'rules' for the participants. Environments and activities acquire meanings and symbolisms which the majority of people in any given culture are likely to recognize and respond to in a similar way. The context changes the nature of the interaction, even when it is between the same people but in different situations.

When the therapist wishes to form a therapeutic relationship, or to use that relationship in a particular way, he selects the environment and activity with demands which are most likely to provoke the quality of interaction which is required. The activity can either facilitate communication and personal disclosure, or inhibit it. It may help to trigger emotions or memories, or to assist in the control of them.

Many examples could be quoted here of the inhibiting or releasing nature of activity in relation to interpersonal communication. I have frequently observed how concrete constructional activities inhibit conversation, whereas unstructured activities do not. I have seen social behaviour change dramatically for the better when the patient was taken out of the hospital setting to participate in an activity in the community where 'best behaviour' was required. I have had many confidences imparted to me while assisting a disabled person in a toilet, and am certain that the intimacy of that particular activity and environment promotes disclosure, provided that the patient knows and trusts the therapist.

The occupational therapist does not, therefore, promote a relationship as an end in itself, but as a means of engaging the patient in an activity, and through the interactions engendered by that activity of promoting the aims of therapy. The skill lies in selecting an activity and environment which will promote interaction with the therapist or others and in selecting a therapeutic approach geared to gaining rapport, and consciously using personal communication skills, to promote interaction and engagement.

8

The prescription of activities as therapy

FOCUSES FOR THE THERAPEUTIC USE OF ACTIVITY

In the preceding chapters occupational therapy has been variously defined, and its core content and primary components discussed. It is clear that the practice of occupational therapists covers a very wide area, and that it is difficult to encapsulate. Taking one of the simpler definitions:

Occupational therapy is the treatment of physical and psychiatric conditions through specific activities to help people to reach their maximum level of function and independence in daily life. (WFOT)

There is some consensus that occupational therapy is *prescribed*, that it uses specific (and often *purposeful*) activities, and that it is concerned with *independence in daily life*.

There are, therefore, two distinct, but overlapping, forms of occupational therapy: using activities as remedial agents to enable, enhance or empower occupational performance, and adapting the materials and processes of activities or the content of the physical and social environments, in order to promote independence or enhance the quality of life. The former is the provision of therapy – treatment (or education) of the patient to achieve specific objectives – and the latter requires intervention by the therapist in some aspect of the daily life of the individual. Although intervention is very important, and may indeed be the primary role for some therapists, e.g. when working in the community, this chapter is concerned primarily with the prescription of activities as therapy.

As has been described in the previous chapters, therapists are concerned with occupations as the organizing framework of a person's life, but activities are the focus of therapy. Activities are viewed from two perspectives: as essential to an individual in the competent performance of his daily life, and as potential remedial, developmental or educational media.

The personal pattern of occupations and activities of an individual are affected by biological and environmental factors and by the competencies or dysfunctions which that individual experiences. The therapist may use activities as a means of exploring and identifying dysfunction, or to promote learning by providing practice and instruction relevant to the individual. The therapist can also, by means of applied analysis and environmental analysis, identify and remove barriers to performance, whether in the environment, in the nature of the activity, or in the abilities of the individual.

The word 'prescription', may jar on some as derived from the 'medical model'. I believe that therapists should use it deliberately and unapologetically when speaking of the use of remedial activities because, fundamentally, occupational therapy in this context *is* a prescribed treatment, however loosely one wishes to maintain the connection.

Therapeutic activities, whether used to meet rehabilitative, developmental or educational goals, or for the purposes of enabling, enhancing or empowering, are not selected casually or without purpose. Selection will certainly involve the patient or client, but it is the business of the therapist to ensure that effective therapy occurs. This implies that some element of prescriptive control must be retained, however gently and empathetically exercised and however carefully negotiated with the client. Of course, choices should be offered, but at the discretion of the therapist.

Why use activities as therapeutic media? The difficulties of explaining the concept which is at one level so simple, and at others so very complex, have beset generations of therapists, and continue to lead to misunderstandings about the nature of occupational therapy (Creek 1992a, Stewart 1992).

We do not, we affirm angrily, simply occupy or 'keep people busy' with activities, and yet the casual observer of therapy in progress may at times see something which looks superficially like 'busy occupation'. Hurried explanations by harassed therapists about the value of process or the key importance of daily activities, like all hasty half-truths, obscure as much as they explain. The individual therapist's personal conceptualization of the rationale for the use of activities is, in any case, likely to vary depending on the model or approach being used.

There are five focuses for the applied use of activities which have alternated in influence over recent decades:

Focus on product

The product of an activity provides a motivation for participation, through intrinsic or extrinsic rewards. Completion of a product or outcome which is valued by the producer, or by others, provides meaning and purpose and promotes engagement in the activity.

Focus on process

Activities possess intrinsic characteristics, derived from the nature of their procedures, practical requirements and performance demands which may be used to achieve precise therapeutic goals and to improve competence in skilled performance.

Focus on competent performance

The individual needs to achieve and maintain competent performance of roles, occupations and activities. Successful participation in an activity and completion of a product or outcome valued by the participant teaches skills and produces subjective experiences of competence, achievement and control. This can enable an individual to return to a positive cycle of competent performance and consequent well-being in the context of his own lifestyle and environment.

Focus on the individual interacting with others by means of activities

Individuals require a repertoire of roles and interactions to live independent, meaningful lives within their physical and social environments. Activities can provide opportunities and experiences by means of which the person can explore relevant roles, reactions and interactions, with the therapist, or with others, and can move from unproductive or maladaptive patterns of participation into new, adaptive and satisfying ones.

Focus on the individual interacting with the environment by means of activities

Activities are the means through which the individual experiences, and reacts to the environment, and designs, adapts or controls it, in order to maintain personal well-being and to achieve goals, satisfaction and quality of life.

FOCUS ON PRODUCT

Early views

Early writers tended to emphasize that while process, not product, was the most important part of therapy, the product should, ideally, be saleable and relevant to the patient. The following quotations from the principles of the American Occupational Therapy Association (O'Sullivan 1955) are typical:

Inferior workmanship, or employment in an occupation which would be trivial for the healthy, may be attended with the greatest benefits to the sick or injured, but standards worthy of entirely normal persons must be maintained for proper mental stimulation.

The production of a well-made, useful and attractive article, or the accomplishment of a useful task, requires healthy exercise of mind and body, gives the greatest satisfaction and thus produces the most beneficial effects.

Novelty, variety, individuality and utility of the products enhance the value of an occupation as a treatment measure.

Quantity, quality and saleability of the products may prove beneficial by satisfying and stimulating the patient, but should never be permitted to obscure the main purpose.

It is interesting that here 'purpose' is plainly the purpose of the *therapist* not that of the patient, but the benefit of patient satisfaction is noted.

A decade later in Britain, the standard textbook of the day (MacDonald 1964) stated:

There has been a tendency, in the last few years to swing away from the use of art and craftwork for treatment. This has in part been brought about by a mistaken interpretation of occupational therapy as 'giving the patients something to do', resulting in a series of unattractive rugs, unoriginal and badly made felt toys, or baskets or embroidery of poor design or in poor quality materials. The swing has gone over almost too far to production, and 'industrial work' or 'out work' on contract is considered a more up to date form of treatment. It cannot be claimed that one or other activity is more therapeutic and/or economic. Problems and abuses arise in the use of either . . . in both cases care must be taken that patients are not exploited, in the former by making things for staff or hospital sales; in the latter by providing cheap labour for concerns outside the hospital. . . . There is a tendency however, to use the therapeutic emphasis as an excuse for accepting a low standard of work which *could* be better. This is a poor compliment to, and poor business for, a patient who genuinely needs to earn and who needs the stimulation of finding that his goods are in demand.

These concerns of 30 years ago, together with changing patterns of health care which resulted in restricted treatment time, combined by the mid-1970s to make many therapists regard the use of anything resulting in a 'craft-type' product with grave suspicion. As previously described, this resulted in a 'natural' purpose and product being replaced by the contrived ones of 'gaining therapy' and 'getting better'. While this may be motivating, it now seems at odds with the philosophy of occupational therapy. The patient might better be referred to a different form of treatment.

Creativity

The innate capacity of human beings to produce artefacts of aesthetic rather than practical use has been mentioned. Humans are creative, inventive and adaptive; but how far is creativity – even specific talent such as the ability to paint – innate and genetically determined, and how far is it the result of opportunity, education and cultural influence?

Views have changed in synchrony with the development of scientific hypotheses and research, and occupational therapy has changed perspective accordingly; but therapists have generally valued creative activities.

Does every individual have some capacity for creativity? Therapists would probably argue that this is the case. How important, then, is it that this should find expression in the life of the individual? Is creativity so fundamental that people who are deprived of the opportunity of self-expression through creative activity will become dysfunctional? What, in any case, do we mean by creativity? Is the production of a good meal for a family as creative as the production of a poem or painting?

The views of cultures and of individuals are very subjective when it comes to such judgements, and it is not a topic which lends itself readily to research. Is creativity related to the process or to the product, or to both? It is probably impossible to separate these two elements, but process often seems significant to the participant; once the picture is painted, the play performed, the meal consumed, the creative person moves on to the next project, for which the last product simply served as a stepping stone.

In occupational therapy, views of creativity have changed over the years. The use of creativity in physical rehabilitation has been reduced to a minimum in favour of a more pragmatic, functional approach. In mental health, creative activities such as music, art and drama have been used projectively, to enable the individual to gain insights into his situation; the product is frequently still of less value than the process, except insofar as it may provide insights into the patient's problems or needs. The focus on leisure may renew the interest in promoting creativity as part of a balanced life, especially for people who are unable to work.

If creative work is to be undertaken the con-cerns with standards, meaning for the patient and quality of materials and design remain as relevant today as they were 30 years ago. There is nothing therapeutic in the production of tacky items, and nothing compounds failure more than spurious approval which convinces neither patient nor therapist.

What is meant by product?

It is a mistake to limit the discussion of 'product' to artefacts or art-objects. Products can be intangible and ephemeral – in the case of many recreational and social activities, for example, enjoyment of the 'process' *is* the product. You party for the sake of partying; you enjoyed it, but it is over – perhaps the pleasant memory, or the new friendship counts as a product? Similarly, many activities of daily living do not have a specific product except in the sense that something necessary is achieved; you wash, bath, dress and eat because you need to; some degree of discomfort or social disapproval results if you do not.

However, subjective views of the product will also be affected by a variety of sociocultural factors and learned attitudes and values. For this reason, while the product *may* be the motivation for participation, it may equally be incidental to a host of contingent or extrinsic rewards, e.g. social approval, financial gain, enhanced status or sexual identity. Due to the individual nature of experience and learning, these factors are not easy to predict with certainty.

The narrow perception of the meaning of 'product' and a general discomfort with the term has led to a view of activity as 'purposeful' rather than 'productive'. There seems to be a consensus that activities used as therapy should be purposeful, although it is difficult to envisage activities which are totally purposeless. This leaves the question of 'whose purpose'. Is the purpose that of the participating patient, or that of the prescribing therapist, or is it a negotiated amalgam of the two?

There remains the paradox that it may be the completion of the product that motivates the patient, and the therapeutic benefits of process which motivate the therapist. How far is it ethical for the therapist to manipulate the patient into making an object or participating in an event by convincing him that he would like to have the product or experience for its own sake, when she realizes that this is, essentially, a confidence trick designed to obtain participation in a therapeutic process? It may be that in some cases the patient's knowledge of that fact itself inhibits participation or lessen beneficial effects, or that the patient is unable to comprehend the concept of therapy – but this applies to a minority of patients.

Although the intentions of the therapist are undoubtedly to 'do good' to the patient, a manipulative approach shows signs of the ancient philosophical argument about 'the ends justifying the means'. Pragmatically, perhaps, they sometimes do; but it is better, if possible, that both therapist and patient are fully aware of both sides of the process/product equation, and value both appropriately.

FOCUS ON PROCESS
Intrinsic characteristics of activities

Past views

Early practitioners were struck by the benefits of active participation in purposeful activity – any activity – for those with mental or physical illness. The benefits were clear: improved physical stamina or ability, improved mood, improved concentration, enhanced sense of well-being and reduction in symptoms. If engagement in productive occupation was normal and healthy, it followed that patients who were deprived of occupational opportunities and constructive routines would add inactivity, boredom, and consequent general physical and mental malaise to their problems. It gradually became clear that institutionalization was frequently responsible for as many problems as the illness which precipitated admission.

What began as an important, but relatively simplistic, observation that 'work is good for you', developed into an appreciation that some activities were better, or more appropriate than others. But why? And how could these benefits be harnessed to provide therapy? Could occupations have intrinsic characteristics which could be used therapeutically? Early occupational analysis proposed that occupations had general performance attributes, e.g. active, sedentary, heavy, light, manual, dexterous, complex and simple. The nature of the activity or task should be matched to the needs of the patient.

Because much of this work took place in psychiatric settings where the emotional reactions and behaviours of patients were significant, the idea of intrinsic characteristics was extended to include suppositions about the affective impact of various activities. Crafts were described as 'sedative' or 'stimulating' in accordance with the type of movements required and the degree of stimulation provided by materials (O'Sullivan 1955). Fidler & Fidler (1958) stated:

The physical activity which is employed can in some cases be roughly correlated with emotional states and can be used to bring out such expression or can be avoided to escape such expression.

The need for sensory, motor and cognitive and interactive responses was also considered.

In the 1950s crafts and productive activities in physical rehabilitation were subjected to detailed analysis of muscle work and joint movement so that they could be matched precisely to a patient's condition and the aims of therapy. This was a comparatively simple matter, since physical actions and effort can be analysed by observation. The concept of grading a therapeutic programme of activities to meet the changing needs and improved physical competence of the patient was well established by the mid-1950s (Colson 1944, Jones 1960, MacDonald 1964).

However, by the late 1960s in the UK this approach was already being challenged as too 'unscientific' to provide effective physical rehabilitation. Such activities were difficult to prescribe and control accurately; too much of the activity might be non-specific. More purpose-designed rehabilitation equipment, which could be precisely controlled and graded, was needed. As I was fresh from training which emphasized biomechanical and behavioural theories, my article 'Our techniques and apparatus are often out of date' reflected the 'new thinking' (Hagedorn 1969). I spent much of the mid-1970s testing and reporting on prototypes of such equipment.

Although I personally continued to believe in the importance of product completion, the reductive attitude to activity analysis, which valued the process to the exclusion of other features, led eventually to the retention of specific activity, but the removal of product, e.g. repetitive use of an elevated sander to smooth down a piece of wood which never became incorporated into an end-product, swinging an arm in a sprung sling or moving adapted solitaire pieces without actually playing a game. The purpose of engaging in the activity became 'to obtain therapy' rather than 'to make or complete something'. Occupational therapists in physical practice became increasingly indistinguishable from physiotherapists.

The current view

It would be surprising if, after 50 or more years, this view of the intrinsic characteristics of occupations or activities were to remain unchanged. In fact, although some of this early theory has been discarded, the concept of activities having intrinsic features which can be analysed, identified and related to therapeutic need remains a cornerstone of therapy. The process of 'doing' still has therapeutic value, although there are now differing interpretations of the rationale for this.

In current practice in mental health, analysis of physical, and especially of cognitive–perceptual and psychosocial, components of activity continues. Affective analysis, however, does not because it has been recognized that the problem with designating affective characteristics to an activity is that emotional reactions and values are not intrinsic, but are brought to the situation by the participant. One person's enjoyable activity is neutral or even unpleasant for another; what one person perceives as intricate and satisfying, another may find frustratingly laborious and tedious (Young & Quinn 1992; Turner 1992).

A good example is that of wedging clay: this used to be described as providing an outlet for aggression because of the necessity for heavy thumping and banging of the clay to remove air bubbles. In practice a few patients may find it so; others, however, may describe it as a soothing activity, like making dough; some may find it pointless, and others will find it highly unpleasant because of the cold, sticky, tactile qualities of the clay. These reactions may be significant; the material has triggered them, but they cannot be assumed or predicted in advance, except as hypotheses based on an understanding of the patient.

Current views of the affective aspects of activities therefore consider the subjective individual reactions of the patient, and the meaning, or lack of meaning or personal associations which the activity may have for him, attributing the affective response to the *person* rather than to some innate characteristic of the activity. Nonetheless it is a commonsense observation that activities do have some innate characteristics which promote broad affective responses, e.g. boredom, excitement or irritation. This is an area in which very little research has been conducted, and it is therefore impossible to do more than conjecture.

In physical practice the current trend, under the influence of the American theoreticians of the past decade, seems to be towards restoring purpose and meaning to activity. However, while physical and cognitive activity analysis continues and is still relevant, the decreasing need for physical rehabilitation and the very short time available for it in the majority of acute conditions greatly constrains the scope and relevance of the specific therapeutic use of activities in physical practice.

Activity analysis and microanalysis – separating out the observable performance skills and other attributes of an activity and its component tasks – remains one of the core skills of occupational therapy; but there is a greater awareness of the importance of the 'total process' (including purpose and product), of the impact of environmental factors and situational elements, and of the difficulty of predicting individual responses to an activity.

Flow

Some activities have the capacity to draw the participant into a state of flow or focused engagement in which awareness of extraneous external or even internal stimuli is greatly decreased, and the participant is unaware of the passage of time, personal concerns, or discomfort.

Flow is an attribute of process as a gestalt, rather than of its component parts. It, like affective response, is an unpredictable and situational attribute, although it is possible to identify some activities which produce flow more reliably than others.

These activities are usually those which require the sustained use of skill, judgement, attention, problem-solving or creativity, presenting continued challenges (Csikszentmihalyi 1993) and which require, in fact, the integrated use of all the higher level cognitive, process and sensorimotor skills. The activity is typically one which the participant finds meaningful, relevant and motivating. To 'lose oneself' in an absorbing activity leaves one with the experience of satisfaction and a sense of refreshment rather than fatigue.

The therapeutic benefits of flow were recognized by early practitioners, but have become somewhat neglected over the years. Diversional occupation – selected by the patient and used to relieve boredom, provide interest or maintain ability – fell sharply from favour in the UK during the 1960s, partly as a consequence of the move towards specific and scientific application of activities described above. The rejection of the value of diversion may have contaminated the view of intensely focused engagement as a beneficial attribute.

Is it wrong, however, to provide the patient with the chance to do something he enjoys simply for the sake of enjoying it, and of losing himself and his concerns for a while? Is it not therapeutic to participate in an activity so totally absorbing that discomfort, anxiety or disturbing thoughts are diminished, and concentration, perseverance, standing tolerance, range of movement, (or whatever performance is wanted) are automatically brought into use and sustained long past the normal thresholds?

Csikszentmihalyi reports that research into the incidence of flow showed that opportunities for the occurence of flow at work and in leisure are limited in modern western lifestyles. Although people dislike the idea of work, the typical working adult in the USA was said to 'experience flow on the job three times as often as in free time'. In free time occupations, researchers were surprised to find that 'driving a car is the most constant source of flow experiences, followed by conversations with friends and family'. Creative, constructive projects also achieved high ratings, but few people performed these. Surprisingly, watching TV was rated as enjoyable, although rarely producing flow; Csikszentmihalyi hypothesizes that this is related either to the lack of effort required to participate or to the majority of people's impoverished expectations and opportunities for productive personal leisure.

The difficulty of predicting flow and ensuring that it will occur, and the very practical problem of the length of time and the facilities required to give a person a challenging and involving experience, have perhaps added to the problem. Csikszentmihalyi proposes that this supports the argument for pure research into occupations, in other words, more occupational science.

It would certainly help if we understood better the complexities of performance at the effective level. It also provides a valuable argument against reductionism in the prescription of activity; when fully engaged in an activity the patient cannot help but utilize the total range of skills. An attempt to isolate one or other performance component can render the whole activity artificial, and is bound to limit the experience of flow.

It is interesting that those occupations which have been developed as 'mono-therapies', such as art, music, drama and horticulture, are those which have a high capacity to provoke engagement. If only we could capture, distil and bottle the elusive essence of flow we might better appreciate its therapeutic potential.

FOCUS ON COMPETENT PERFORMANCE

The functional approach

When viewing activities as therapy one asks the

question 'how can experiences and activities which will benefit this person best be constructed?' The process of matching an activity to therapeutic objectives may be viewed, in some respects, as artifical.

In the functional approach the questions become 'what does this person need to do in order to function as a competent and independent individual? What are his roles, his obligations, his needs and wishes, and how do these relate to the pattern of his life? What can he currently do; what can he not do? How can I enable him to do more? What physical, social, or pathological barriers exist to prevent his enablement?' The answer to these questions may or may not involve engagement in therapeutic activities.

Objective assessment of the patient's current performance is related to the history of past performance, his current condition and his future needs, in the context of his physical and sociocultural environment. The functional approach is associated with the view that occupations are divisible into work, leisure/play and activities of daily living. However, much of the focus in the past tended to be on work and activities of daily living, for the functional approach is essentially practical, and can at times verge on the utilitarian.

More recent models, such as occupational performance (CAOT 1983), while maintaining a general emphasis on function, have restated the approach in terms of individual need – whether the client 'needs to, wants to or is expected to perform' any given activity, and then whether he 'can perform, does perform and is satisfied with his performance' (Law et al 1990).

The occupational therapist is concerned with the individual as an actor on his own special stage, with his own requirement to play many parts. These parts require competence in activities which enable the individual to meet those needs for survival, safety and affiliation which Maslow includes at the base of his hierarchy. These are the activities which a person *must* perform if he is to remain healthy. If he is unable to perform them someone else must offer assistance; if performance is impaired other more complex and meaningful activities involved in work or leisure are likely to be impaired or impossible.

In the functional approach, intervention is aimed at restoring or enhancing performance by therapy or provision of aids, enabling by provision of environmental adaptation, or by teaching new skills or providing new information. All of these goals may be achieved by means of participation in selected relevant activities – the key word here is *relevant*, for such activities are usually those in which the patient will actually need to participate, or those utilizing directly relevant skills.

While the importance of this 'holistic' approach, considering all aspects of the patient's life, is always emphasized, the functional approach may in practice become reductive, focusing on a narrow range of abilities or performance deficits. Is this wrong? It may depend on the specialty in which the therapist is working, and on the frame of reference being used.

If a woman attends an occupational therapy clinic to request a solution to the problem of picking up things from the floor it may be pragmatic simply to offer her a long-handled pick-up stick. Further exploration of her patterns of occupation and psychosocial needs could indicate the need for further intervention, or might be viewed as intrusive. On the other hand, the therapist who treats a woman who is unable to leave her home solely for the difficulty she has going through the front door is likely to be ignoring significant other needs.

The competent self

The concept of the competent self differs from the functional view of the competent performer, although the two are closely related. In the functional view it is the fact of performance (or failure to perform) which is important; this tends to be related to the therapist's observations and judgements about the patient's performance in relation to his needs.

In the view of the competent self it is the individual's personal perception of himself as a competent or incompetent actor or performer in his own life which is significant. This view acknowledges the essential feedback link between the person evaluating his own actions as successful, gaining improved perceptions of the self as competent, and therefore achieving subsequent competent performance.

It is interesting that this open system view of the person seems at first sight to have some deterministic features reminiscent of operant conditioning, with its language of input, feedback and reinforcement, and yet its proponents are strongly humanistic. Despite the system's language, it is essentially the cognitive–affective meaning which this feedback has and its effect in building self-concept which are important, rather than the fact that behaviour is likely to be reinforced by perceptions of efficacy.

Kielhofner (1985) holds the view that the individual explores and masters his environment through his occupations; competence and mastery feed back into a benign cycle, while helplessness and incompetence fuel perceptions of the self as incapable, controlled and enhanced in a vicious cycle of dysfunction. Reed & Sanderson (1983) describe how the individual adapts through occupational performance, controlling, exploring and adapting the environment by means of this performance.

This active, reciprocal, cognitive–developmental view of the individual growing, changing and modifying his life and environment by means of his skills in occupations, and in turn being modified by them has been highly influential, placing priority on the examination of motivation and meaning as the driving forces of individual behaviour and choices. Loss of function becomes one factor in the dynamics of behaviour rather than the prime focus.

Client-centred views, based on humanistic theories (Rogers, Maslow) concerning self-actualization and the ability of the individual to steer his own destiny have also been influential, in particular in swinging the 'balance of power' away from the prescriptive medical model and towards a model of partnership and client-centred therapy, emphasizing the importance of client choice and a social model of disability.

Mocellin (1992a,b), while also emphasizing the therapeutic benefits of perceptions of efficacy and control is a particularly strong advocate of client involvement in directing the therapeutic process. He criticizes the model of human occupation as 'highly prescriptive and controlling' and questions whether within it 'patients are allowed to choose their therapeutic occupation or whether it is prescribed for them, whether they decide on priorities and whether they are also formally involved in evaluating the therapeutic outcome'. He seems to favour a more strongly sociological and educational model of therapy with a client-centred or partnership-style of relationship.

The net result of these theories is that the focus of therapy turns from considering any intrinsic characteristics of the occupation towards the opportunities it offers the individual to experience the physical and human environment and to gain perceptions of competence and control. What is done becomes of less importance than that it is done to a standard which pleases and satisfies the patient, and that it is meaningful to him and enhances his self-concept and self-confidence.

FOCUS ON THE INDIVIDUAL INTERACTING WITH OTHER PEOPLE

Humans are 'social animals'. Although most people value and need a portion of privacy in their lives, few are truly reclusive to the point of avoiding all contact with others. The framework of daily life involves a myriad of different levels of encounter, from the transient and casual to the long-term and intimate. A person who is unable to cope with the intricacies of acceptable sociable behaviour is seriously disadvantaged.

Much of this network of interaction and communication is mediated by activities. Activities are a vehicle for both primary and secondary socialization. They enable people to meet others and provide a social or cultural context for communication and cooperation. Shared participation in activities promotes bonding and provides experience of affiliation or cultural affirmation. Activities shared and enjoyed by people who have a close and intimate relationship often become laden with additional meaning, and become vehicles for deepening the relationship. The interactionist view of activities as symbols is also important here.

The therapist's use of self is frequently mediated by activities which can build confidence, trust and respect between therapist and patient. Returning to a more process-related view of activity, therapists use activities to assess interactive skills and can structure experiences which will facilitate communication, role-taking and the building of relationships. These activities do not need to be overtly social – many activities can be modified to promote and teach social behaviours such as sharing, cooperation and conversation.

FOCUS ON PERSON–ENVIRONMENTAL INTERACTIONS

The importance of person–environmental interactions has already been mentioned in the context of the competent self. A person is able to influence the environment only by taking action to effect change. Activities may use elements of the environment, add to it, or remove from it. Environmental factors in turn trigger appropriate engagement in activity.

Activities enable the person to exist safely in what might otherwise be a hostile setting, and to create things for use and pleasure. In order to be able to explore and master the environment the person needs a wide repertoire of activities. Enabling a person to be safe and competent within his own special situation is an important aspect of occupational therapy. These ideas are developed further in Chapter 9.

APPROACHES IN RELATION TO ACTIVITIES

The focuses that have been discussed are highlighted to a greater or lesser extent by various frames of reference or models which affect the view of activities and their place in therapy. Some of the main differences in perspective between a selection of approaches are summarized in Box 8.1.

Box 8.1	Approaches in relation to activities
Approach	*View of activity*
Behavioural	Activity is learned by interaction with environment. Product acts as a reinforcer. Purpose relates to the desire to obtain the reinforcer. Procedure is a chain of learned responses.
Biomechanical	Activity is carried out by means of sensorimotor skills. Product serves as a motivation to produce the required movements. Purpose of participation is to obtain therapy for specific muscles, joints or aspects of sensory reception. Procedure provides the required movements, resistence, endurance, etc.
Developmental	Activity aids development of skill, exploration of and adaptation of, or to, the environment. Products and purposes relate to these goals as sought by the individual. Procedures are adaptive responses requiring learned abilities achieved in a developmental sequence.
Analytical	Activity is motivated by unconscious purposes and processes which colour views of objective purpose, procedure and product.
Interactive	Activity is the means whereby the individual carries out roles and conducts social and personal relationships. Purposes, procedures and products all relate to interpersonal transactions which may be symbolic in nature.
Client-centred	Activity is the means whereby the individual achieves self-actualization. It is motivated by personal choices and perceptions. Products are valued in accordance with personal relevance, choices and meanings. Procedures are the means whereby a person exerts control over his present life.
Cognitive	Activity is the means whereby the individual creates meaning and structure in his world. It is the observable result of cognitive–affective processes. Cognitive interpretation of feedback from the results and products of activity enhances or inhibits future performance. Products are valued for their meaning to the individual and the degree to which they match internal constructs or schemata and satisfy personal imperatives. Procedures require cognitive–perceptual organization.

SUMMARY OF FOCUSES

The five focuses which have been explored in this chapter illustrate a philosophical development in occupational therapy, the stages of which are:

1. an original concern with useful productivity
2. a concern with the process of engagement as a therapeutic agent
3. the promotion of functional competence in necessary activities
4. the use of activities as a means of interacting with other people or the environment
5. the perception of the self as competent through the performance of activities.

It is clear that tensions exist between these focuses: the emphasis on product versus process, the view of competence as objective or subjective and the degree to which the therapist should or should not be prescriptive. There seems currently to be some uncertainty whether these focuses, some of which stem from the early years of the profession, all remain legitimate and valid. Are they simply different focuses, or are they symptomatic of an evolutionary stage in which new ideas have been added on to older ones, although the older ones have not yet been rejected?

The ideas discussed in this chapter are summarized in Box 8.2.

Box 8.2   Therapeutic activities

1. Activities possess intrinsic characteristics which combine to produce performance demand which requires the participant to possess particular knowledge, skills, attitudes and personal abilities in order to achieve a successful outcome or product.
2. This performance demand defines the requirements for participation and indicates whether or not the activity has therapeutic potential, and whether the individual is capable of engaging in it.
3. The therapist can adjust performance demand by adapting features of the activity in order to enable or enhance overall performance or selected skills, or to provide therapy or opportunities for assessment.
4. The situational elements of an activity combine to produce subjective, affective, cognitive or perceptual responses. These are highly individual in nature, but a therapist may encourage such responses by providing appropriate situational elements.
5. Successful participation in an activity and completion of a product or outcome valued by the participant produces subjective experiences of competence, achievement and control. This can enable an individual to return to a positive cycle of performance and well-being.
6. Activities are the means whereby a person engages in interactions with others. Activities can provide opportunities and experiences by means of which a person can explore relevant roles, reactions and interactions, with the therapist or with others, and can move from unproductive or maladaptive patterns of participation into new, adaptive and satisfying ones.
7. Activities are the means through which an individual interacts with the environment, changes it, and is reciprocally changed by it.

COMPETENT PERFORMANCE AND OCCUPATIONAL THERAPY

In the preceding chapters a number of quite complex ideas have been expressed concerning the nature of occupations, environments and personal skills and responses, and consequent perspectives on occupational therapy.

Competent performance is the ability of the individual to cope effectively, consistently and to his own satisfaction, with the roles, occupations and activities which have priority within his life. The ability to do this depends on a balance between three elements: the response of the individual, the performance demands of the activity and the demands of the environment.

The response of the individual depends on self-concept, performance and process skills, experience, knowledge, values and meanings. Performance demand is the knowledge, attitudes, skills and abilities required to complete an activity or task. Environmental demand is created by sociocultural context, other people, expectations, cues, constructs, materials and tools.

When these are synchronous and compatible, with each element in harmony with the others, optimum performance can occur. When one or other of the elements is 'out of step', problems and dysfunctions arise.

The contribution of the occupational therapist lies in assisting the individual to define what he needs or wants to do, and then in analysing the points where performance is unbalanced by lack of experience or skill, inappropriate response or inappropriate demand.

When the problem area has been defined the therapist can intervene to improve the person's response, to alter the performance demand of the activity, or to change environmental demand in order to enable or enhance competent performance within relevant aspects of daily life. These concepts can be expressed as a diagram (Fig. 8.1).

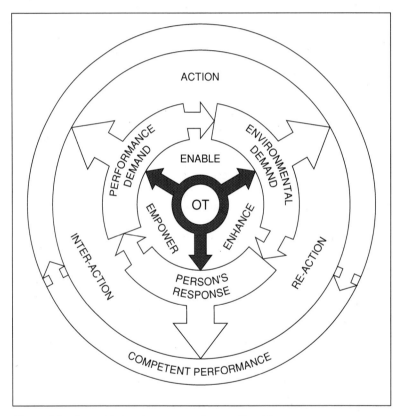

Figure 8.1 Competent performance and occupational therapy.

9

Occupational therapy: macroanalysis

I proposed in Chapter 4 that an occupation has a title and its participant a role title, and that occupations have nine attributes: principles, positions, possessions, purposes, processes, products, patterns, practical requirements and performance demands. Macroanalysis uses these headings to describe and define an occupation. Since occupational therapy is itself an occupation it seems logical to use this '10P' structure to analyse professional concerns and practice.

PARTICIPANTS

In the UK the primary participant is the appropriately qualified State Registered occupational therapist, holding either a Diploma of the College of Occupational Therapists or a BSc in occupational therapy, or a practitioner trained abroad in a college which satisfies the requirements of the World Federation of Occupational Therapists, Assistants may be graded as helpers, aides or technicians with appropriate trade or technical qualifications, and with variable amounts of health-related training.

PRINCIPLES

The philosophy, values and knowledge base of occupational therapy have been described in the preceding chapters. A summary seldom does justice to the richness of such a complex tapestry of ideas and beliefs, and risks being reductive.

Nonetheless, some fundamental principles are listed below:

1. Engagement in roles, occupations and activities is a defining characteristic of humanity.

2. Failure to engage in necessary and meaningful roles, occupations and activities has serious consequences for the well-being and health of an individual.

3. The individual must respond adaptively to environmental and performance demands in order to perform roles, occupations and activities successfully.

4. Engagement in prescribed activities can enable and enhance performance, health and well-being, and can empower the individual to take an active part in shaping her future life.

5. Alteration of environmental or performance demands by the therapist can facilitate functional performance and promote positive perceptions and emotions in the participant.

POSITIONS

Occupational therapy may be classified as work (not leisure or self-care); it is generally recognized as a profession – certainly therapists view themselves as professionals. While in the past being 'professional' brought automatic status and respect this is now less likely to be the case. In the past decade there has been a noticeable political reaction against specialists and 'professional experts' who seem to have become regarded as operating some kind of elitist 'closed shop' or monopolistic cartel. Professionals are now required to justify their actions by more than the time-hallowed phrase 'in my professional opinion'.

In the UK, occupational therapy retains the image of a middle-class occupation for well-educated white women, and despite active efforts to broaden the social and ethnic base of the profession and the inclusion of more male participants this is probably still an accurate description of the majority of practitioners in Britain. This may be viewed as a matter of concern, since it does not reflect the current social and ethnic mix of the population in the UK, members of all groups are consumers of the service. It is difficult to prove whether or not the service provided suffers in consequence. This is a problem shared with other professions.

Assistant grades of staff come from a much wider socioeconomic and educational range and include more men, and since these workers often have close contact with patients (sometimes, it must be said, closer contact than therapists), this probably serves to counterbalance any social bias.

Health care professions are generally well-regarded as making a positive contribution to society, but occupational therapy still suffers from misconceptions in the minds of the public (and other health care professionals), concerning its purposes and processes. These views can serve to promote an image of a service which is perhaps somewhat trivial in nature and more of a luxury than a necessity. Such attitudes are changing, if only slowly in some quarters.

POSSESSIONS

Occupational therapists have claimed the identification of occupational dysfunction and the prescription of activities for therapeutic purposes as their central possession. The latter is probably still the one area where 'border disputes' are rare. In almost all of the other traditional areas of occupational therapy – social training, activities of daily living, provision of adaptations, orthotics, functional assessment, creative activities – a small army of psychologists, social workers, educationalists, nurses, physiotherapists and others can make counterclaims of ownership. Pieces of 'occupational therapy territory' have been broken off and turned into specialist therapies, e.g. social and recreational therapies and art, music, drama and horticultural therapies; therapists in all of these now have recognized qualifications, many at diploma or degree level.

Occupational therapists have also been quick to invade the territory of others, taking on roles as, for example, counsellors, psychotherapists, educators and social workers.

The blurring of boundaries can be important in close multidisciplinary teamwork, but it does not aid professional identity. Therapists may be in danger of becoming too compliant when border invasions occur. Defining and defending the borders of our territory may soon become as important as defining and defending the professional core when therapists are faced with being edged out of practice by the competition. Equally, when therapists engage in forms of therapy which other professions already 'own', this reduces the perceived value of occupational therapy.

This is not an argument for becoming negatively or aggressively defensive, but for much improved communication about, and marketing of, occupational therapy services, together with insistence on high quality practice. The best defence against intruders is evidence that occupational therapists perform at a higher level of competence.

PURPOSES

Occupational therapy has three purposes:

- Enabling
- Enhancing
- Empowering

Enabling

- Enabling the individual to become more proficient in occupations, activities and role performance, thus maintaining her independence and meeting her personal, social and cultural needs, especially when proficiency has been lost due to injury, illness or environmental barriers.

Enhancing

- Enhancing the performance of an individual in roles, occupation and activities, by developing skills and removing barriers, in order to use potential to achieve optimum function and personal satisfaction in all aspects of life.

- Enhancing the environment and the individual's capacity to interact with it through activities, in order to provide interest, stimulation and quality of life for the user or inhabitant.

Empowering

- Empowering the individual, through participation in occupations, activities and roles, to take choices, to accept responsibility, to benefit from and exercise normal human rights, and to achieve meaningful and realistic life goals through roles, occupations and activities.
- Empowering the individual to take informed decisions and actions concerning personal health by providing information and explanation.
- Empowering the individual to accept her personal value, abilities, and fallible humanity, and to accept these things in others.

PROCESSES

In order to enable, enhance and empower, occupational therapists engage in core processes which are central to the profession, but which may be modified by the selection of a practice model or frame of reference.

CORE PROCESSES OF OCCUPATIONAL THERAPY

Metaprocesses

Case management

This is the central, organizing and coordinating process of therapy, the purpose of which is to identify and provide the intervention needed by the individual referred for therapy, and to achieve a satisfactory outcome (product).

Actions include: data management; assessment, analysis and evaluation; planning and providing therapy or intervention; selection of therapeutic approach/media; recording and reporting; evaluating outcomes; maintaining standards and quality of services; and effective use of personal and other resources.

Problem analysis and clinical/ethical reasoning

The purpose is to define problems and solutions in order to take decisions concerning the priorities, aims, objectives, approaches and methods of treatment or intervention in relation to the unique situation and needs of an individual.

The products are clinical decisions and goals resulting in consequent interventions, and the selection of appropriate frame of reference techniques and media.

Actions include: obtaining and analysing data; defining problems and issues; reflection; finding patterns; utilizing experience; making predictions and hypotheses; setting priorities; taking decisions; and initiating and undertaking research.

Implementation of therapy or intervention

The purpose is to carry out treatment of a patient or to implement an action plan to achieve agreed goals to meet the identified needs of the patient. Implementation must be consistent with the individual's rights and wishes and must promote the general health, safety and well-being of the individual.

The product is an observable positive change in the patient, or the patient's environment or pattern of participation, or the patient's reported feelings or perceptions.

Actions include: program design and organization; modification of performance or environmental demand; use of personal, technical, creative, constructive or social skills; engaging patient in activity which meets therapeutic goals; teaching; problem-solving; monitoring; documentation; reporting; liaison with others; using correct physical handling when required; maintaining a safe therapeutic environment; adhering to local policies and procedures; obtaining equipment, adaptations or services; referring to other services or agencies; altering intervention as required; terminating intervention when completed; and making appropriate discharge or follow-up arrangements.

Service management

The purpose is to maintain the efficient, economical and effective provision of occupational therapy services, and to ensure the maintenance of professional standards and the quality of service provision.

The product is an effective, high quality, service.

Actions include: planning; timetabling; obtaining and monitoring resources; documentation; liaison; communication; administration; organization; supervision and deployment of staff; organization of self; reporting; appraising; auditing; monitoring; policy creation and review; setting standards; budgeting, obtaining and analysing performance indicators and statistical data; and researching.

These processes will be described in Part 2.

The integrative processes

Therapeutic use of self

The purpose is to to use interactions between therapist and patient to enhance, enable and empower the autonomous performance of the patient.

The products include positive reactions on behalf of the patient such as exhibiting trust, confidence, insight, improved performance.

Actions include: use of self as therapeutic agent; maintenance of professional standards and ethics; personal development; verbal and non-verbal communication; showing empathy; giving support; and seeking and using supervision.

Assessment and evaluation of individual potential and needs

The purpose is to ascertain the abilities of the patient and her current condition and potential.

The product is a baseline for therapy or intervention, and for review and evaluation of progress, and consequent continuation or discontinuation of interventions.

Actions include: selection of appropriate assessment; interviewing; measuring; testing; observing; recording data; analysing data; comparison with other data or norms; identifying and quantifying dysfunctions or needs; communicating data to patient or others; setting goals for consequent therapy or intervention.

Occupational analysis and adaptation

The purposes include: obtaining knowledge of occupations, activities and tasks; understanding and evaluating the performance of an individual; analysing performance demand and matching this to the therapeutic needs of the patient; and adapting purposes, products, procedures, practical requirements and performance demand to provide therapy or to enable, enhance and empower the individual.

Products include: data concerning occupations, activities and tasks; data concerning patient abilities and dysfunctions; records of analysis; treatment plans incorporating the outcomes of analysis; and action plans leading to adaptations of activities or tasks.

Environmental analysis and adaptation

The purpose is to identify environmental elements and demands, in order to make adaptations for therapeutic purposes or to enhance performance.

The products include: data concerning an environment; records of analysis; treatment plans incorporating adaptations to environment; and adaptations to tools, furniture or buildings used by a patient to enable, enhance or empower autonomous performance.

Each process involves competence in a number of activities which could be analysed further into tasks. Activity and task analysis would provide data on specific performance skills. In view of the complexity of the profession a comprehensive study would be impractically lengthy. Nonetheless, general analyses of the activities performed and skills used by differing grades of practitioner (e.g. the standards produced by the AOTA, or standards of good practice produced by the COT) are illuminating, and improve curriculum development and the creation of appropriate practice standards.

It may be felt that the above section excludes some important occupational therapy processes, procedures or techniques. The point is that the processes listed are part of the professional core. Others, or variations, are derived by adopting one of the frames of reference from the conceptual belt. This has been described in Chapter 2.

PRODUCTS

Definition of the products, or outcomes, of occupational therapy is difficult because these relate to the purposes and goals of individual therapy, which vary according to the circumstances.

In general terms a product, whether tangible or intangible, must be something which can be identified as a change, which can be reported objectively, or subjectively, which has resulted from an occupational therapist's intervention, and which should correspond to the aims or goals which were set by patient and therapist at the start of therapy. It is clearly much easier to deal with observable, measurable, products than with those which are subjective and intangible.

Observable products relate to changes in the patient's occupational or social competence resulting from therapy, and/or changes in the patient's environment resulting from intervention by the therapist.

Examples of changes in the patient might be:

- improved physical function, e.g. range or power of movement; stamina
- improved competence in performing a task
- return to social or work roles
- removal of the symptoms of medical or psychological illness
- decreased behaviour relating to anxiety, phobia or obsession
- greater ability to communicate with or relate to others.

Examples of changes in the patient's environment might be:

- provision of an orthosis

- adaptation of personal clothing
- provision of adaptive equipment in the home or workplace
- provision of structural alterations or additions to the home
- provision of stimulating materials and opportunities
- removal of architectural barriers.

Subjectively reported products might include:

- feelings of improved well-being and enhanced quality of life
- removal of, or reduction in, unpleasant, anxious or obsessive thoughts
- improved perceptions of self as a competent and effective person
- positive feelings concerning roles or relationships
- improved understanding of personal needs or motivations
- feelings of purpose and enjoyment when participating in activities.

PATTERNS OF PERFORMANCE

Historically, occupational therapy has been a 9.00–5.00, Monday–Friday profession, and much clinical practice remains locked into this format, especially in physical settings.

The appropriateness of such patterns may well be increasingly questioned. The basic fact is that people's occupational behaviour takes up the greater portion of each 24-hour period, 7 days a week, and that the behaviours which occur before and after the '9.00–5.00 slot' are frequently markedly different from those which occur during it. Perhaps this is another inheritance from the concern of occupational therapy with work, although even this sphere of activity is not limited to the standard day.

Although few therapists yet work over weekends, flexitime working is more frequent, and some therapists are now on hand at 7.00 a.m. when patients get up, and in the evenings when they are at leisure or going to bed. Evening clinics are still the exception but are sometimes offered. The value of artificial patterns of activity enforced by the rigidity of programme timetabling is questionable, e.g. does a patient regard getting undressed and dressed again in the middle of the afternoon as a meaningful activity (except, perhaps, in the context of obtaining therapy)?

PRACTICAL REQUIREMENTS

Practical requirements relate to the need for tools, materials and physical or sociocultural environmental factors. A full list of these requirements for occupational therapy would be extremely long, especially as different lists would be required for each specialty. However, it is perhaps useful to consider how far occupational therapy can be practised in the absence of appropriate environments, tools and materials?

Since the therapist's central concern is the patient's competence in practical, physical and social activities, there is a requirement for realistic situations, materials and environments with which to explore and practise these activities.

This may be achieved in numerous ways, e.g. in special facilities within an occupational therapy department or clinic, in the patient's own home or workplace or in the everyday environment. However, there is a trend, especially in community practice, for the therapist to be obliged to work from an office desk, with few other resources; it must be questioned how far it is possible for a therapist in such a situation to offer clients a sufficiently rich experience of activities to achieve all the purposes and processes of therapy.

PERFORMANCE DEMANDS

In order to perform any occupational process a combination of specific knowledge and skills, together with appropriate attitudes is required, and the participant must have the personal abilities and attributes be able to meet these demands.

A detailed analysis of the performance demands of occupational therapy would be lengthy, and research evidence is disparate and hard to coordinate into a total picture.

However, to encourage the debate and to stimulate further research, a brief and incomplete analysis is given below.

Personal attributes of participant

- physical and psychological health and stamina
- emotional stability
- well-integrated personality with good insight
- intelligence and broadly-based education
- good problem-analysing abilities
- creative, adaptive and lateral thinking
- highly developed communication and interpersonal skills.

Attitudes

1. Optimism and a positive expectation of being able to intervene to improve the situation of most individuals under most circumstances.

2. Valuing each individual as unique, and possessing potential, irrespective of any disadvantage, disability, or other adverse circumstance.

3. Providing an equal and non-discriminatory service to all individuals under all circumstances.

4. Seeking, through a partnership with the individual, to enable and empower her to participate actively in the processes of therapy to achieve goals which are desired by, and relevant to, that individual.

5. Valuing participation in activity as a means of promoting health and well-being.

6. Considering the experience of meaning in, and quality of, life to be essential, and viewing participation in activity as a means of achieving this.

7. Respecting, non-judgementally, the subjective nature of personal experiences, thoughts and wishes.

8. Valuing the provision of high quality, efficient and effective services, maintaining and seeking to improve standards of service delivery and practice within an ethical framework.

9. Valuing and retaining a lifelong commitment to personal and professional development.

10. Valuing colleagues, students and other health care workers, and actively seeking to share knowledge and contribute to their endeavours.

Knowledge

- theory, philosophy, values, ethics and principles of occupational therapy
- models of practice and frames of reference
- theories of problem analysis and clinical/ethical reasoning
- biological, social, psychological, medical sciences
- health promotion
- ergonomics and anthropometrics
- health and social policy and legal framework for practice
- case management process and techniques
- theory and practice of prescription of activities as therapy
- theory and practice of occupational analysis and adaptation
- theory and practice of environmental analysis and adaptation
- theory and practice of assessment and evaluation
- theory and practice of therapeutic use of self
- theory and techniques of resource management
- research techniques
- practical techniques: creative, craft, trade, technical, activities of daily living
- specialist techniques associated with: physical or psychological rehabilitation, physical, psychological or social development, education

Skills

The skills used by occupational therapists are at the highest level of integration and complexity (Allen's level 6 (Allen 1985)) and it is difficult to separate and analyse them.

The chief skill of a therapist is 'being a therapist' i.e. being able to carry out the numerous actions previously described in a competent, coordinated and effective manner. In addition, the therapist will gain expertise in a selection of skills appropriate to the area of practice.

To produce a detailed list of all these competencies would require a small book – as can be seen by looking at examples of occupational therapy curricula – and this is an exercise beyond the scope of this text. This complexity does, however, raise an important educational issue. How can competencies be assessed to ensure that the student is sufficiently proficient to practise? At what level should this be done? If each separate task were to be evaluated the list would become unmanageably long and the time required for training impractically extended.

Is it more necessary to know that a therapist can perform a quantity of specific actions and skills, or to know that he can pull together a complex array of knowledge and skills, and, through clinical reasoning, deliver appropriate therapy? The dilemma is that both are necessary; the student must demonstrate not only theoretical knowledge of what should be done, when, how and why, but also the skill of actually doing it, in a real situation with real stresses.

Once again, occupational therapy is not alone in having this problem, other practice-based professions have a similar difficulty. Given the pressure to condense and accelerate courses, educationalists will continue to be faced with challenging decisions about how best to ensure theoretical breadth, depth and practical competence.

10

The productive self

INTRODUCTION

There are many ways of describing the human condition. In Part 1 of this book, perspectives relevant to the core components of occupational therapy, the person, the occupation, the therapist and the environment have been explored.

Central to occupational therapy is a view of the individual engaging in roles, occupations and activities. Through activities the person expresses personal wishes, needs and abilities, maintains well-being, gains knowledge, experiences emotions and produces observable effects on the environment.

Models of occupational performance such as those constructed by Reed & Sanderson, Kielhofner or Cynkin & Robinson, all attempt to convey this understanding of the self as essentially *productive*.

These descriptions of human performance are not in themselves models of *occupational therapy*; they do not tell the therapist what treatment to give. They are models of the *occupational nature of humanity* which serve as a means of conceptualizing and organizing therapy by means of compatible models or frames of reference.

Originality is difficult to achieve in the construction of integrative models of this kind, for the basic concepts are derived from existing life sciences. Variations are due to the different 'packaging' and selection of the available information and its interpretation within the core philosophy and principles of occupational therapy.

It is probably inevitable that, having spent much time immersed in these principles, I have arrived at a personal construct which unites and interprets the information concerning the nature of human performance. I have named this model 'the productive self'. Although it is not greatly different from existing models in some respects, in others it includes concepts which have not previously been expressed in quite this form. For this reason the model is included so that it may, together with other models, aid in theory building.

The model is developmental in that it places importance on the interaction between the innate potential of the individual and his experiences, actions, and environment. It also draws strongly on cognitive and humanistic psychology. There are, however, elements of both analytical and physiological frames of reference. I see no incompatibility in this duality, for the individual is both a physical and a psychological being, part constrained and part able to choose, living partly in a tangible world, and partly in one composed of abstract images, symbols and dreams. Different frames of reference are needed to describe these differing aspects.

Note: To save repetition 'he' will be used to convey both he and she in the following text. As noted, the model draws on cognitive and developmental theory and is a synthesis of many ideas; it would become tedious to both author and reader if every possible source were to be cross-referenced, therefore only a few references to specific theorists will be included.

TWO WORLDS, TWO SELVES

Central to this model is the view that the self, by which I mean the elements which combine to give us our identity, is divisible into two areas, public self and private self, and that the environment is similarly divisible into the external environment and the internal environment. These environments have no direct connection, but are united by the person's activities and experiences within, and interpretations of, each area.

COMPOSITION OF THE MODEL

To gain a preliminary mental image of the model, think first of a set of shapes – circle, triangle, circle, square and circle – nesting one inside the other, like a Russion doll (Fig. 10.1).

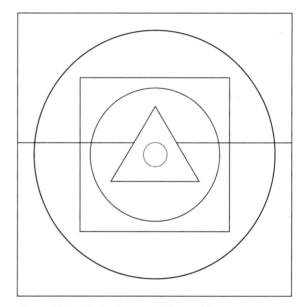

Figure 10.1 Basic structure of the model.

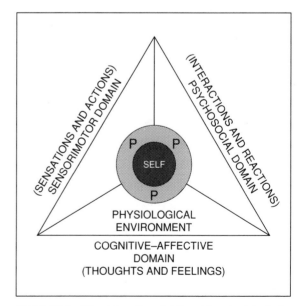

Figure 10.2 Three domains of skill and the physiological environment.

In the very centre of the set the small circle contains the inner core of the self, and a package of potential (P) with which a person is born. This in turn is surrounded by a triangle, the boundary of which indicates the three domains of skill: sensorimotor components (sensations and actions), psychosocial components (interactions and reactions) and cognitive–affective components (thoughts and feelings) (Fig. 10.2).

Within the triangle is the physiological environment. This is where physical reactions and demands are generated by the need to maintain homeostasis, and where the individual's sense of self as a physical being is located.

Now see this triangle surrounded by a circle (Fig. 10.3). This is the area of life space in which roles, occupations, activities and tasks are performed.

Surrounding this is a square, representing the resource area within the environment, the things, people, and knowledge which the individual uses when engaged in occupational performance. This area, although defined, is capable of gaining and losing content, and the boundary is therefore again shown with a broken line.

Finally, the larger circle represents the remainder of the known and unknown world. The circles are bisected by a line which divides both life space and environment into two sectors. This line represents the outer boundary of the body, the skin, which separates the inner and outer worlds from each other.

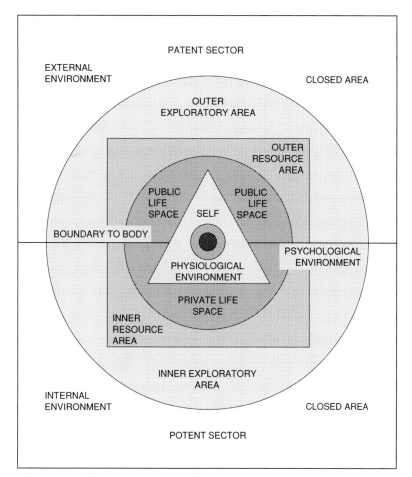

Figure 10.3 The internal and external environments.

The upper portion of this model is the patent sector, that which is open to view, where observable actions and interactions take place. The lower portion is the potent sector, of which only the individual can be aware – potent because it is the powerful source of intention and action. This is the realm of sensations, thoughts and feelings, and reactions to others.

These two 'worlds' are separate, but are united by the sensory receptors and processors in the body through which information must be received, passed inwards, perceived, coded, stored and processed, and by the motor effectors, by means of which actions can be taken in the outer world.

The external and internal environments

The content of the external environment is within the physical world. The internal environment has two parts, the physiological environment and the psychological environment. The latter is an abstract mental construct created by the individual. The environment in each sector is divided into three areas (Fig. 10.4).

The outer resource area is the known and familiar world inhabited by the individual containing the information and materials within his daily experience, which are required for occupational performance. The inner resource area is the personal storehouse of information and memories. The outer exploratory area represents the rest of the world, containing more remote, but potentially accessible resources. The inner exploratory area is equivalent to the subconscious. The outer closed area is the rest of the universe, and the inner closed area may be equated with the unconscious. Both these areas are inaccessible and their contents are unknown: they are therefore indicated outside the model.

Life space

Life space is the area indicated within the dotted circle (Fig. 10.3). The concept of life space, which is adapted from an idea originated by Lewin (1951), is complex, and needs some explanation. Although for convenience it has been drawn as a circle, it is really a dynamic and constantly

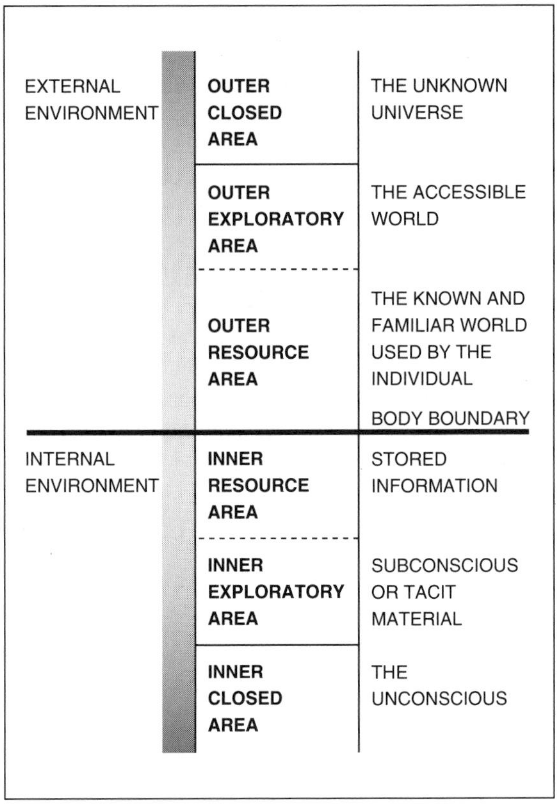

EXTERNAL ENVIRONMENT	OUTER CLOSED AREA	THE UNKNOWN UNIVERSE
	OUTER EXPLORATORY AREA	THE ACCESSIBLE WORLD
	OUTER RESOURCE AREA	THE KNOWN AND FAMILIAR WORLD USED BY THE INDIVIDUAL
		BODY BOUNDARY
INTERNAL ENVIRONMENT	INNER RESOURCE AREA	STORED INFORMATION
	INNER EXPLORATORY AREA	SUBCONSCIOUS OR TACIT MATERIAL
	INNER CLOSED AREA	THE UNCONSCIOUS

Figure 10.4 Divisions of the internal and external environments.

changing space which has no fixed physical form, since it exists only in the consciousness of the individual. It is defined by the extent to which the person is, at any moment, aware of portions of his physiological or psychological environment or of his external environment.

Private life space is the portion of the inner world to which the person is, for the moment, paying attention, and public life space is a similar area in the outer world. Although the person usually remains conscious of the existence of both life spaces, awareness is continually fluctuating, extending, narrowing, changing focus and switching from inner to outer environments. Life space is where the person is, at any one moment, living his life, thinking feeling, acting and interacting.

The person cannot be aware of elements which are, at that moment, outside his life space, nor can he ever be aware of the totality of these environments and, indeed, he needs to protect himself from the enormity of such awareness by focusing his attention within a defined area.

Life space might also be conceptualized as a 'balloon' surrounding each part of the self. Imagine that each part of the self is able to swing like a pendulum through the internal or external environment, thus moving life space with it into and out of the available areas. Alternatively, think of the self sitting within life space and pulling into it, or pushing out of it things wanted or unwanted. Neither of these similes is exact, for the process I am trying to describe is much more complex; but for the moment some notion of self and life space changing shape and focus within accessible inner or outer space will

suffice. It is always difficult to represent a dynamic concept within the confines of a two-dimensional diagram.

Box 10.1 The self		
Portion of self	*Component of self*	*Environment*
Public self	Known to others but not to self	External environment
	Known to self and others	
Private self	Known to self, unknown to others	Internal environment
	Unknown to self or others	

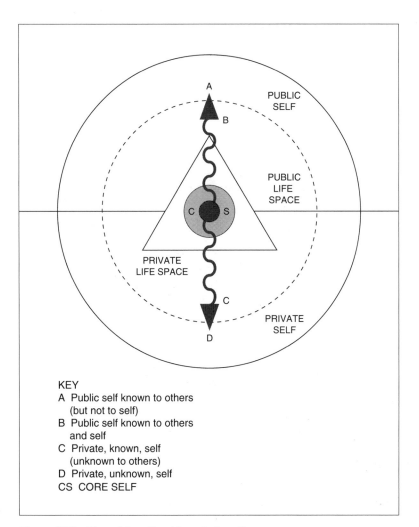

KEY
A Public self known to others (but not to self)
B Public self known to others and self
C Private, known, self (unknown to others)
D Private, unknown, self
CS CORE SELF

Figure 10.5   The public self and the private self.

The public self and the private self

The self can be described as having four components which exist in these interdependent but separate environments, and which are, to differing degrees, known to the individual or to others (Box 10.1) (Johari window, Hargie 1994).

The public self and the private self can be depicted as small arrows extending outwards into life space in the external and internal environments respectively. In each case the outer tip extends into an area of which the individual is unaware, so portions of the self remain unknown (Fig. 10.5). The central core of the self remains aware of both parts of the self, as a composite total identity, and may sometimes act consciously to keep the elements of the self in balance; however, rather as life space changes focus, so does central consciousness of the public or private self.

Any overwhelming event within a part of the environment – pain within the physiological environment, a strong emotion in the psychological environment, some stress or threat in the external environment – can temporarily monopolize attention and may have long-lasting effects on the central perception of identity.

Application to occupational therapy

For the occupational therapist, the essential feature of this view of the person and environment as divisible into these two parts, is that the only means of communication between the two worlds which the individual inhabits, is action which is initiated by the private self in private life space, using cognitive–affective skills, and is actualized by the public self in public life space using sensorimotor and psychosocial skills.

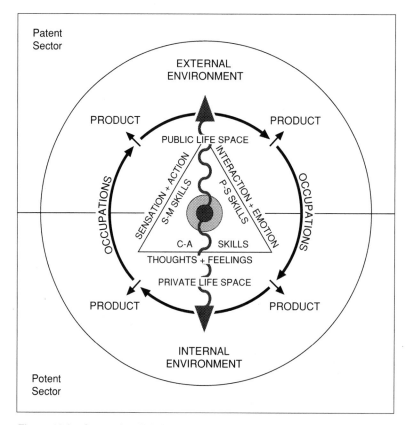

Figure 10.6 Occupations link the potent and patent sectors.

Thus occupations are the means of linking the 'inner' and 'outer' worlds. Since the private self is, by definition, invisible to others, it is made manifest only in the person's external actions. Equally, the results (products) of actions and experiences in the outer world, in public life space, are the only means which the person has of understanding or influencing his external environment or of gaining understanding of himself, as reflected by his actions within it and his interactions with others.

Occupations are represented by the circling arrows at the interface between life space and the environment (Fig. 10.6). If this interface is magnified it can be seen to consist of the hierarchy of tasks, activities and occupations as described in Ch. 5 (Fig. 10.7). The relationship between levels is not precisely linear, however, since the elements of the hierarchy have differing relationships and functions within the passage of time.

Put simply, therefore, occupations bridge the gap between public life space and private life space, between the inner and outer words. For this reason, occupations can be used as therapy.

SUMMARY OF THE MODEL

The introduction of a number of new concepts simultaneously can be indigestible, so it may be helpful to summarize the material which has been presented so far.

To return to the original image of shapes nesting inside each other like a Russian doll, the model of the productive self can be presented in simplified form as shown in Figure 10.8. The person exists within an external environment, and also within an internal physiological environment and a psychological environment which he constructs within his mind. He develops a personal identify or selfhood, which has public and private aspects.

The self is born with potential and develops skills, which are combined within life space using material from the resource areas, in order to perform activities which result in some

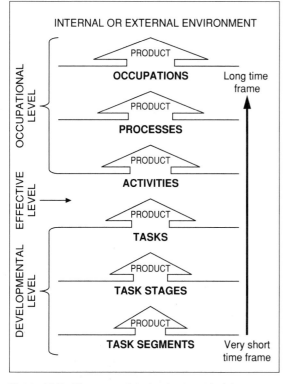

Figure 10.7   The occupations/environment interface.

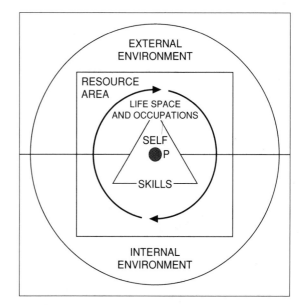

Figure 10.8   Simplifed version of the model.

change to an aspect of objective reality, or the nature of subjective experience, in other words, a product.

The whole model is shown in Figure 10.9. The concepts will now be presented in more detail.

THE POTENT SECTOR

THE PRIVATE SELF

The private self is composed of a person's conscious awareness of his mind and body. It contains his sensations, inner thoughts, ideas, dreams, memories, emotions, attitudes and values. It contains his beliefs about his own capabilities and his power to make choices and to take effective action. It includes his concepts of other people and of the external world insofar as they relate to his identity, and his ideas about what others may think of him.

The private self is not accessible to others. We may try to communicate, but we are each locked into our own being, and however close we may come to another individual, ultimately we are unable fully to express that experience.

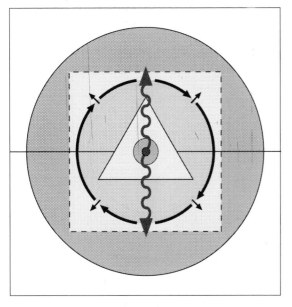

Figure 10.9 The productive self.

The private self is known to the individual only in part. Some individuals have very well-developed insight and can understand and honestly acknowledge much of the private self, others may have very poorly-developed concepts or strong defence mechanisms which mean that much of the inner self is unknown.

A portion of this unknown self may be seen as protruding into the deeper layers of the psychological environment into which, as will be explained, the individual has only partial access.

The privare self is the powerhouse which generates the individual's goals, purposes, actions and interactions, which are then expressed in the real world. It is continually modified by the outcomes of these productive actions and interactions and by the events which are experienced in the outer world. Reciprocally, events within private life space, e.g. an emotional crisis or a strong desire or powerful idea, will influence what happens in the world outside.

THE INTERNAL ENVIRONMENT

This is a mental construct, a personal world, derived partly from our perceptions and interpretations of internal and external reality, and partly from the inner landscape of thoughts, memories, dreams and desires. As will be described, it has depths and layers.

Boundaries between the 'real' and 'unreal' elements in the internal environment are often blurred, and the content of this environment is far more unstable and changeable than that of the external world.

The physiological environment

The individual has a biological identity, composed of an awareness of his body shape and mass together with an incomplete understanding of what he looks like 'on the surface'. His package of genetic potential endows him with various skills in varying proportions. His perceptual and spatial sensations locate his body and being in time and space.

Most of the mechanisms which maintain homeostasis in the basic systems, and react to stressors, are automatic and unconscious. For the most part, awareness of them intrudes only as a feeling of well-being when things are in balance, and a feeling of discomfort or ill-health when they are not.

However, the awareness of basic physiological survival need does intrude intermittently, and demands attention in direct proportion to the strength of the need. Hunger, thirst, avoidance of pain and need for sexual release all produce responses in the form of activities designed to satisfy these needs or, in some circumstances, to divert the mind from the need to satisfy them.

Physical illness, trauma or the more insidious effects of physiological stress, are experienced by the private self and resonate deep into the layers of the psychological environment.

The psychological environment

The content of the psychological environment is subjective and abstract. The individual commences construction of it from the moment of birth, or perhaps even earlier. It reflects both events and experiences in the 'real' world, and those which are purely internal and which have not nor, in some cases, ever could, exist in the external environment.

Because material in this environment is abstract it is hard for the individual to become aware of it. Material may take many forms, e.g. words, numbers, colours, symbols, images, pictures; feelings; remembered sensations; memories of real people, things or events; or constructs of imaginary images and fantasies. This environment also contains images of the past and of future events, both of which can exist only in the inner experience of the individual.

The psychological environment can be visualized as having three layers, the resource area, the exploratory area and the closed area. This should not be taken too literally; it is merely a simplified model of what is probably a subtle gradation in accessibility. It mirrors the layers of the external environment.

The inner resource area and private life space

The inner resource area contains the individual's store of accessible memories, concepts, attitudes, values, feelings, associations, information, knowledge and patterns for the organizations and use of skill. The person can mentally bring parts of this store into his private life space so that he can 'walk around' in this store, examining the contents at will, and selecting what to use.

As with any tangible 'storecupboard' in the outer world, effective organization of this storage area and of the mechanisms for retrieval are essential for effective performance of activities within private life space.

It is necessary also to acquire the skill of excluding unwanted material which might distract from the task in hand; both inner and outer life space are subject to invasions from the environment, inner or outer, which change their focus and distract from the task in hand.

Private life space is the area to which the person is currently paying attention and in which tasks or activities may be performed.

In a well-ordered mind, material from the resource area can be shifted in and out of life space at will. Material such as previous learning, a memory, the location of a thing or place, a feeling about a person, or a visualization of a person or object, can be brought into focus, while unwanted material can be re-stored or rejected. No matter how well-organized people are, however, few can maintain a totally ordered private life space and resource area, or do so for extended periods, for the nature of the psychological environment is intensely subjective, fluid and unstructured, and follows a logic different from that in the physical world.

The concept that activities can be performed in private life space is important. In this inner space the individual experiences conscious identity and thinks, plans, dreams, meditates, prays, manipulates ideas, experiences emotions and conducts the activities of the inner life. These activities are often pre-occupational, both in the sense of being necessary precursors to action, and in the sense of engaging attention within private life space and excluding awareness of much that is happening in the outer world. Such activities may be related to work, to recreation or play, or to self-care in the form of 'mental housework' to maintain the self.

Products within private life space are necessarily abstract, but include ideas, plans, inventions, calculations, sentences, poems, decisions, feelings and creative design processes. However, none of this inner 'work' (or play) can have significant external effect unless transferred into public life space to be actioned.

Conscious activities within private life space require the use of skills within the domains of sensation, thought and feeling, and reaction to others. Skill components within these domains have to be developed as the individual matures. It is by means of these skills that the products of the inner world can be translated into actions through sensorimotor and psychomotor skills in public life space.

Just as one can, through the automated processes of the body, continue to perform actions of which one is unaware, so one can within the resource area, but outside the conscious focus of life space, the mind may continue to 'do work' of which the private self is not conscious at the time. (Personal experience suggests that much planning, problem-solving and creativity operates in this way).

The inner exploratory area

This includes repressed and suppressed material, dreams, symbols and buried memories. It may also contain material which can be released to trigger creativity.

The desire to journey into this 'inner space' has led to the development of meditative, contemplative and transcendental techniques, and to the use (and misuse) of substances which may 'open the gates' to this layer.

Voyaging into inner space is difficult, but may provide insight concerning personal abilities and the dynamics of personal behaviour and relationships. However, these are dangerous waters, for some of the material is there because the individual does not wish to be confronted with it.

Intrusion of unwanted material from this area into private life space can be very stressful and may lead to anxieties, guilt, and doubts about self-worth. It can also, as it were, bulge against the walls of private life space, causing an internal pressure which results in discomfort, although the cause is unknown.

The inner closed area

In analytical terms, the unconscious is inaccessible to the individual. It contains memories which are buried too deeply to recall, and the deepest cupboards in which our most gruesome skeletons are locked. It may perhaps contain the 'shadow self' – the areas of personal identity unknown to the self or others, and those which the person is unable to accept and acknowledge. Like its equivalent in the external world, the person may be vaguely aware that the area exists, but can only speculate on the content.

Material may sometimes be released from this area by some internal or external trigger to filter back into the exploratory area, causing discomfort as described earlier. On rare occasions where material from this buried layer erupts suddenly into consciousness the results can be explosive, although this may result in either positive or negative outcomes.

THE PATENT SECTOR

THE PUBLIC SELF

The visible part of the individual within the external environment is the public self. This is made up of the external appearance of the physical body and its apparent personality, roles, actions and reactions. It is both how the individual appears and how he chooses to appear. A portion of this self protrudes into the area outside life space so that the person is unaware of it, but so that others may observe it.

The self is contained within the skin, the envelope of the physical body, which can be indicated on the model by the thick line dividing the potent and patent sectors (see Fig. 10.6), and this is the area which can most readily be damaged by some intrusion from the external environment – be it by accident, virus, or the surgeon's knife.

It is the 'tip of the triangle', the active and interactive portions of the body which can be seen by others. People interact when their public selves come close to each other and their public life spaces overlap. One may be physically near someone, yet not include him in one's life space; at that moment he does not, for you, exist. Interaction does not, however, require physical proximity, simply a conjunction of life spaces, as might be the case down a telephone line. Close relationships develop as increasingly intense awareness of public selves, sharing of life space, and disclosures concerning private selves occur.

Public self mirrors aspects of the private self, but the degree of congruence is variable, both from one situation to another in the same individual, and between individuals. Some people are able to adapt to and accept many roles, others are more rigid. Where large gaps develop between public self and private self the individual is liable to become dysfunctional.

PUBLIC LIFE SPACE

Public life space is the individual's area of operation within the external environment at any given moment, as effected by sensorimotor or psychosocial skills. It contains only those people, objects, tools, materials or sensory information of which the person is currently aware. It is these factors which generate the external demand for occupational engagement.

As with private life space, the focus of awareness can shift from moment to moment to expand or contract the area attended to, and to include or exclude items. When too much material is pushed into life space than can comfortably be dealt with or attended to, the individual experiences stress. A life space which is barren and featureless is equally stressful.

THE EXTERNAL ENVIRONMENT

This contains the elements of the physical world which are relatively permanent and stable and which can be studied objectively. The degree of objectivity may be subject to philosophical debate, but that is not the issue here. Even accepting that the experience of the external world is individual and in that sense subjective, its subjectivity is of a very different nature to that which affects experiences of the internal environment.

The characteristics of things which can be touched, heard, seen and tasted do not normally alter impetuously or unpredictably. The experience of one person can be compared with that of another and, under normal circumstances, will be very similar. The physical world appears to obey rules; scientific laws can be formulated. The external environment is experienced exclusively in the present.

The outer resource area

The resource area is the known and familiar world inhabited by the individual. It contains all the people, places and objects he commonly relates to, encounters and uses. These are not all, at any one time, within his public life space, but can be brought within it at will.

The individual may expand and contract his attention to include more or less of this resource area and is able physically to move around within it. He may scan a table top for a needed tool, move from area to area within a room, walk from room to room, or travel to the shops or to work.

The richness of the resources in this area is relevant developmentally, occupationally, socially and educationally. An impoverished resource area limits occupational scope and in severe cases may restrict the development of skills within all three domains.

The outer exploratory area

The outer exploratory area is the world beyond the known and familiar. It is far larger than any one individual is able to know well. Parts of this area can quite easily be reached, e.g. travel in one's own country or holidays abroad. Other parts are relatively inaccessible and are unlikely to be reached except by a minority, e.g. the Amazon rainforest or the peak of Everest.

The individual can choose to bring some part of this unknown territory into his life space, both by actually entering it and vicariously, by reading about or viewing the adventures of others. Given the human desire for adventure, delight in novelty and fascination with the unknown, this uncharted but accessible territory is very important both symbolically and as a resource.

Humankind seems to possess the urge to push the boundaries of this area as far as possible into the inaccessible; why else do we climb mountains, reach for the moon, or attempt to number and name the infinitesimal building blocks of the universe? It is tempting to see this journeying as a metaphor or symbol of the equally difficult but rewarding inner exploration, and it is interesting that lone explorers frequently mention that such insights result from their experiences.

The outer closed area

The outer closed area of the external environment is the solar system and universe. This may be partially perceived, but is incompletely understood and can never be fully known, however far the boundaries of human exploration are extended.

OCCUPATIONS AND THE PRODUCTIVE SELF

Occupations have already been described as bridging the gap between the inner and outer worlds which the individual inhabits. The simplest way to explain this is by using a developmental model.

When an individual is born he is a small package of potentials whose awareness of the inner environment is low and of the external environment is even more limited. The resource area is almost non-existent; the exploratory area is restricted to immediate surroundings or strong internal sensations or emotions. The rest of the inner and outer world is closed and unknown.

As maturation and development takes place the person identifies the boundaries of his physiological environment and acquires skills – cognitive and affective, sensorimotor and psychosocial – through which both inner and outer environments can be explored.

To begin with he must distinguish between the things which comprise the self and things which do not, between physical sensations and emotions, and between the realities of the inner life space and the outer life space. For a child this is difficult: both worlds seem very real; inner dreams and fantasies are as powerful as, or often more powerful than, experiences in the external environment.

Gradually the infant builds and extends his inner and outer resource areas, learns to differentiate between them and finds names for the things which they contain. Through this exploration he develops the ability to concentrate on and attend to things of interest to him, and to integrate his public and private life spaces, and begins to develop a sense of public self and private self.

He finds that by using all his skills he can exert influence and control on the outer world, and through this process he can make his desires, which are at first merely abstractions in his inner world, real. To begin with he strives only to be comfortable, to get what he wants when he wants it. Then he discovers that he can find pleasure in manipulating and exploring objects; simultaneously he discovers the frustration of finding that he cannot master and control all the elements in his world. Nonetheless, there are areas where control is possible and where skills have effects. He begins to perform simple task segments, task stages and finally tasks; he has begun to be productive.

As the child's repertoire of knowledge, skill, and attitudes expands, so does the size of the inner and outer resource areas. Other people's life spaces coincide with his, sometimes pleasantly and sometimes painfully. Tasks lead to routines; routines build up to activities, activities chain to form processes. Finally, a rich repertoire of roles and occupations is developed as the individual leaves childhood and becomes an adult.

The components of occupations are stored within the inner and outer resource areas, waiting to be used. In the inner resource area lie the memories of what is learned and experienced, patterns and sequences of skill, feelings about what is done, and images of the self as a competent or incompetent performer of each occupation. In the outer resource area, the individual has access to the tools, materials, people or other things or circumstances which are needed to perform the occupation.

The trigger for occupational engagement is some kind of event in either the internal or external environment. The person may decide that something is to be done, move his private life space into the appropriate part of the inner resource area and make the preliminary plans or decisions. He can then shift the focus into his public life space, find what is required and perform the activity.

Alternatively, something may intrude into his public life space which makes him aware that action is needed; he will then find the necessary information in the inner resource area and respond appropriately. If necessary this reaction may be very fast, using reflex pathways without conscious thought, as in the case of actions to avoid dangers and ensure survival.

LEVELS OF MEANING

Within this model the concept of balance does not relate to work, leisure and self-care, but to a harmony between utility and meaning in the life of the individual.

The person must be able to do, or to have done, what is necessary, but also needs to do that which has meaning and brings fulfilment. Perceptions of meaning are intensely personal; it does not matter what others may think, the individual's subjective experience of meaning, or lack of meaning, in his life is the only criterion.

Meaning is derived from a complex of cognitive–affective attributes, memories, experiences, rewards, successes and other positive factors which confirm and validate personal experience of efficacy and selfhood.

The degree to which an individual can describe engagement in meaningful, fulfilling activities is an index of 'occupational health'. The richer the pattern the better, but a little meaning can go a long way to counterbalance the effects of an otherwise restricted or mundane life. Lack of meaning is both a symptom and a cause of dysfunction.

At the proto-occupational level, tasks and routines are often value-neutral and bring only low-level satisfaction; this may be at a simple, almost physiological level, e.g. a pleasant taste or sound, a comforting hug, avoidance of discomfort, or may be the cognitive satisfaction of task completion, i.e. a job done, so that something more interesting or personally important can be tackled.

Meaning is more readily found at the effective level, through engagement in activities which are part of valued occupations or roles which give shape to a person's life.

It is therefore highly important to identify the areas of meaning within a person's life, and to give priority to enabling participation in these activities to continue, or, where this is impossible, to enable the person to find an alternative.

THE PRODUCTIVE SELF AND THE NATURE OF DYSFUNCTION

Given this model of the person, it becomes possible to describe occupational dysfunction within the terms and structure of the model. It soon becomes apparent why it is so difficult to unravel dysfunction; there are so many places where things may break down.

Potential

Most people are born with far more potential than is ever likely to be used. This means that there is 'spare capacity' which may help the individual to adapt to adverse circumstances.

A person may be born with the disadvantage

of having very little potential, or may become damaged in such a way that potential is reduced. Lost or missing potential cannot be regained. The smaller the quantity of potential which is there to begin with, the less it will be possible for adaptation to occur.

Physiological environment

Many stressors may upset the delicate balance of homeostasis with consequent effects on physical or psychological function. Stressors may be internal, and relatively minor, e.g. high blood pressure, slight pain or unpleasant thoughts, or more extreme, e.g. poisoning, infection, injury or surgical intervention. External stressors include heat, cold, loud noises or lack of oxygen.

Severe damage to the body changes the size and shape of the physiological environment with consequent effects on the person's perceptions of his physical self, and on his inner sense of well-being. Such damage may also remove the potential for skill.

Skills

The three domains of skill must be developed through experience and coordinated to produce smooth performance. This process may break down in many ways: a skill area may be undeveloped, skills may be lost or skill coordination may be poor. Internal or external environmental conditions may limit skill use or development.

The resource areas

The outer resource area provides the necessities for productivity; if these are unavailable activities cannot be performed.

The inner 'storecupboard' must be well-stocked if it is to be useful. Material is generated within the inner resource area through the use of cognitive and affective skills, and transferred into it from the external resource area via sensorimotor and psychosocial skills.

Material may not be generated, may not be useful, may be badly stored, or may not be stored at all. The person cannot use what he does not possess, or is unaware of having. Retrieval systems may break down. Other material from, or events in, the psychological or external environments may affect this process.

Occupational repertoire

The developmental process of skill acquisition and performance of tasks, activities, occupations and roles may be disrupted in many ways. The store of occupational performance may be inadequate, due to poor learning, faulty storage or lack of opportunity for practice. External resources may be insufficient. The ability to initiate actions in either private or public life space may be faulty or absent. Motivation may be affected by numerous factors in both the patent and potent sectors, but especially by perceptions of the self as a competent actor in the external environment.

Exploratory areas

All material in the resource area was once in the exploratory area. The person has to find what is needed and transfer it into the resource area. If the person is unable to explore, the area explored does not contain what is needed, or for some reason the transfer into the resource area cannot be made, then performance will be affected.

The exploratory area also contains stresses and dangers, e.g. an accident, toxin, or other inhabitant of the external area, or a highly stressful thought or emotion from the inner area. These may damage the person.

Life space

The person may be unable to construct his life space and to move it freely around the resource areas as required. He may find it impossible to focus, or to exclude unwanted and intrusive material. He may equally exclude material which would be useful and will therefore be unable to perform well. Anything that is not found within life space cannot be attended to, therefore learning may be poor.

The self

Problems affecting the self lie at the root of much dysfunction. Examples include:

- Failure to develop self concept.
- Lack of insight into public or private self: the area of known self is small.
- Lack of congruence between public and private self; tension is developed between the actions of each part of the self.
- Mistaken beliefs about the way others see one's public or private self.
- Mistaken beliefs about the ability or lack of ability to exercise control on the external environment.
- Withdrawal into the inner world; or attempt to retreat from it into the external environment by being over-busy in the public life space.
- Confusion of material from the inner environment with that from the outer environment (or the reverse).
- Fear of allowing the self to venture into the exploratory areas.
- Damage to self by some person or thing in the external environment.

These examples should be sufficient to indicate the applicability of the model, but there are many more interpretations.

APPLICABILITY OF APPROACHES WITHIN THE MODEL

Within the problem-based process of case management the therapist may use this model to identify the likely origin of dysfunction. The model does not suggest what action should be taken but it does help to direct the therapist towards appropriate approaches and processes. Although any voluntary action must involve the operation of all domains and both sectors, some approaches are more relevant to the potent sector, and some apply mainly to the patent sector.

Central to this process of problem identification is the analysis of which skills need to be developed, gained, regained or adapted, which occupational level dysfunction is located in, and performance demands and environmental demands in relationship to individual potential and skill.

The therapist cannot affect the internal environment directly; in order to do so she must operate within the external environment, bringing herself and her own life space within the patient's public life space, and affecting the content of his resource area and his actions within it. She may enable him to become aware of material in his exploratory areas both internal and external by means of exploratory activities. Through actions and interactions within the public life space which she temporarily shares with the patient, he may be empowered to act and explore in ways he was previously unable to manage. By enriching or enhancing the content of the resource areas, performance may be enabled.

Skills which are observable within the hidden domains of sensation, thought and feeling, as well as in the domains of action and interaction, can be developed, and the repertoire of occupations within the inner resource area can be enlarged.

By noting changes in the public self and the actions and reactions within the patent sector, the therapist may be able to infer the changes and events within the invisible potent sector.

The central premise of occupational therapy is its ability to affect the operations of the potent sector, by means of productive actions within the patent sector, utilizing the integrative nature of performance to achieve this.

The approaches that can be used within the model are illustrated in Table 10.1.

The inclusion of both holistic and reductionist approaches is not incompatible because these are not used simultaneously but as options and as relevant to the domain of concern. Where all domains are involved, the more holistic approaches become more relevant.

BODY, MIND AND SPIRIT: PHILOSOPHICAL IMPLICATIONS

The philosophical debate over whether body and mind are the same thing or separate entities

Table 10.1 Use of approaches within the model

Area of problem	Approach	Occupational level
Patent sector		
Outer resource area	Environmental analysis and adaptation	All
	Occupational analysis and adaptation	All
Sensorimotor domain	Biomechanical approach	Effective/developmental
	Neurodevelopmental approaches	Developmental
	Sensory integration	Developmental
	Behavioural approaches	Developmental
	Educational approaches	All
	Rehabilitative approaches	Effective
	Adaptive approaches	All
Psychosocial domain	Behavioural approaches	Developmental
	Interactive approaches	Effective
	Humanistic approaches	All
	Educational approaches	All
	Rehabilitative approaches	Effective
	Developmental approaches	Developmental
	Adaptive approaches	All
Potent sector		
Inner resource area	Education	All
Cognitive–affective domain	Cognitive–behavioural approaches	Developmental
	Cognitive–perceptual approaches	Developmental
	Cognitive–developmental approaches	Effective/developmental
	Cognitive–affective approaches	Effective/developmental
	Humanistic approaches	All
	Psychotherapeutic approaches	Effective
	Analytical approaches	Effective
	Developmental approaches	Developmental
	Educational approaches	All
	Rehabilitative approaches	Effective
	Adaptive approaches	All

is interesting but insoluble. From the point of view of occupational performance, mind and body may both have their own role but must operate in an integrated manner.

The model is existential in that it emphasizes the importance of consciousness, choice and purpose, and of awareness of both inner and outer worlds and the operations carried out within them.

Human experience is intensely subjective, whether the self explores the abstract landscape of the inner world, or travels bodily through the tangible external environment. The fact that my own inner world can never be entered by anyone else does not diminish my sense of its reality. Although I have no means of proving that this experience is the same for other people, I cannot personally accept that it is possible to

provide therapy on the basis of the external, observable features of behaviour alone. This is not to dismiss behaviourism, it is simply one approach, of limited application within the patent sector, and related to learning of skills and task stages at proto-occupational level.

The protective envelope of the body contains the internal environment and provides the visible part of the person's public self. In physiological terms, health is the maintenance of homeostasis which enables all aspects of body and mind to function in harmony. The internal environment is a product of both body and mind and is affected by the health of both. Personal identity is developed by interaction of body and mind, through the activities of the self, within the external and internal environments.

The self is central to the model, since a

person's sense of individual identity is central to his experience of life. The search for self, for self-actualization and for the integration of all aspects of self into a balanced whole has been the focus of much recent philosophical thought. However, many religions have expressed the need to *lose* the sense of self.

It is a paradox of human experience that joyfully losing the sense of self in a greater whole, in a state where knowing, feeling, doing and being are as one, is felt to be a momentous experience. Historically, this has been achieved by two routes; through submersion of the self in *action*, e.g. the experience of flow during a creative activity, through disciplined routine, ritual, extreme physical effort, or during sex, and through submersion of the self in *inaction*, via trance, meditation and other mental or physical disciplines such as some forms of yoga.

If the occupational therapist is to be at all concerned with this need to lose the sense of self – and that is debatable – it must be through the medium of action, of losing the self in activity. The journey into the depths of quiet inner space, where identity is relinquished however important, is not within the scope of the occupational therapist.

What then, of the spirit? It is not necessary to include such a concept within the model; it can function quite well in an atheistic or humanistic version of the human condition, although if a spiritual dimension exists within the mind of the client, it should not be dismissed or ignored. If, however, a person is to be given a soul, or is to acknowledge a deity, I must leave it to the discretion of the reader to discern where, within the model, these may be located.

Most religions have some concept of the soul being *inside*, within the potent sector, and of the deity being either *outside*, in the patent sector, or in some way present in both sectors. If pressed, I would prefer to include the soul as a kind of attribute, manifestation or energizing force within the central core of the self, perhaps a part of potential. However, the question of whether the soul acquires or produces personal identity, or whether it is something different is beyond the scope of this text.

PART 2

Processes

11

Case management

THE CASE MANAGEMENT PROCESS

Effective use of the case management process is the key to effective therapy, and a thorough understanding of it is essential. The process is problem-based and problem analysis occurs at various stages. Clinical reasoning takes place throughout, as judgements are made continually concerning the relevance of information, consequent conclusions, decisions and actions. It is these latter processes which make the generic process of case management applicable to each individual. Although these processes are distinct, they are so closely integrated that they need to be described together.

Various writers include different stages in the case management process. For simplicity the process can be viewed as starting with referral, leading on to intervention and ending with discharge. The process of intervention can be compressed into four stages which can be repeated as a cycle until the outcome is satisfactory or no further action is possible. Each stage is linked by exploration, discovery and action (indicated by the arrows) by means of which the therapist and client, through the structure of the process, form a partnership to direct, drive and implement therapy or intervention (Fig. 11.1).

The other five processes: assessment and evaluation, occupational analysis and adaptation, environmental analysis and adaptation, therapeutic self and resource management are drawn into use during intervention, and are coordinated

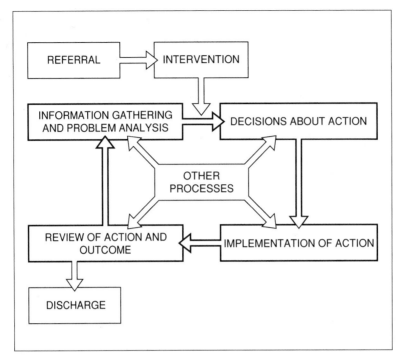

Figure 11.1 The case management process.

and organized by the overall process of case management.

The structure and sequence of the process is no more than a skeleton on which to hang the 'muscles and nerves' of therapy. It is an asset to the therapist as it assists him to order thoughts and actions. In order to understand how the case management process 'drives' therapy or intervention it is necessary to understand how clinical reasoning, problem-analysis and problem-solving take place.

The cognitive processing of the therapist is the key to effective therapy, although the patient must be included. It is the means whereby the therapist makes sense of the case for himself, in the light of what the patient and others contribute, and of his own objective observations, and it helps the patient to collaborate in the development of that shared understanding, and the consequent decisions and actions.

Clinical reasoning, in all its forms, is a core process, because *only* an occupational therapist can *think* like an occupational therapist.

REASONING

Reasoning is the cognitive process whereby conclusions can be reached on the basis of information available. There are logical rules by which deductive reasoning can take place on an 'if so, then this follows' basis. Other rules can be used in inductive reasoning where probabilities are weighed up in order to reach a likely answer.

The problem with these reasoning processes is that, unless we have trained as logicians, we are not accustomed to using the rules consciously and critically. Cognitive processes develop, more or less effectively, as a child learns and experiments with living. While all humans use similar basic cognitive strategies, each individual develops idiosyncratic patterns and 'rules of thumb' based on experience.

For example, when trying to make sense of other people and situations, we tend to use mental short-cuts known as heuristics. A heuristic is a strategy that can be applied to a number of problems which usually, but not always, yield a correct solution (Atkinson et al 1993). Therapists use several of these heuristics in clinical reasoning, as will be explained. Unfortunately, human mental processing is also subject to a number of errors, fallacies and biases of which we tend to be unaware. Some of these will be described in the following section.

An awareness of these mental mechanisms and potential biases can greatly improve the quality of clinical reasoning. Readers who have not recently read books on cognitive psychology and social psychology are recommended to do so, as many new findings concerning cognition and information processing can improve understanding of the reasoning process. Schwartz (1991), for example, describes the, still controversial, view of multiple intelligences in relation to occupational therapy reasoning, and suggests that the therapist must learn and practise many modes of reasoning, including logic, scientific analysis and also more phenomenological modes.

CLINICAL REASONING

Clinical reasoning has been mentioned in Chapter 6. The term has become an accepted shorthand for a complex set of cognitive processes. It has been called 'explicating complexity' and 'how therapists put the science and art of practice together' (Cohn 1991). Each time a new patient or client presents for therapy, the therapist must begin anew to develop a therapeutic relationship, to understand the unique features of the case, to relate it to similar cases and to design a course of action. But how is this done? We are only just beginning to understand the process, and to realize how essential it is that we should appreciate its elegance and learn to use it more effectively.

Research and literature

Burke & DePoy (1991) express the issue succinctly:

An understanding of the clinical reasoning process may reveal the unique ways that occupational therapists come to assess and seek solutions to patients' problems and to delimit the scope of their practice to what is uniquely occupational therapy. Clinical reasoning addresses many of the unstated thoughts and formulations that therapists develop when they work with patients.

The key words in this passage are 'unique' and 'unstated', for they encapsulate our professional dilemma. How can we express, to ourselves or others, the unique nature of our cognitive processing, when the processing is not only unstated, but frequently occurs so rapidly that it appears intuitive. The therapist thinks, judges and acts, but cannot readily explain how these judgements and decisions were reached.

Occupational therapists are not alone in this problem; Schon (1983) states that:

Professionals have been disturbed to find that they cannot account for the processes which they have come to see as central to professional competence. It is difficult for them to imagine how to describe and teach what might be meant by making sense of uncertainty, performing artistically, setting problems, and choosing among competing professional paradigms, when these processes seem mysterious in the light of the prevailing model of professional knowledge.

He adds that:

In some professions, awareness of uncertainty, complexity, instability, uniqueness and value conflict has led to the emergence of professional pluralism. Competing views of professional practice – competing images of the professional role, the central values of the profession and the relevant knowledge and skills – have come into good currency.

These words were not written specifically for occupational therapists, but their relevance is clear. It may be comforting to know that we are not alone – at least it removes one cause of professional anxiety – but it does not remove the obligation to do something about the situation.

Schell & Cervero (1993) 'found more than 23 articles in occupational therapy literature since 1982 that address some aspect of clinical reasoning'; 23 articles within a decade does not seem a very great amount, but the authors listed only articles of American origin. The topic may be of great importance, but it is certainly not an easy one to analyse.

Research has been conducted to see if it is possible to describe therapists' reasoning processes. This has been attempted by exploring the differences between various grades of practitioner, from novice to expert (Burke & DePoy 1991, Slater & Cohn 1991), and by investigating practice (Fleming 1991, Mattingly 1994). It is not surprising that those most interested in understanding the process are those who have to teach it, so several papers refer to clinical education.

Any therapist who acts as a supervisor to students will realize that there are differences in the ways in which first year students and final year students think, and between the reasoning of newly qualified and experienced therapists.

The study by Slater & Cohn (1991) explored these differences. They found that 'Novice clinicians focused primarily on objective findings, observable signs, and rules by which to make decisions. They focused on context-free elements, that is, the disease process, free from the context of the patients who have these diseases.' In other words, new students 'do it by the book', using the strategies of surface learning to find rules to help them to order facts and make decisions.

Advanced beginners 'recognized the presence and absence of behaviour but were not yet able to attach meaning to it'. They were still unable to determine priorities and did not yet see the entire picture. It takes time for students to develop and use strategies of deep learning which connect disparate information and provide comprehensive understanding of complex issues and relationships.

The competent practitioners 'saw the situation as a set of facts'. They could identify which facts and observations were relevant and 'could handle multiple patient care demands with a feeling of mastery'. However, 'they lacked the creativity and flexibility which characterized more experienced therapists' work'.

The proficient or experienced practitioners generated increasing numbers of hypotheses, even before meeting the patient, and were able to revise and adapt treatment plans. They 'perceived a situation as a whole ... had a sense of direction and a vision of where the patient should go, and were able to take steps towards that goal.' Significantly, the experienced therapist is able 'to think analytically by combining rules and guidelines to make decisions' and can modify plans and expectations as treatment progresses or as a situation changes. 'No deliberation occurs – it appears just to happen as the therapist draws from similar experiences that trigger plans which have worked in the past and may be re-applied to new situations.'

Experienced practitioners can 'think on their feet' and use what Schon refers to as 'reflecting in action', by which he means both 'knowing more than we can say' while engaged in action, and being able to re-shape the action while doing it, thus acting and thinking simultaneously.

This inability consciously to track the stages of the reasoning process, or to express tacit knowledge, is a difficulty which increases in direct proportion to the experience and competence of the practitioner, and forms a considerable barrier to the study of the reasoning process in action.

Mattingly (1991a) writes pithily that 'clinical reasoning is more that having a reason', and proceeds to state:

Much of the fluidity and ease that we associate with the competent, experienced professional is a result of knowledge that has become habitual and automatic, that is, the professional does not have to stop and think of what to do next.

To return to Cohn & Slater's study, expert practitioners appear to work intuitively, but 'Intuition is not irrational, unconscious or guesswork, but rather the product of situational involvement and recognition of similarity.' Experts are aware of rules, but are able to 'move beyond a rigid application of these guidelines based on an inner sense of knowing what to do next'. Burke & DePoy (1991) add to this picture the idea that 'Mastery and excellence seem to be linked by vision. For the master clinician, the internal vision of practice provides the motive for and goal of practice.'

These descriptions show the value of experience in building the therapist's mental 'database'. The more experienced therapist is able to seek similarities to past situations and solutions, and to adapt these for the current case, and, importantly is able to predict the direction that the case will take. He has a sound cognitive construct of occupational therapy and is able to visualize a possible sequence of events, or alternative sequences, ahead of time, and to make multiple hypotheses to explain the case. Ryan's research (1991) indicates the richness of the thinking of experienced practitioners.

These findings connect with the view of clinical reasoning which Fleming (1993) proposes. She describes several forms of reasoning which work together to make sense of the case.

Reasoning includes, but is not limited to, hypothetical reasoning, pattern recognition, intuitive reasoning, ethical reasoning, interactive reasoning, and procedural reasoning. Therapists use particular forms of reasoning to interpret and analyze various aspects of the whole problem complex . . . The profession's unique approach to treating patients, which therapists call *individualizing*, causes therapists to take the phenomenological perspective toward the patient, the clinical condition, and the patient's family and social context.

Mattingly (1991a) stresses the importance of narrative reasoning. 'Therapists think with stories in two distinct, but equally important ways – through storytelling and story creation. . . . therapists not only listen to the stories that their patients tell them, but also tell stories about their patients'. By this she means that the therapist can take the patient's story on into the future, or back into the past, and thereby gain understanding of the options and outcomes. She calls this process of creative thinking 'therapeutic employment'.

Schell & Cervero (1993) adopt narrative reasoning as one of three primary forms of reasoning used by therapists. 'Scientific reasoning implies a logical process based on hypothesis testing. Narrative reasoning reflects a phenomenological process in which stories are used to give meaning to therapeutic events.'

To these they add a third form, which they have called 'pragmatic reasoning'. This is based on the concept of *situated cognition* in which 'mental activities are inherently shaped by the situation: learning that occurs in one context is not necessarily transferable to another

context.' The authors speculate that this theory 'may explain concerns raised by educators and managers about the difficulty new therapists have in using school-based knowledge in the clinic', and conclude that 'it seems obvious that contextual factors that inhibit or facilitate therapy (e.g. hospital setting, patient population, departmental tradition) are themselves part of the clinical reasoning process.'

Rogers & Holm (1991) add the idea of 'diagnostic reasoning', i.e. the process whereby the occupational therapist produces 'a problem statement or a series of statements that describe the functional deficits towards which occupational therapy intervention is directed.' They explain that diagnostic reasoning encompasses problem-sensing and problem definition, and link it to the process of developing and testing hypotheses concerning the patient.

Several authors have added ethical reasoning to the list as an indispensable part of decision-making. In her wide-ranging and carefully crafted lecture, Rogers (1983) summarizes her view of professional practice as follows:

Without science, clinical enquiry is not systematic; without ethics, it is not responsible; without art, it is not convincing. The intentions and potentials of chronically disabled patients are difficult to discern, but a therapist of understanding will elicit them, and use them to help patients discover health within themselves.

It is surely not news that human thinking is a complex process. We should not therefore be surprised to discover that clinical reasoning, which is both science and art, is also complex and multifaceted.

Role of the therapist

Exploration of the process of reasoning has to take account of the fact that, as therapists, we appear not only to think in different modes, but even to switch between these modes with great rapidity, or worse, at times to operate in more than one mode simultaneously.

There is also, and this is a theme running throughout the practice of occupational therapy, a tension between 'analytical–quantitative–scientific–medical model' thinking, and 'intuitive–creative–qualitative–phenomenological' thinking. The former takes evidence, applies logical analysis, tests, proves and comes up with justified results. The latter jumps about in time, place and person, makes leaps and connections, invents scenarios, and takes note of gut reaction and impression. Is this the result of multiple intelligences, or of a 'left-brain/right-brain' dichotomy in action?

Those who do not accept the validity of a non-scientific approach may argue that this plurality is a sign of a profession which is confused about its scientific base, and which therefore resorts to intuition. However, there is an equally strong body of opinion that views occupational therapy as a social science and believes that, for a profession which deals with people, meanings and situations, a clinically logical approach which fails to consider the phenomenological aspects is inadequate.

It is equally arguable that all reductive analysis of cognition is unsatisfactory, because in practice we 'think' as a whole person in a whole situation, utilizing a wide spectrum of sensory, perceptual and cognitive inputs and processing.

It is at least clear that therapists must try to understand the processes of clinical reasoning better in order to use them more effectively. It is also clear that increased understanding is likely to lead us further away from any view of a 'formula' approach to therapy.

The most important factors in reasoning may turn out to be the situational ones – the fact that on each occasion there is an individual therapist with personal ideas, values, cognitive strategies and view of therapy, who is working in a particular setting, at a particular time, under certain conditions, in partnership with another individual who is also unique.

In the following section, various styles of reasoning will be described. In very broad terms it is possible to divide these forms of reasoning into two main groups: 'convergent modes' – those which tend towards scientific, 'straight line', logical processing; and 'divergent modes' – those which employ lateral thinking, intuitive or creative processing and a generally pheno-menological approach. There is, however, some overlap and, as already mentioned, therapists appear to shift in and out of different modes quite rapidly.

CONVERGENT MODES

Diagnostic reasoning

From the occupational therapy perspective, 'diagnosis' does not refer to 'what is wrong with the patient', but rather to the interpretation of the patient's situation in terms of the concerns and therapeutic methods of occupational therapy. Diagnostic reasoning employs a problem-based, information processing mode of thinking. It involves 'four basic processes: cue acquisition, hypothesis generation, cue interpretation and hypothesis evaluation' (Rogers & Holm 1991).

The result of this process is, according to Rogers & Holm, descriptive, explanatory, cue and pathological. The descriptive element relates to deficits or problems in occupational perform-ance. The explanatory element gives hypotheses to account for the deficit. The cues are those sig-nificant observations and pieces of information which, cumulatively, lead to the formation of the description and hypothesis and could be used to justify these. Pathological elements give the medical basis or causation of problems and indicate prognosis.

Hypothetical reasoning

When using hypothetical reasoning the therapist constructs statements which may explain and connect the available data. These statements express suppositions rather than defined facts, and can be tested, accepted or rejected. Hypoth-eses do not have to be written down, although this may help, as they are stored in memory: 'this could be caused by . . .'; 'I wonder if x and y are connected?'; 'If I do this, will the result be that . . .'; 'It looks as if the main problem is going to be . . .'.

There is a fine distinction between a hypothesis and an assumption. An assumption is an idea which is *accepted as true* (COD) for the purposes of action. We all make assumptions in daily life, because if we did not, action would continually be inhibited.

Since it is impractical to test every idea or theory which a therapist may use, some assumptions have to be made. These may concern the prognosis, the nature of the condition or certain aspects of therapy. As discussed in Part 1, there will be basic assumptions concerning the nature of occupational therapy and the occupational nature of an individual. Other assumptions will be accepted when a particular model or frame of reference is adopted. The point about an assumption is that, once accepted, it is not usually questioned actively, unless very clear evidence is obtained to contradict it.

The kinds of assumption which the therapist must avoid are those 'snap judgements' concerning the needs and wishes of a patient which then serve to close the mind to further investigation. The danger is that assumptions, rather than hypotheses, can be made too early, thus producing a restrictive mental set which eliminates further consideration.

Humans are cognitively programmed to make assumptions. We intuitively observe and collect data, try to detect covariation or correlation, and attempt to infer cause and effect (Atkinson et al 1993) We naturally attribute motivations to people and interpret situations in certain ways. We create cognitive schemata – patterns or 'mini-theories' – often based on limited information, which gives us the mental satisfaction of putting the thing, or the person, tidily 'into a box'. We dislike mental 'loose ends' but tend to take the easy route to tying them up. We create stereotypes, knowingly or unknowingly.

In particular, the hidden rules of social interaction are developed on the basis of assumptions, which may not be correct, but which tend to be powerful and persistent in their effects. The patterns of thinking generated by assumptions can become automatic so that we are no longer even aware of them and do not question them.

All of these mechanisms are subjective and liable to bias. If we are to take an objective view of the patient we must be acutely aware of these cognitive traps. It is essential to differentiate between objectively testable data, the therapist's personal view of the situation and the subjective reality experienced by the patient. Part of professional development is becoming aware of one's habitual patterns of thought, and one's tendency to use stereotypes or assumptions.

In clinical reasoning we ought to be dealing not with assumptions, but with hypotheses – statements about things which are proposed as suppositions which must be actively explored and tested. In order to form a hypothesis, data must be gathered, cues found and interpreted, and alternative hypotheses considered and evaluated. As a therapist reads through an initial referral, or scans case notes for the first time, hypotheses are generated, reviewed, rejected or put aside for further consideration at a suprising rate. One of the uses of a frame of reference is to give a defined structure for, and limits to, the generation of hypotheses. The more experience the therapist has of similar cases or situations the more hypotheses will be generated.

A hypothesis which has been tested and judged correct may then become an assumption upon which therapy can be based, at least until something occurs to disprove it.

Pattern recognition

Although every patient is a unique person, the situation in which she finds herself is not unique, for much of human experience is shared. Indeed, as Schon (1983) points out, if every situation were unique a professional would simply proceed each time by trial and error and expertise would scarcely enter into the equation. Medical diagnosis is based essentially on the recognition of patterns of signs and symptoms, and pattern recognition is accepted as an important reasoning mechanism in other professions.

Interestingly, such discussion may be presented in the context of qualitative research methods, rather than simply as a clinical strategy. May (1994) (a nurse educator), for example, distinguishes between pattern acquisition – 'the ability to know where to look'; and pattern recognition – 'the ability to know similarities and differences based on previous experience'. May continues:

These processes cannot be observed or understood directly; they can only be understood by the product. Expert analysts cannot tell you how a pattern was seen; they can tell you how their procedures set up the conditions in which the pattern was discerned, what attracted their attention, and, after the fact, how the pattern is evidenced in the data. Pattern recognition is instantaneous and can be substantiated in retrospect, but cannot be predicted.

The problems of tacit knowing and the role of experience are again emphasized.

Pattern recognition is not a simple matter. The difficulty is that people refuse to conform to textbook descriptions of life. Their conditions are atypical, their pathology is mixed, and their life situations are tangled and untidy. The therapist must make sense of this in terms of his scientific knowledge and practical experience, and must also help the patient to make sense of her own situation. This is analogous with a detective trying to make sense of a crime; one starts with too much information, or too little; one seeks clues, tries to sort the relevant from the irrelevant, and gradually builds a possible picture, or even several alternative pictures, which might explain or connect the facts.

Miss Marple, Agatha Christie's famous elderly sleuth 'with a mind like a bacon slicer', makes frequent use of pattern recognition. At some point in the story she will make some cryptic comment concerning something which the parlourmaid did several years ago; this will turn out to have been a pattern of behaviour similar to that of the murderer. Miss Marple has made the connection between the present pattern and a previous one. It is, however, essential to retain an open mind, even when a pattern seems established, for it may mask others. It is also unwise to assume that the behaviour or reactions of one person can automatically be generalized to another, even in a similar situation.

The mind continually looks for patterns, matching the current situation with schemata of previous ones, searching memories of textbooks for templates of matching information and recalling previous similar patients. Using the 'representativeness heuristic' means making a 'best guess' judgement or inference based on resemblance to a typical case (Baron & Byrne 1987).

All these pattern-matching strategies can be illuminating, but, like premature adoption of an assumption, there may be dangers: the mind is too anxious to find the pattern and make the match, and too content to accept a pattern once detected; it may find patterns where none exist, or try to 'fit the patient to the pattern'. Seeing patterns that are not there is called *illusory correlation*.

Thinking may also be biased by the 'availability heuristic' – judgements tend to be based on how easily things come to mind (Baron & Byrne 1987), by the vividness of a piece of information, and by the primacy effect – the first information we receive has the greatest impact on our overall impressions (Atkinson et al 1993). People also tend to notice and recall things that support their beliefs more than things which confute them, i.e. 'confirmation bias'. This is similar to the Rosenthal effect, whereby you 'see what you expect to see'. If your referral card tells you that your patient is a schizophrenic you *see* a schizophrenic.

DIVERGENT MODES

Interactive reasoning

Fleming describes interactive reasoning as follows: it 'takes place during face-to-face encounters between therapist and patient. It is a form of reasoning therapists employ when they want to better understand a patient as a person.'

Interactive reasoning involves the therapist in talking, listening and actively processing the information received. As the interaction progresses the conversation is steered in a direction which will help to obtain more information, pursue issues, explore feelings, stimulate participation, examine problems and reach solutions. The techniques which a therapist may use to achieve this are those derived from the process of therapeutic use of self, which will be described in Chapter ••, and include verbal and non-verbal strategies.

Fleming, quoting research by others, lists reasons for interactive reasoning:

- to engage the person in the treatment session
- to use humour to relieve tension

- to get to know the person as a person
- to understand the disability (situation/problem) from the patient's point of view
- to understand the patient's 'story'
- to fine-tune treatment to match individual needs
- to communicate a sense of acceptance, trust or hope to the patient
- to construct a shared language of actions and meanings
- to determine whether a treatment session is going well.

(Adapted from Fleming 1993)

Although it is possible to observe the results of this process in action, and to describe its purposes, it is difficult to describe the under-lying reasoning process. A student therapist struggled to explain this to me midway through her training by describing the experience of interacting with a patient, while being simul-taneously aware that another part of her thera-peutic identity stood back from the situation and commented, interpreted and directed. This 'inner therapist' conducting a mental dialogue is surely a personification of an internal reasoning pro-cess, and conscious monitoring of this dialogue or sharing it with others is very helpful.

Narrative reasoning

Mattingly (1989, 1991) is especially interested in the narrative nature of the process whereby we help a patient to tell his or her story, unravel the meanings and implications, and jointly work towards a desired outcome of the 'story'. She believes that 'clinical reasoning in occupational therapy is primarily directed not to a biological world of disease, but to a human world of motives, values and beliefs – a world of human meaning' (Mattingly 1991a).

During the interactive process described above, the therapist encourages and facilitates the patient to tell his story – from the trivia of what happened at the weekend to the significant life events which may underlie his problems. The therapist is able to use this story-telling in many

ways: as a means of developing rapport, for assessment, to understand the personal meanings situations may have for the patient and to predict outcomes.

In the course of hearing the patient tell his story other forms of reasoning – hypothesizing, intuition and pattern recognition – will be brought into play. The mental monitor in the mind of the therapist continually evaluates data making notes such as 'I recognize that ...'; 'I must ask more about that ...'; 'that could be important ... '; 'that does not ring true ...' or 'something is missing here ...'.

The therapist not only helps the patient to tell the story and understand it, but also, through activities and interactions, writes 'scripts' where-by the outcome may be changed to a more positive one. This process is improvizational; both therapist and patient are actors in this 'mini-drama' and can take advantage of occurrences or build on fortuitious circumstances. There may be many routes to the desired 'ending' of the story.

Kielhofner (1992) describes how he drew upon his theoretical framework:

To create a narrative explanation of (the patient's) circumstances and to imagine a better direction for his life to unfold ... within this larger story I constructed smaller stories that I expected to unfold in particular sessions ... the therapy session was, as Mattingly described it, an opportunity for him to remake his life story.

Kielhofner emphasizes the link between this process and the use of models or frames of reference as a means of providing interpre-tations of the story and constructing potential outcomes.

Since we are concerned here with both acting and interaction, it is not surprising that these concepts are similar to those used by inter-actionists such as Goffman, who 'adopt a dramaturgical model of social interaction. Social life, like a play, is made up: it is a human construction that has the meaning and reality that human beings give it' (O'Donnell 1992). This view of life casts us all as actors in the dramas of our own lives. The therapist, there-fore, has a key role in constructing and acting out situations and meanings which are relevant to the patient.

Intuition

Intuition is defined as 'immediate apprehension by the mind *without* reasoning' (COD). It seems inappropriate, therefore, to talk of 'intuitive *reasoning*'. Most therapists experience the occasional sensation of a flash of knowing, a surge of gut reaction or an instant connection being made. However, intuition is most likely the result of lightning-fast processing of information and subliminal cues, especially concerning body language and emotions. Some therapists are highly intuitive, and, as already noted, intuition is a characteristic of very experienced and expert therapists, which supports the idea that experience is used as a basis for intuition. In the sense of insight, intuition is also a part of problem-solving; it is a basic mental capability.

Heuristic inquiry

The term 'heuristic' has already been mentioned; in its simplest form heuristic inquiry is a cognitive mechanism providing useful patterns of thought and action, formed through personal experience.

However, the term *heuristics* also applies to 'a way of engaging in scientific search through methods and processes aimed at discovery; a way of self-inquiry and dialogue with others aimed at finding the underlying meanings of important human experiences' (Moustakas 1990).

As a form of research this is an intense, passionate and single-minded process which would be impractical as a reasoning mechanism in day-to-day therapy. However, the concepts and processes of heuristic research and inquiry, as outlined by Moustakas, do have resonances for the methods sometimes used by therapists during clinical reasoning.

The stages of heuristic inquiry include:

- Identifying with the focus of inquiry – in a clinical setting, putting oneself imaginatively into the patient's situation, temporarily be-

coming the person and seeing her problems in her way.
- Self-dialogue – a conscious conversation with oneself, mentally discussing the situation and one's ideas about it.
- Tacit knowing – here we return to the theme of knowing more than we can tell – 'tacit knowing gives birth to the hunches and vague formless insights that characterize heuristic discovery' (Moustakas 1990). Tacit knowledge is, by its nature, both mysterious and inexplicable.
- Intuition is seen as the bridge between the tacit and the explicit. It is linked to pattern recognition – 'intuition makes immediate knowledge possible without the intervening steps of logic and reasoning ... in the intuitive process one draws on clues; one senses a pattern or underlying condition that enables one to imagine and to characterize the reality, state of mind or condition.' (Moustakas 1990.)
- Indwelling and focusing are forms of concentrated reflection and rumination.
- Understanding the internal frame of reference – only the individual concerned can explain the meanings of her own experience.

Armed with these techniques, which are innate, but honed by use and experience, the inquirer can proceed through phases of inquiry: engaging with the problem; immersing herself in it; allowing time for incubation (that useful process where the mind, if left to do so, will produce the idea or information without the conscious need for searching); reaching the stage of illumination or understanding; explicating the situation in terms of the knowledge and understandings gained; and finally forming a creative synthesis which 'usually takes the form of a narrative, but may be expressed as a poem, drawing, painting or by some other form' (Moustakas 1990).

Although it must be stressed that this description relates to an intensive research process, there are clear analogies with reasoning in occupational therapy, and especially with expressive or interpretive techniques used with patients. It seems likely that therapists may use forms of heuristic search in addition to other methods, especially when delving into personal meanings or emotions, and may also facilitate heuristic discovery in their patients. Interestingly, Moustakas ends his book with an account of a humanistic psychotherapist using heuristic methods in his therapy.

Pragmatic reasoning

Thinking is influenced not only by the situation, but also by the individual doing the thinking. Schell & Cervero (1993) draw attention to effects on clinical reasoning of circumstances unconnected with the patient.

The concerns of pragmatic reasoning include both the therapist's personal and practice contexts. Examples of therapist contexts are repertoire of therapy skills, ability to read the practice culture, negotiation skills and personal motivation. Examples of the practice context are the power relationships of occupational therapy within the organization, reimbursement resources for treatment services and the kinds of available space and equipment. Therapists reason about all of these issues when they plan for, supervise, implement and reflect on occupational therapy services.

A part of this type of reasoning is therefore a practical evaluation of available resources and constraints, but another part is far more nebulous, concerning prevailing values and ethos, and the knowledge, skills and attitudes of the individual therapist.

THE CASE MANAGEMENT SEQUENCE

PROBLEM ANALYSIS

All of the reasoning modes that have been described in this chapter contribute to the process of problem analysis. The sequence of case management provides the structure for problem analysis, and reasoning occurs continually as the problems are identified and framed, and as solutions or actions are proposed. It is helpful to understand that the process has a sequence and structure, especially when one is learning to be an effective problem manager. However, in practice these stages may become condensed or blurred and, as with the processes of clinical reasoning, the therapist may find it difficult to explain how he arrived at his conclusion, and may remain largely unconscious of the intricacies of the problem analysis process.

Some therapists dislike the use of the term 'problem', but if there is no problem, why is the patient referred? There must be some need which can be met by therapy, otherwise the referral is unnecessary. In one sense, the problem to be analysed and solved is not that of the patient, but that of the therapist in negotiating with the patient to define the need and decide on action. The term 'problem' should not imply only negative aspects of a situation, but rather that a situation exists that requires therapy or intervention. In order to understand a problem, both positive and negative sides of the situation must be considered.

The therapist begins by identifying whether the difficulties which the patient is experiencing are within the remit of the therapist. This involves exploration of function, competencies in relationships, roles, occupations or activities, presence of dysfunction, and ability to use or relate to the physical or social environment. The therapist will also consider the positive features in the patient's current or past life in relation to this information, and will seek to identify strengths and abilities which may be used or built upon.

The process of problem 'naming and framing' means being able to say 'I know what is going on in this patient's life; I can list several problem areas. I can make some firm, or tentative, hypotheses about the reasons for these. Depending on what the patient and I negotiate as priorities, I can see some ways in which the situations could be improved, and I know ways of achieving this.'

The problem list may be clearly defined or inconclusive. Defining the problem may sometimes *be* the problem, for once it is clear it becomes possible to do something about it. Defining the problem and causes of it may take up the major part of some interventions.

A problem situation is one of uncertainty. If one knew precisely 'what is wrong', 'what to do' and 'how to do it', there would be no problem. If solutions to the problems which therapists encounter could be found in neatly described formulae on the pages of a textbook, therapists would soon become redundant. Problems which require the use of clinical reasoning occur in the indeterminate zones of practice and share the characteristics of 'uncertainty, uniqueness and conflict' (Schon 1987).

The term 'problem analysis' is used deliberately because it is all too easy to become locked into 'problem solving'. Apart from the very obvious fact that a problem cannot be solved effectively until the nature of it is understood, some problems do not have clear-cut 'solutions'.

Schon (1983) describes the process of problem analysis as 'problem setting': 'a process in which, interactively, we name the things to which we will attend and frame the context in which we will attend to them.' The words 'naming' and 'framing' have become current terminology in describing this process.

There are three main stages: data collection and analysis; problem definition and solution development. (Refer to Figure 11.1 and Tables 12.1–12.4 to see how this relates to the case management process.)

DATA COLLECTION

It is important to be aware of the quality, reliability and degree of objectivity of the data. This is not to imply that only objective data is useful, for subjective data can be very important, but it is necessary to distinguish between the two. It is equally important to separate the therapist's own interpretation of facts from the raw data.

It is also necessary to be aware of whether one is breaking new ground or following a well-trodden path. Once captured, data can (within the constraints of permission and confidentiality) be shared; nothing is more irritating to a client, and time-wasting for all concerned, than continual visits from professionals all asking the same questions.

DATA ANALYSIS

The analysis of data concerning a patient is no simple matter. It requires clinical reasoning, and tests the deductive, logical, problem-analysing skills of the therapist, who must find the relevant cues and relate the information concerning *this* patient to his previous experience and knowledge, without falling into the trap of stereotyping either the patient or the required action because something superficially similar has been encountered before.

The first rule of data analysis is that it is only as good as the data. If the therapist has gathered insufficient information, a full analysis cannot be carried out. This part of the process is primarily a matter of asking questions and deciding which of the answers are relevant. Having too much information can be as much of a nuisance as having too little. Inexperienced therapists typically find it hard to 'see the wood for the trees'.

As has been noted, students and newly qualified therapists typically find it harder to ask the 'right' questions, ask fewer of them and rely on textbook interpretations to a much greater extent than do experienced or expert practitioners.

A number of basic questions will help to steer the process of information gathering and analysis:

- How much do I need to know about this person? This will be somewhere along a continuum from basic data to a full medical, social, environmental and occupational history.
- Where can I obtain this information? Has anyone else already captured it? Does it matter if I duplicate this?
- Why am I asking these questions? Examples may be: legal recording requirements, to expand on an area which may be significant, to define a problem area or to gain a rapport with the patient.
- Which parts of this information seem to be significant, of possible significance, probably insignificant or definitely irrelevant?
- What is the 'occupational therapy focus' on this patient? Is it a specific referral with a clear-cut need or something more nebulous? Does it concern occupational spread, performance skills, environmental factors, roles and relationships,

physical or psychological dysfunction, or several of these?

• What is my objective view of this situation? What is the patient's (or are others') subjective view(s)? Are these at variance? Why, and is this part of the problem?

• What else do I need to know?

As data are analysed, the internal dialogue in which hypotheses are posed and accepted or rejected is established. Mental statements serve to define the need for therapy or intervention and alert the therapist to further issues.

PROBLEM DEFINITION

Although it is clearly necessary to gain an outline view of the problem from the outset, preliminary problem definition must be treated with caution. Identifying the problem can be deceptively simple: it may be easy to state that the patient 'is depressed', 'has a right hemiplegia', 'has been unable to hold down a job'. However, this says little about the problem within the diagnostic terms of occupational therapy.

It is wise to remember that the apparent problem may not be the real, underlying problem, that complex situations involve multiple problems, and that early labelling of a problem can eliminate productive alternative lines of thought, and may result in a reductive approach.

Many complex problems have an 'onion skin' character; as one problem is peeled away, others are revealed below it, so that the process of analysis must be repeated several times.

FRAME ANALYSIS

Frame analysis (Schon 1983) is the process of understanding the nature of the problem. One of the functions of a frame of reference is, as the name implies, the provision of boundaries to and definition of a certain type of problem.

As discussed earlier, the point at which a theoretical structure is adopted affects the whole process. If the conceptual lens is used from the outset, the problem must be seen and interpreted through that lens (the theory-driven pattern). If the nature of the problem is explored through the process of case management (the process-driven pattern), the nature of the problem is defined and various models or frames of reference may then be used as tools to provide explanations of the problem or frameworks for potential action. Both methods are of use, but the danger in the theory-driven pattern is that the problem may be made to fit the model, and wider explanations be discarded; on the other hand, the process-driven pattern may provide too many explanations.

It is interesting to note that Kielhofner (1992) has shifted towards the process-driven approach, listing eight 'models' (among them, human occupation) which provide differing ways of seeing 'normal order' in a system and what happens when something goes wrong. He advocates the benefits of using more than one model: 'the combination of models may enable a therapist to better understand and address the multidimensionality of a therapeutic process in which systemic and personal change may occur simultaneously.' A key function of clinical reasoning is to discriminate between various possible explanations and solutions.

He states that 'problem definition and solution are grounded in the professional's understanding of his or her work, responsibilities and capabilities.' He then proposes that different professions have different understandings, which result in different forms of problem analysis – or rather, in analysis which gives differing interpretations and emphases to the same problem. It is important for the therapist to recognize that others may name and frame a problem differently; Schon (1987) notes that 'those who hold conflicting frames pay attention to different facts and make different sense of the facts they notice.'

A colleague reminded me of the case of a profoundly handicapped young woman who habitually bit staff, which caused added concern since she was a carrier of hepatitis B. Various professions were mustered to give advice. The microbiologist checked that all staff had been immunized and proposed strong protective gloves and sleeves for staff. Nurses suggested that she should wear some kind of restraint when being handled. The psychiatrist recommended increased doses of tranquilisers. The psychologist suggested a behavioural approach, withdrawing any attention or contact if biting took place. The occupational therapist asked questions about who she bit, what she was doing at the time, and what was happening during the pattern of her activities which might contribute to the problem. In each case the problem was framed according to the perception of the profession.

However, there is also a difficulty for a therapist who may be able to frame a problem in a variety of ways and must decide which is most applicable. For example, if a disabled person becomes housebound, it is relatively simple to name the problem – the person does not go out, and the desired outcome – the person should be able to leave the house when she wishes. This might be framed as a problem of access (adaptation model; environmental alteration); however, if recent physical deterioration had increased immobility it might also be a problem of physical dysfunction or of mobility (rehabilitation model; biomechanical frame of reference). If the person is depressed or lacks self-esteem, it might become a problem of motivation (cognitive–behavioural frame of reference or humanistic frame of reference). If the person is being kept in by overprotective relatives, or lacks a supportive social network it could be described as a social problem (interactive frame of reference).

It is possible that several of these frames may apply and a holistic problem-based view would consider how these may interact – does the patient lack motivation because of decreased mobility, or does the lack of mobility stem from disuse due to decreased motivation? Is the lack of motivation due to a lack of opportunity and environmental obstacles, to a repeated experience of failure, or to some more fundamental trait within the client's personality?

The essence of correct framing is that the solutions in each case will be different, e.g. provide a wheelchair or walking aid, build a ramp, provide rehabilitation, group therapy or family counselling, or fix a weekly trip to a suitable club, i.e. provide experiences which have meaning and successful outcomes. Not all of these solutions may be appropriate as occupational therapy intervention; a referral to other agencies may be needed.

The therapist must remain versatile and aware of the pluralistic nature of practice, for, as Kielhofner (1992) points out: 'Models can be used inappropriately to find problems where they do not exist.' They may also serve to 'squeeze' inappropriate problems into a confined frame of reference.

In addition, it is necessary to become aware of who 'owns' the problem. Is the patient aware of it and troubled by it, and if so, how much? One person's problem is another's 'niggle' and a third person's 'catastrophe'. Is the problem in the mind of someone other than the patient, e.g. a relative, the neighbours or the referring agent? The 'something must be done' syndrome is not always the best basis for action. The problem may reside in a family, in an environment, or even in society as a whole, and not in the patient who has been referred. Is the person experiencing a problem, or being experienced *as* one?

The way the therapist sees the problem may differ from the way the patient sees it. Indeed, persuading the patient to accept that there is a problem may *be* the problem. Naming and framing needs to be done by the therapist and client in partnership; they must reach an agreement on the nature of the problem and its existence, before any useful further action can be taken.

IDENTIFICATION OF THE DESIRED OUTCOME

The desired outcome is the state which would be attained if the problem were resolved. This is not the same as the solution, which is the means whereby the outcome will be achieved. It may be relatively easy to decide what is wanted, but deciding how to achieve it may be difficult, or even impossible.

A journey from London to Edinburgh can be used as a simple example. The problem is that you are in London; the desired outcome is that you arrive in Edinburgh. The solutions include flying, driving or going by train. Either walking or cycling are possible, but unlikely choices. Hitch-hiking would be uncertain and hazardous. Your solution will depend on the cost, convenience and length of time of the journey.

However, clinging to the vision of an ideal but unattainable outcome can mean you do not put your energies into achieving a more limited aim. If you are determined to go *only* from London to Edinburgh, but cannot afford to, you may ignore the possibility of having a pleasant day out in Brighton instead. The patient who longs for his hemiplegic arm to be 'better' may reject all attempts to get him to compensate for its loss of function. The patient who thinks his or her problems will vanish 'When I move to another district', 'if I get a divorce', or 'when I change jobs' may be avoiding the exploration of the real nature of the difficulties he or she faces.

There may be several possible outcomes, and the therapist and client must decide on which is best. They may agree on one, but find it unattainable for some reason, and jointly have to re-define the problem, outcome and new solution.

It is worth noting that there are some situations in which the therapist knows what the problem is and what the goal may be, but does not understand all the origins or dynamics of the problem. This does not preclude an attempt to find a solution, but may make it more of a process of trial and error.

SOLUTION DEVELOPMENT

It has been noted that it can be relatively simple to describe a 'desired state' which will occur if the problem can be removed. Identifying the solution may be much harder. Does a solution even exist? In our imperfect world, solutions are often a means to achieve only a partial resolution of the problem, or only a modified version of a desired outcome. The therapist needs to be clear about how far he and the client are prepared to compromise.

Atkinson et al (1993) state that problem solution requires that a goal be divided into subgoals and that the following strategies can then be used:

Reducing differences between the current state and the goal state.

Means–ends analysis – eliminating the most important differences between the current state and the goal state.

Working backwards (from the desired state to the problem).

Atkinson et al describe these strategies as 'weak' because they are generalized; more effective strategies which derive from experience, and distinguish expert problem-solvers from novices include:

Having more representations (mental images of the problem, spatial, visual or in words).

Representing the problem in terms of solution principles rather than surface features (e.g. 'In this sort of situation I know that this kind of action will be effective').

Forming a plan before acting (and mentally testing alternative plans).

Reasoning forwards rather than working backwards.

It is clear from these strategies that pattern recognition and procedural reasoning are brought into use.

The development of clinical solutions often takes time and has to be conducted in stages, especially since the client must be closely involved in developing the solution. Some clients are unable to participate much in this process, at least at first, and it may take a long while for participation to be attained, if it ever is. It may then be impractical to delay action until this stage is reached, and in any case the therapist must decide how to intervene, or else decide not to treat the case. Decisions about action must be taken before the case management process can procede, thus an action plan must be produced.

An action plan is formed by means of the following sequence (see Ch. 12):

1. Decide desired outcome.
2. Set long-term aim(s).
3. Decide general method for achieving outcome, e.g. therapy programme, obtain resources, patient action, refer onwards.

4. Decide priority for action.
5. Set short term goals/objectives to achieve.
6. Set criteria for evaluation of whether objectives are met.
7. Plan detailed action to achieve objectives.

None of these decisions is simple, and selecting a priority for action is often the hardest part. So many factors can be involved, e.g. the patient's wishes, practicalities, time available, therapy resources, consideration of what is likely to be most therapeutically effective, cost-effectiveness or what others are doing. Sometimes therapy has to be conducted by a circuitous route and an obvious priority has to be postponed in favour of action which lays the foundations for it to be tackled later.

The action plan is the means whereby the proposed solution is to be put into practice. The action plan states the aim, and then lists the action to be taken in sequence. It is usually best to break the aim into subgoals, and these may be broken down into specific objectives. Each goal or objective may have an action plan. It is important to have a manageable number of compatible objectives, or the plan will become overloaded. The way in which a plan is evolved and implemented is discussed in Chapter 12.

Once it has been decided what is to be done, it is possible to select appropriate methods of achieving the outcome. There are numerous text-books which give information about treatment of specific physical or psychosocial conditions. The chosen approach will bring with it an armoury of procedures, techniques and media; some approaches are more straightforward and prescriptive than others.

This is where the art and science of therapy combine to form an alchemy which, at its best, works remarkably well. Unfortunately, no-one has yet found a way of describing this process. Other factors aside, it is unlikely that all therapists use an identical conceptual framework to take decisions, especially those of the gut reaction kind which the expert therapist appears to use to match the patient to exactly the right activity at the right time to achieve the desired result.

CASE MANAGEMENT: THE INTEGRATIVE PROCESS

It should be clear by now that the processes of clinical reasoning and problem analysis are those whereby decisions are taken, whereas case management offers the procedural structure to sequence, organize and document these processes, and the subsequent action.

As described at the beginning of this chapter, the case management process starts with referral and ends with discharge. The process of intervention which occurs between these two events is cyclical in nature, and will be described in Chapter 12.

The actions which start and conclude the case management process – accepting a referral, recording the case and discharging the patient or client – require separate consideration.

REFERRAL

A referral can originate from a number of sources: a medical practitioner, another health care professional, a relative or carer, or the patient. The first decision to be made on receipt of a referral is whether it should be accepted. Wherever the referral originates, it is essential to record its receipt, and its acceptance or refusal, following the local policy for this.

Receipt of a referral does not oblige the therapist to accept it. Acceptance is primarily a matter of clinical judgement as to whether it is appropriate for an occupational therapist to intervene, and whether suitable services, of an acceptable standard and efficacy, can be offered. Local policies may mean that certain categories of client are given priority, or that others must be placed on a waiting list. Referrals which are unclear, unattributed or otherwise unsatisfactory may be returned to the sender for clarification.

Medical referral is still probably the most common source, since therapists remain legally tied to the concept of 'profession allied to medicine'. While prescription of therapy rests with the therapist, referral in most situations is still seen, at least nominally, as the province of the doctor.

It is simple to ensure the requirement for access to a medical practitioner in a clinical setting, but in the community, contact with the client's general practitioner (GP) may be tenuous. One solution is for the social services therapist to notify the GP of a referral and intended action, leaving it to the GP to respond if this is not desired. Sanction by a GP becomes a matter of importance if the GP is the budget-holder for the service; the therapist attached to a primary care team would be unwise to initiate intervention without being aware of whether funding for the service was approved.

In the absence of any policy which prevents acceptance, the general presumption must be that a referral should be accepted and acted upon until there is proof to suggest otherwise. The therapist's mind is geared to see potential for therapeutic intervention in most situations; this is admirable, but sometimes results in reluctance to refuse a case which is really inappropriate.

Refusal to accept a referral must be fully justified, and the reasons recorded, and it is the responsibility of the therapist to make a referral to a more appropriate service if necessary. There should be no way in which such a decision could be viewed as having been prejudiced by age, sex, race or any other factor concerning the personal circumstances of the client. The test is clinical efficacy and appropriateness. Where lack of service is caused by limited or deficient resources, any system of prioritizing must be developed with managerial support, and should be explicit. Therapists should report to managers every case in which necessary therapy is prevented or impeded by lack of resources.

'Snap' judgements are best avoided. Inappropriate referrals may indicate simply that the referring person lacks information about the purposes and scope of occupational therapy, and may mask a real need which the therapist could identify and address. It is frequently necessary to accept the referral in order to identify the needs of the patient or client, following which a final decision concerning the necessity of treatment or intervention can be made. This assessment of need should, however, be counted as intervention, however minimal.

CONFIRMATION OF THE PATIENT'S NEED FOR, AND ACCEPTANCE OF, THERAPY

If there is some difficulty in the areas of legitimate concern to the therapist, it is simple to confirm that therapy should be provided. Whether it *can* be may depend on other circumstances and, crucially, on the agreement of the patient. This should be formally obtained and recorded.

A clear refusal by a patient who has received an explicit description of the purposes, processes and benefits of the proposed intervention prohibits further action. The person must be asked directly whether she is refusing the offer of therapy or intervention, and whether this refusal applies to all aspects of the intervention, or to just one area. Any such refusal, together with the reasons, must be documented, and the record should also specify precisely what the patient was told concerning the purposes and methods of intervention. The referring agent must be informed at once.

Acceptance of a referral is usually the point at which a new case-file is started and the case becomes counted for statistical purposes. It sometimes happens that further assessment or information shows that occupational therapy is unnecessary or inappropriate. The reasons for the therapist's decision not to intervene may be based on medical, therapeutic, practical or ethical reasons, but must be clearly justified and recorded.

DOCUMENTATION OF THE CASE MANAGEMENT PROCESS

The importance of clear, accurate recording at all stages of the process cannot be over-emphasized. Good practice is essential, not only for the smooth and effective provision of services to patients, but also to comply with legal requirements, and to protect the therapist. Guidance is given in various COT standards documents, in Hopkins & Smith (1993) and in various texts on service management, and may also be found in local policies and procedures.

Documents include case notes, treatment records, assessments, letters, reports, progress summaries, goal plans, or notes of case discussions or telephone calls. Case records should ideally be written in such a way that, if necessary, a colleague could take the notes and continue the treatment of the patient with relatively little disruption.

Basic principles of documentation include:

• The patient/client must be identified clearly on all documentation, with special care being taken if there is more than one person with the same or a similar name.

• Information concerning a patient must be clear, relevant, written in a professional manner using appropriate terminology, and must specify if there are any special observations, precautions, contraindications or complications of which those dealing with the patient should be aware.

• All documents or entries in records must be dated and signed by the therapist in person.

• Documents must be legible. It is wise to avoid making corrections; if a correction must be made the passage should be crossed through, not erased or covered over. The deletion and the correction should be dated and signed or initialled.

• Documents must be stored safely, access restricted to appropriate people, and confidentiality maintained. A document in transit should be sent in a manner which prevents unauthorized or casual access.

• All action agreed with the patient/client must be recorded, giving full details of what was agreed, when, the expected outcome, any target dates, who is to be responsible, and any other pertinent material. It is particularly important to note agreement to, or refusal of, any therapy, and to make it clear that appropriate and sufficient explanations have been given.

• All action taken on behalf of the patient must be recorded, together with notes on the consequence or outcomes of such action.

• All communication with others concerning the patient must be noted, and copies of correspondence kept where appropriate.

• The patient/client should be aware, at least in general terms, of the content of any records held concerning her, and of her right to access to documentation. Any computerized records must be dealt with in accordance with current legislation.

DISCHARGE

Once all goals have been achieved, or have proved impossible to achieve, treatment or intervention should be ceased. Conclusion of therapy must be proved to have been justified, and not merely expedient. A full case record should be retained on file. A discharge summary or report may be needed.

If further intervention by another agency, a follow-up visit, or a case review is needed, this must be arranged.

12

Intervention

THE NATURE OF INTERVENTION

Strictly speaking, intervention is the process of acting on behalf of the patient or client, whereas therapy indicates the provision of treatment. However, intervention is used in this chapter as a generic term for *all* the actions of the therapist, whether directly involving the patient or client, or taken on his behalf. Both of these aspects of intervention will be described.

Occupational therapists lay claim to a holistic style of intervention which is appropriate at all ages, providing that a problem relative to roles, occupations, activities or skills can be shown to exist.

The therapist is a genericist, a general practitioner, qualified to work with patients from babyhood to extreme old age, whether their condition is psychological, developmental, neurological, medical, orthopaedic or traumatic, or due to the effects of heredity, environment, society, faulty learning, ageing, or almost any other factor.

This is a wide brief. If taken from the standpoint of medical specialisms concerned with diagnosis and remediation, it may seem an overly ambitious mixture. Of course, in practice, most therapists develop expertise in a defined area. However, the therapist is not primarily concerned with illnesses and diagnoses, nor even with effecting 'cures'.

The central concern is with the individual having a personal sense of well-being and efficacy, functioning in a healthy manner, in an environment which provides an appropriate mix of support and challenge, by means of roles, occupations and activities.

To use a wise old medical proverb, the therapist does not need to know what illness the patient has as much as to understand what patient the illness has, and in particular, what roles, occupations and environments the patient possesses or uses. In any event, patients referred for occupational therapy often are not 'ill'; they are suffering from a situation, a problem or a set of circumstances.

Each person presenting for therapy is a 'new beginning'. Each intervention is designed for the individual, and relates to his unique situation. Norms are not irrelevant; they may illuminate understanding of how people in general think or move or react, and provide a useful background, but the therapist must recognize that 'the normal person' is a myth, a mere statistical device.

The continuum of function and dysfunction is not applicable as a yardstick by which to measure each person and decide how, or if, he is deficient in relation to some ideal state. It is an expression of how far an individual is able to manage his life in all aspects from the necessary to the frivolous, to his own satisfaction, and with minimum disruption to others. The goals of intervention are therefore set by patient and therapist working in partnership.

Once this is accepted and understood the process of intervention can be seen as manageable because on each occasion, for each intervention, the therapist is working with a real person, in a real situation, for a limited number of realistic goals, by means of the organizing process of case management. This is of central importance to the question of measuring outcomes.

Intervention is the pivotal part of the case management process; it begins once the referral has been accepted, with the collection of information and initial assessment of the patient, so that the therapist may confirm that intervention is justified.

At that point, the cycle of intervention commences with further gathering of information, assessment, and data analysis, so that the therapist, through clinical reasoning, and in partnership with the patient, can frame the problem, select or confirm the approach and decide on a priority for action. Intervention continues, in the form of setting aims, planning intervention, carrying it out, reassessing, monitoring progress and evaluating the outcomes, until the patient or client is discharged.

There may be one cycle or several, or even overlapping cycles concerned with different problems. This process has been demonstrated in Figure 3.16A but can also be illustrated by a flowchart (see Fig. 14.1).

Intervention is a multivariate phenomenon. There are shelves full of occupational therapy texts explaining the details of therapy within particular specialties, for specific conditions, in certain locations, or using defined techniques. Once again, the purpose of this chapter is not to describe specific procedures, but to indicate general principles.

The difficulty in pinpointing the role of occupational therapists has been described in Chapter 2. Definitions tend to emphasize aims, purposes, scope or outcomes of therapy, rather than actions. The description given in Box 12.1 is an attempt at a generalized statement concerning the nature of intervention and therapy within the frame of a problem-based process-driven pattern.

It is likely to be easier to describe practice in a particular area of occupational therapy, since the nature of intervention or therapy will clearly be dictated by situational circumstances such as choice of approach, location of therapy and the nature of the patient's condition; these can be described in the relevant context.

It is the duty of occupational therapists to explain their services to employers, managers, purchasers, professional colleagues, clients and the general public. The profession must become more adept at doing this succinctly and in comprehensible terms.

STAGES IN THE INTERVENTION PROCESS

As shown in Figure 11.1, the process of intervention can be condensed into four stages, each

Box 12.1 The role of the occupational therapist

1. The therapist will, through therapeutic use of self, develop a professional relationship with the client/patient, and use this relationship to decide with the individual the nature of the problem, personal priorities and the aims of intervention/therapy.

2. The therapist will set goals and objectives for the provision of intervention or therapy, as negotiated with the patient/client, and in liaison with others where necessary. These will describe personal outcomes for the individual, related to roles, occupations or activities, in the areas of work, leisure, or personal and domestic activities. Intervention will deal with problems in one or more of the following areas: rehabilitation, education, development or adaptation.

3. Written case records will be kept: in particular, aims, goals and objectives, action to achieve these and subsequent assessments, progress and outcomes will be recorded by the therapist, and communicated to others as appropriate, respecting confidentiality and professional ethics.

4. The therapist will design a treatment plan/action plan to meet aims, goals and objectives.

5. Where appropriate the therapist may enable and empower the client to act on his own behalf.

6. The therapist may use skills of environmental and occupational analysis and adaptation to adapt environments and occupations, to remove occupational barriers and to enable and enhance performance or to provide beneficial activities and experiences.

7. The therapist may use special techniques derived from relevant frames of reference to provide specific physical, cognitive or psychosocial therapy.

8. The therapist may instruct the patient in skills or adaptive techniques, or provide information, or practice and experience in skills, tasks, activities, occupations or roles.

9. The therapist may intervene on behalf of the client to obtain items, resources, services or access which the client requires. This may involve direct provision by the therapist or communication with, and coordination of action by, other professionals, voluntary and statutory agencies, commercial organizations, carers, and other providers.

10. The therapist may visit the client's home, workplace or other relevant environment to assess, advise, teach, treat, adapt, or provide other intervention.

11. The therapist will continually monitor, assess and evaluate progress towards defined objectives and outcomes, evaluate the effects of therapy/intervention, modify and progress therapy, to ensure that actions taken are appropriate and efficacious.

12. The therapist will ensure that all necessary action has been taken before discharge and that appropriate arrangements for discharge are made.

13. The therapist will work actively towards personal and professional development, seeking to maintain the standards of currently accepted good practice and of professional and ethical behaviour.

14. The therapist will manage human and physical resources to ensure effective, efficient and economical provision of a high quality service.

of which has a number of subsidiary activities. These can be summarized in the form of tables which demonstrate that the quality of the thinking and decision-taking in the initial stages is crucial to the success of later intervention, and that time must be allowed for both this and final evaluation (see Tables 12.1–12.4).

STAGE 1: INFORMATION GATHERING AND PROBLEM ANALYSIS (Table 12.1)

Information gathering and recording

This preliminary stage is crucial because at this point the therapist must, with the patient/client, confirm whether there is a valid reason for occupational therapy to be provided, and, if so, the general nature of the need/problem. This is a kind of preliminary filtration process in which the therapist tries to extract the important, relevant information.

Having accepted the case, the information-gathering process can be conducted in relation to a specific need or problem, or to decide what the precise nature of the problem is, what solutions may be available or what action should be taken.

The case record for an individual referred for occupational therapy contains the details of this process as relevant to that individual, and should include all information, decisions, plans, actions,

Table 12.1   Stage 1: information gathering and problem analysis

Procedure	Examples of reasoning
Information gathering and recording	What? How much? Where from?
Initial assessment	Of what? For what purpose? How?
Data analysis	Determine relevance, validity, quality and reliability. Sufficient? So what? Conclusions.
Initial problem and asset identification	Needs? Strengths? Assets? Person's wishes? Where/whose is the problem? Problem list.
Confirmation of patient's acceptance of and need for therapy	Person will/will not benefit from occupational therapy, Person does/does not wish to receive occupational therapy, Need for other intervention? Justify.
Select, or confirm selection of, model or frame of reference	How to frame the problem? Consequent approach? Suitable? Relevant? Helpful? Effect on subsequent action/thinking? Compatibility with that used by others? Acceptability to patient?
Frame problem(s), desired outcome and possible solutions	Is case sufficiently understood for action to be initiated? Does patient share your understanding of problem and outcomes? If more than one solution, which is best?

progress and outcomes. The first section of a case record usually contains the personal details of the patient, and relevant social, environmental, occupational and medical history.

Information may be obtained from the patient during an interview, from records, from other professionals, or from relative or carers. It is helpful to make a distinction between subjective data – personal feelings and opinions of the patient and others, and objective data – formally recorded facts or things which the therapist has personally observed and recorded. The SOAP system (A problem-based method of recording which uses the headings Subjective, Objective, Assessment, Planning (Kings Fund Centre 1988)) formalizes this method. It is usually necessary to support reported information by at least some preliminary assessment by means of personal observation.

Information gathering may be repeated subsequently as often as required as part of the cycle of the case management process.

Initial assessment

This moves away from intervention towards the process of assessment and evaluation. Initial assessment is a further scanning and elimination exercise in order to define the problem and obtain a baseline for intervention or therapy.

Assessment may focus on the person, (see Ch. 13) or on aspects of the person's social or physical environment (see Ch. 15).

Data analysis

Data analysis is where clinical reasoning and problem analysis are used to evaluate the case (see Ch. 11). The therapist may undertake part of this analysis privately, but at some point must discuss and test ideas with the patient in order to discover whether the understanding of the situation is shared by the patient, and whether the patient is prepared to participate in setting goals and cooperate with intervention or therapy on this basis. Analysis should be a reciprocal exercise in which the patient/client takes an active part whenever possible.

Initial problem and asset identification

The result of this dialogue should be a mutual agreement about the nature of the problem and the need for therapy or intervention. This is sometimes straightforward, but is frequently tentative at this early stage. The first point of agreement may simply be that further investigation of the situation is required.

Confirmation of patient's acceptance of, and need for, therapy

The patient must agree to participate in the process, with a clear understanding of what is involved and what the outcomes, (insofar as they are known at this stage) may be. At this point, alternative action may be recommended if occupational therapy is agreed to be inappropriate.

Select, or confirm selection of, model or frame of reference

This is a matter for the therapist's professional judgement, in which the majority of patients are unable to participate since they lack the information and expertise to do so. This should not prevent the therapist from explaining options to the patient and involving him in choices where these are available.

In a theory-driven situation it is wise for the therapist to check, once enough information has been gathered, that the theory is compatible with the facts and needs of the case.

In a process-driven pattern, it is only at this stage, when the problem has been adequately understood, that an appropriate problem-based model and approach can be chosen to frame the problem. Framing the problem provides explanations of dysfunction, aetiology and consequent action.

Frame problem(s), desired outcome and possible solutions

This is a checking stage, reviewing the sum of information to date, and confirming framing of the problem, outcome and outline solution within the scope of the selected model or frame of reference.

A summary of these decisions should be clearly recorded as this is the basis for action.

STAGE 2: DECISIONS ABOUT ACTION (Table 12.2)

Although listed in the table as a sequence these actions are closely linked and happen in an integrated manner often almost simultaneously. Sometimes decisions are clear, obvious, and taken so rapidly that the whole process is compressed into a very short time in which the end result appears without conscious awareness of the intervening stages. At at other times it may take a considerable amount of time and thought to untangle a complex situation sufficiently to make these decisions.

Table 12.2   Stage 2: decisions about action

Procedure	Examples of reasoning
Select priorities	What is to be done first? Practicalities, e.g. time, resources? Effectiveness? Patient's wishes? Influence of theory? (Balance this patient's priorities with those of others – management of overall caseload).
Decide on agreed aim(s) and goals	Main aim and consequent goals. Agreed with all involved? Compatible with those of others? Realistic?
Break goals into objectives	Clarity? Timescale? Manageable and with reasonable change of being attained? How will outcome be measured?
Decide on method to achieve objectives	Action needed? Therapy programme? Nature and sequence of programme? Techniques? Media? Frequency/intensity of therapy? Rationale of therapy? Use of theory?
Produce action plan	How is plan to be carried out? Sequence of events or actions? Who does what, where, when how, to and with whom? What is needed? How will it be obtained?
Define means of measuring outcome of plan	How can success/completion/effectiveness be evaluated? Goals and objectives attained? Outcomes described – as expected? Progress towards overall aim?

Select priorities

What is to be done first? This is another point where clinical reasoning must be used and possibly conflicting priorities balanced. Another minefield of questions is raised, concerning chiefly who has the power of decision – the therapist, the patient or someone else.

Does the therapist do first what the patient wants? If this is the same as the therapist's own priority it presents no difficulty, but what if it is different? Wants and needs may not be the same. The therapist's willingness to persuade, direct and prescribe may depend both on the therapeutic relationship and on the approach being used. If the therapist is working biomechanically or behaviourally she may wish to be relatively directive. If she is using a client-centred approach, she must start from the point at which intervention is acceptable, and work round to other issues which she sees as important, but which the client does not.

How far is the selection of priorities influenced by others? The priorities of the doctor who is short of beds, the stressed relative, the anxious neighbour or the insistent co-professional, may not be compatible with the first choice of either the patient or the therapist.

Can the root cause be dealt with, or must intervention be symptomatic because it is impossible or impractical to tackle the cause? It is frustrating for a therapist to have to spend time on palliatives knowing that, if only more time were available, the problem could be sorted out once and for all.

It is essential to evaluate whether intervention is likely to be effective. It may be preferable to do nothing than to do something which is a waste of time or resources.

In general, there is currently a trend in favour of cooperative planning between the informed patient and the therapist. When the patient is unable for some reason to participate in this process the therapist must be more careful than ever to act in a reasoned, ethical and well-justified manner.

Decide on agreed aims and goals; break goals into objectives

The words 'aim', 'goal' and 'objective', can be used rather vaguely. It is helpful to distinguish between them.

Aim: A brief general statement of the agreed intention of intervention. Intervention will end when the aim has been accomplished.

Goal: A concise statement of a defined outcome to be attained at a stage in intervention. Goals may be long-term or short-term.

Objective: A very precise definition of an outcome to be achieved within a defined, short timeframe, including a statement of how it will be carried out, by whom, by when, and a means of evaluating the degree to which it has been achieved.

In the journey on which therapist and patient embark, the aim is the eventual destination. It may take a short time, or very long time, to reach it, but if it is so far into the future as to be out of sight it is unlikely to be relevant. It is best to split wide-ranging aims – there is nothing wrong with having two or three long-term aims, but if there are too many, they will not be achieved.

Goals are stages along the way, and it is best if they are well-defined and have an inbuilt time scale. It also helps if distinct problems are given specific goals. Short-term goals relate to, and build into, a long-term goal.

Objectives are usually very specific, tightly-worded sentences which tell the therapist precisely what the outcome will be for the patient, and how, and by when, this will happen. There should be an inbuilt measure to show when the objective has been attained. Objectives help to make therapy relevant and to move the treatment plan along, changing as each individual objective is achieved, and new ones are set.

There are various styles of documenting aims, goals or objectives. This is influenced by local custom and practice, policies, and the model or frame of reference which may bring its own format and language.

Useful general rules include:

- make a clear statement of the eventual outcome of therapy
- select an outcome which has a realistic prospect of being achieved
- if necessary work towards it in defined stages using specific objectives
- specify the outcome in a way which enables progress to be assessed
- review objectives regularly in relation to goals and overall aim(s).

Produce an action plan

An action plan is a formal record of what the therapist intends to do in the course of providing the patient with therapy. In the case of intervention – when the therapist is taking action on behalf of the patient or client, rather than offering direct treatment – it may be useful to write an action plan stating what is to be achieved, how, when and by whom. The basic principles have been described in the description of the problem-solving process (Chapter 9).

The plan must state briefly:

- what is to be done
- when
- in what sequence
- By whom.

The plan should have a defined timescale and a means of review. A plan may need modification as it is implemented, and these changes should be noted. Once the plan has been carried out a new plan should evolve, or intervention be ended.

An action plan may relate to therapy, indicating how a treatment plan is to be implemented, or to intervention, showing actions the therapist will take on the patient's behalf, e.g. talking to others, phone calls or obtaining resources. Action planning can also be used with the client to provide him with a structure for taking action to solve his own problem.

Define a means of measuring the outcome of the plan

Outcome measures are contentious and are discussed later in this chapter (p. 188). Defining a measurable outcome is not a simple matter. Even where the outcome relates to some measurable physical change or change in performance or behaviour there may be difficulties in specifying the desired change and in measuring if it has occurred. Where the outcome relates to a subjective aspect of the patient's life the difficulties are compounded. How does one measure the 'feel good' factor?

Measures which are purely quantitative may become reductive and mechanistic; measures which are qualitative rely on subjective reporting which is inevitably biased to some extent.

It is hard enough to provide an outcome measure which can show that something has changed. Proving that the change was due to the intervention of the occupational therapist may be even more difficult, if not impossible.

This should not be taken as a negative and pessimistic view which dismisses outcome measures as impossible, but as a realistic appraisal of the difficulties and the need for much more research to be undertaken.

STAGE 3: IMPLEMENTATION OF ACTION (Table 12.3)

Put the plan into action

At this point therapy is provided or intervention is begun. If the preceding description has seemed lengthy this must be seen in relation to its importance as part of the process, rather than to the time it takes. As previously noted, the time required for the essential procedures of data gathering and planning is variable.

Providing therapy

Given the wide variation in type of patient and location of therapy, it would be impractical to attempt to describe the infinitely variable range of potential action taken by a therapist. This is covered in many other textbooks related to applied occupational therapy.

Table 12.3 Stage 3: implementation of action

Procedure	Examples of reasoning/action
Put plan into action	Talk, treat, 'phone, write, liaise, visit, meet, discuss, counsel, advise, set up, install, design, experiment, develop. All actions are taken with reference to the patient and others involved with the case. The therapist engages in a continued inner dialogue concerning the patient and the process and progress of therapy.
Obtain further information or assessment data if required	Are there aspects of the case which need more investigation? Confusions, puzzles? Things which do not 'add up'. What can be done to acquire more information? Any special assessment required? How can hypotheses best be tested?
Continuous review of progress	Is the plan working? Timescale slipping? Treatment producing or not producing expected results? Other people doing what is needed? Patient's views?

Description becomes detailed and complex if therapy is viewed only as observed action, but therapy also involves thought. As previously discussed, there is still much research to be done on clinical reasoning – how therapists think during the treatment process – yet it seems to me that it is this reasoning process which is likely to be the more stable factor. What is done may vary, but how the occupational therapist uses clinical reasoning to monitor and adapt these actions is a core part of professional practice and identity, and should be what distinguishes occupational therapy practice from that of any other, similar, profession.

One of the essential features of occupational therapy (with a few exceptions involving the use of very structured techniques) is its dynamic, improvisational quality. Although a session may be carefully planned, with both activity and environment structured and adapted, what happens when the therapist and patient interact through the medium of the activity – when the central triad comes into operation – is essentially spontaneous and unpredictable.

The occupational therapist may 'script' an event, but the script is for guidance only; it is not a blueprint which must be adhered to without deviation. The therapy session relies on the therapist's ability, through therapeutic use of self and personal skills, to adapt, improvise, and react to and make use of circumstances and the reality of the quality of action and interaction. This is true whether the therapy is aimed at improving physical, cognitive, or psychosocial aspects of function.

This is where the therapist's internal monitor, the 'therapist of the mind' plays, its part so that while the therapist is acting and interacting, there is a simultaneous cognitive dialogue which observes, corrects, adjusts, tweaks, cues, prompts, moves therapy in the desired direction, gets it back on track, problem-solves and capitalizes on events which contribute to the process. This is the process of 'thinking in action' which Schon (1983) describes. Much of it becomes swift and automatic, so that it seems intuitive.

The starting points for therapy are the goals and objectives which have been negotiated with the patient. The therapist must combine both managerial and clinical skills. Listing these actions as a kind of checklist risks reduction of a complex process into a mechanistic sequence and may seem like a simplistic statement of the obvious. In reality the process is complex, interactive and may take a variable length of time. The following list relates only to the preliminary actions needed to set up a therapy session (Box 12.2). It is included principally as a reminder that for each and every patient a continuous sequence of managerial and clinical decisions and actions must be taken.

For the experienced therapist such actions become routine and flow smoothly, but for a student or novice practitioner they may seem daunting, and the sequence appears neither simple nor obvious. Service managers from other disciplines may also not appreciate the time involved in setting up and delivering the process of therapy.

Actions required to initiate therapy

Actions, all of which should be recorded, include those listed in Box 12.2.

The crucial actions are deciding on the precise nature of therapy, which requires the use of clinical reasoning in conjunction with occupational and environmental analysis (as described in Chs 14 and 15), and then critically testing these decisions to ensure that therapy is relevant, acceptable to the patient, likely to be effective, and compatible with the basic philosophy of occupational therapy as modified by any chosen approach.

Each therapy session requires thought and preparation, and the time needed for this must not be underestimated. It can be difficult to convey the importance of such preparation to non-therapists, just as it can be difficult to justify time spent on reflection following therapy, yet both are essential parts of good practice and the provision of a quality service. Occupational therapy cannot be provided on a 'conveyer belt' basis to a continuous flow of patients. This being the case, it is even more incumbent on the therapist to justify therapy and give evidence of efficacy.

Box 12.2   Actions required to initiate therapy

1. Decide what type of therapy is required to achieve the objective(s).
2. Decide the precise nature of treatment for the next week – medium, activity, technique, location and personnel involved.
3. Decide the intensity of treatment required and relate this to the urgency and priority of the case and consequent timescale.
4. Note resource implications – personnel, costs and time.
5. Initiate preparations for specific activities, groups or experiences.
6. Note other therapy or interventions which the patient currently receives and implications for therapy.
7. Make appointments or draw up treatment programme. Arrange transport if required.
8. Note the people with whom decisions must be communicated; ensure this is done. Delegate actions as required.
9. Note how this patient integrates with, or conflicts with, the existing caseload; make any consequent alterations to this or other treatment plans.
10. Check that decisions can be justified and that objective(s) are being met; check that suitable outcome measures have been included so that effectiveness of therapy can be measured. Set a date for review.
11. Take time to explain the intentions and process of therapy to the patient (and others if necessary).

Intervention on behalf of the client

Planning and carrying out intervention – action by the therapist on behalf of the client – is primarily a managerial process. Once the objective has been jointly decided on, the therapist will:

1. Decide what actions are required to achieve the objective.
2. Decide the order in which the actions should be taken.
3. Decide the urgency, priority and consequent timescale.
4. Note resource implications – personnel, costs and time.

These decisions are recorded as part of the action plan. The plan is then carried out and action taken is recorded as it occurs, together with any problems or consequences which are relevant. Once all the required actions have been successfully completed the therapist can either move to another intervention or close the case. This may not be a simple as it sounds, bearing in mind that the therapist is normally dealing with many such action plans for a whole caseload.

Obtain further information or assessment data if required and review progress

Ongoing assessment is part of therapy and is built into the treatment process as both formal and informal procedures.

As intervention or therapy progresses there may well be the need for more information to provide facts about performance, or more background to the case. Confusions and puzzles need exploration; sometimes things do not 'add up' in the therapist's mind and contradictions or anomalies must be explored. Changes must be quantified and described clearly. Assessment in the sense of a continuous monitoring and review of progress of the process and results of therapy is essential, and the results must be recorded.

STAGE 4: REVIEW OF ACTION AND OUTCOMES (Table 12.4)

The question of reviewing outcomes and evaluating intervention is so crucial that it will be discussed separately in the next section.

Revision of plan

Unless the objective was simple and easily achieved the treatment plan will require continuous revision to ensure progress. It is often difficult for an inexperienced therapist to know how fast progress should be. Does the patient require 'pushing' or is he being put under too much pressure? Rates of progress are intensely individual and there is no simple formula.

Table 12.4 Stage 4: review of action and outcome

Procedure	Examples of reasoning
Review outcomes in relation to goals and objectives	Have objectives been met? How well? Clinically effective? Cost-effective? Speed of progress/ action? Objective measures? Subjective measures? What next? Patient's views? Others' views?
Adapt/revise plan if required	Changes; what is the next stage? How to move things in direction of desired outcome? New problems? New solutions? Has aim been attained? Is intervention completed?

Even slow progress may be worthwhile, but if progress has ceased, the therapist must consider whether this is simply a plateau before the next improvement, or whether the ceiling of achievement has been reached. Nothing at all is gained by recording a static condition for an extended period of time: either treatment is ineffective and should be ended, or a different goal or objective should be chosen.

EVALUATION OF THE OUTCOMES OF INTERVENTION

Evaluation is carried out both formally and informally, but it is the formal, structured methods, described as audit, which are most valid and relevant. The term 'audit' is derived from the process of critically checking accounts which is carried out by an independent auditor. It implies that something is scrutinized, quantified and measured; this is relatively easy when it concerns figures or materials, but is very hard when it refers to evaluating people and the processes and outcomes of therapy.

The measurement of outcomes is an integral part of quality assurance (QA) which has been adopted into health care services from industry. Donabedian's approach to QA in health care (1980) is often quoted; he uses three headings, structure, process and outcomes, to define the three main components of a service. WHO (1988) defines the objectives of QA as improving 'the outcome of all health care in terms of health, functional ability, patient well-being and consumer satisfaction.' Whalley Hammell (1994) defines outcome measures in occupational therapy as referring to 'an end product in terms of health, performance and satisfaction'.

Evaluation of outcomes is a complex process but one which is essential. Unfortunately it is beset by controversial issues, by imprecise and still-evolving methodology and terminology, and by the conflicting interests of service providers, users and managers, who tend to interpret it in different ways.

Austin & Clark (1993), in discussing outcome measures, write that:

Each perspective will yield different priorities . . . in brief, the patient values subjective qualitative measures that summarize personal experiences, the manager requires reliable quantitative measures that summarize collective experiences, and therapists need both types of measures.

Therapists additionally need information for evaluation and development of practice.

Quality assurance requires a mixture of professional and managerial skills and knowledge, and has connections with both intervention and resource management, but since it should be an integral part of intervention it is introduced in this chapter.

I find it most helpful to consider QA as being conducted by means of three linked and overlapping forms of audit: clinical audit, quality audit and service audit.

CLINICAL AUDIT

Clinical audit is derived from medical audit which is defined in *Working for Patients* (NHS 1988) as 'a systematic critical analysis of the quality of medical care including the procedures used for diagnosis and treatment, the use of resources, and the resulting outcome for patients'.

Clinical audit requires standards to be set, and some means of measuring the outcomes of intervention. Because it is an audit of clinical practice, much may depend on professional judgement, and it therefore needs to be carried out primarily by the profession involved.

Informal clinical audit is a continuing process in every intervention, as the individual therapist evaluates what she is doing with and on behalf of the client, and asks whether her interventions are having the required effect, and what might need to be changed to improve the outcome.

Formal clinical audit provides the therapist with the means of evaluating personal practice against an accepted criterion of what is 'good'. It provides evidence that therapy is effective, and leads to the development of improved therapeutic techniques, or to personal development for the therapist. It may raise research questions.

It provides managers with evidence that the services which are purchased are worth purchasing, and the client with evidence that the process of therapy is worth engaging in, and that results have been achieved in line with the outcomes which he and the therapist have agreed.

QUALITY AUDIT

This is concerned both with what was done, and also, crucially, how well it was done. Again, the implication is that there are standards which have been set, and a procedure whereby the degree to which they have been met can be evaluated. Quality audit has both managerial and professional components.

Quality audit may be undertaken by means of case review, questionnaires, surveys and structured interviews. Typical questions may include: has this intervention been carried out to the set standard? Is the user (patient/client/consumer) satisfied? Could it have been done better? How can the service be improved?

User satisfaction may further be gauged by appraising the content of complaints, or by informal meetings, interviews, or quality circles in which both staff and users participate. Comment from those external to the system, such as the Health Advisory Service, management consultants or pressure groups of various kinds may be considered. Surveys or questionnaires may be used.

Quality audit provides the client with standards against which service provision can be evaluated, and a means whereby opinions on the service may be relayed back to the providers. It provides

managers with evidence that resources are being used for high quality services. It provides therapists with feedback on actual provision, and an incentive to strive to continually improve service provision.

SERVICE AUDIT

This is primarily a managerial exercise concerned with quantifying the manner in which the process of intervention has been delivered. It typically involves setting standards, policies and procedures for efficient service provision, and then checking that these have been adhered to, e.g. that each patient referred will be interviewed within 3 days of receipt of referral, that a waiting list should have a set limit or that records should be kept in a particular form. It may include statistical records which quantify service use and check cost-effectiveness or the use of resources.

The production of 'league tables' featuring a 'star rating system' by means of which aspects of service in different hospitals may be compared is an example of service audit.

Because it deals with quantifiable aspects of service structure and process it is, in comparison with clinical or quality audit, easier to undertake, and can unfortunately sometimes be seen as a substitute for these more nebulous, but ultimately more significant forms of audit.

This process may be undertaken by clinicians, but, provided that relevant standards have been set, may be carried out by managers or administrators.

Service audit provides managers with evidence that intervention is efficient and cost-effective, and is meeting set objectives or priorities. It provides therapists with feedback on organizational aspects of the service. It may provide the client with information concerning service standards and the use of public resources.

SUMMARY OF FORMS OF AUDIT

There are three overlapping forms of audit, which consider different aspects of intervention; each is of interest to managers, therapists and clients from differing perspectives.

Clinical audit evaluates the outcomes of intervention, in relation to set objectives or criteria, and accepted standards of good professional practice.

Quality audit evaluates structure, process and outcomes, focusing on how well intervention was provided, and suggests ways in which it might be improved.

Service audit measures quantifiable aspects of the structure and process of intervention, against set targets.

Since quality audit and service audit are, to a large extent, concerned with the management of resources they will be discussed in Chapter 17.

CLINICAL AUDIT

OBJECTIVES OF CLINICAL AUDIT

Clinical audit has three main objectives:

- ensuring that good standards of practice are maintained
- evaluating outcomes of interventions
- developing good practice.

It has to be recognized that clinical audit (indeed, all forms of audit) take time and resources, which need to be allocated and not simply 'stolen' from an already busy working schedule.

Clinical audit depends on access to standards and outcome measures which can be used as criteria of evaluation. A standard is a statement defining one aspect of the methods, circumstances and resources of a level of provision. Standards may be set nationally, by government departments or professional bodies, locally by health providers and purchasers, and by individual therapists.

A standard ought to be attainable; there is little point in having over-idealized standards, and there are usually resource implications for standard maintenance and development. For this reason standards may be 'minimum', defining levels below which the service should not be permitted to slip, rather than a target to be achieved.

Standards are not fixed and permanent; they change as expectations and techniques develop. In any system of standards the essential feature is a method of regular review and revision, to see that 'goal-posts' are appropriate, and, when necessary, are moved. It is especially important for individual practitioners to remain abreast of current research and the development of good practice, and to ensure that personal standards match these.

There is some confusion between the objectives and outcomes of intervention. This is best resolved by regarding an objective as an expression of intention, and an outcome as the actual result. An outcome may also be a wider result, dealing with cost-effective use of resources, individual patient satisfaction, well-being or health, or wider socioeconomic implications. It may be helpful to use the term 'clinical outcome' or 'intervention outcome', when describing the results of intervention for an individual.

An outcome measure is a means whereby the final result can be evaluated and, where possible, quantified. This may be in relation to a set standard or procedure, an objective, a functional attainment, patient satisfaction, the known normal efficacy of an intervention, or any one of numerous other measures.

ENSURING GOOD STANDARDS OF PRACTICE

THERAPY PROTOCOLS

Earlier in this chapter I emphasized the individual improvisational nature of occupational therapy, which cannot, and should not, be reduced to a formula. While this is true in respect of an individual treatment plan and a single therapy session, it would be misleading to conclude that there are no constants when planning therapy for a given type of patient.

There is usually, in each situation, a set of actions which may be appropriate and other actions which are not. For a given treatment location it should be possible to define certain standard approaches or procedures and to describe the occupational therapy service, albeit in generalized terms, without falling into the trap of devising stereotyped treatment formulae. There are groups of patients with relatively homogenous characteristics and needs, and where these can be identified it may be possible to describe the principles of therapy.

Managers will, rightly, require information on the treatment that is being offered, to whom, by whom, when, where, why, how, how often, to what aim and at what cost. These simple headings, translated into applicable professional terminology, form the basis of a protocol, which can have many uses.

Occupational therapy protocols state what occupational therapy does or intends to do in given situations. They can be used for service planning, and negotiating for resources, setting standards, research, education and training and role definition. (Warren 1993)

To this list may be added marketing of services and development of outcome measures.

A protocol, as described by Warren, may be either a managerial or a clinical document, or both. Managerially, it is a more limited version of service documents which may be called operational policies, mission statements, business plans, or various other titles which tend to change with managerial fashion! These are useful documents, but are somewhat beyond the scope of this text.

The more interesting use of protocols is as clinical guidelines which define a service to a target group of patients. Warren points out that, apart from the usefulness of the completed document, the act of producing it is itself very instructive, and concludes:

The protocol is simply a tool to help occupational therapists to clarify thoughts and ideas, to commit these to paper in an organized way, and to present them coherently. Protocols allow the exchange and sharing of information and experience.

A protocol may be presented as text or by using a grid or flowchart. The chief requirements are brevity, clarity, simplicity and avoidance of excessive jargon. The protocol should be specific to its area of use and should describe what is actually done, not some idealized version of this which cannot be sustained in practice. A protocol may represent good practice, but may

not necessarily be transferable or replicable without adaptation.

Protocols have their drawbacks. For one thing, they are frequently diagnosis-based – they describe 'how to treat × condition'. Bearing in mind that therapists treat *people* and not conditions, and that therapy ought to be occupationally referenced, it becomes much harder to write a relevant protocol. A protocol can easily become tight and prescriptive and can be seen as 'holy writ' from which deviation is impossible. This can be avoided by resisting the temptation to describe therapy routines or procedures in exhaustive detail.

It may, however, be difficult to write a protocol for occupational therapy which is not diagnosis-linked and which is, at the same time, sufficiently prescriptive to satisfy a purchaser who wants to know what he is getting, how long it will take and what it will cost, as opposed to a long list of 'ifs, buts and maybes'.

AUDIT BY OTHER THERAPISTS

One approach to ensuring good standards is to allow one's cases to be examined at intervals by experienced therapists who can comment on what was done in terms of relevance, compliance with good practice and effectiveness.

There are various ways in which this can be done: by means of regular supervision, through case presentations and discussions and by peer group audit. As a collective procedure this often has rapid results in crystallizing ideas about practice within a particular service location, smoothing procedures, and sharing information and expertise.

Peer group audit has the following objectives (Johnson 1992):

- to identify common patterns and changes in health and social care
- to monitor the delivery of occupational therapy, including intervention and outcomes
- to develop intervention models and strategies which ensure resources are used to best effect and meet clients' needs
- to aid research.

Audit must take place against a background of

set standards, up-to-date information on research and intervention techniques, and case records which are kept in a manner which facilitates audit.

During audit, it is important to consider both positive and negative outcomes, to explore strengths and weaknesses of intervention and to make consequent improvements in service delivery.

It is important that clinical audit is carried out in an atmosphere of mutual respect, trust and exploration, not in a defensive or protective manner.

OUTCOME MEASURES

An outcome means that something has changed because of the action taken by the therapist with or on behalf of the client, or by the client as part of his therapy. Deciding whether change has occurred and quantifying the degree to which this has happened sounds straightforward, but it is not.

There has been much discussion concerning outcome measures most applicable to occupational therapy. An outcome measure needs to compare progress over time, in relation to intervention.

Austin & Clark (1993) list three types of outcome measures:

- Measures of health status: functional assessment and well-being
- Clinical indicators and measures: treatment aims and clinical observations
- Patient satisfaction: perceptions of process and outcomes

Jeffrey (1993) lists the following classifications of outcome measures:

- disorder-specific measures, demonstrating changes in the clinical condition of the patient
- functional status measures, illustrating changes in ADL or IADL (synonymous with DADL)
- mental health status measures, e.g. social adjustment, dependency/independence, role effectiveness

- global health status measures
- quality of life measures
- comprehensive rehabilitation measures
- consumer satisfaction outcomes.

She further describes the purpose of outcome measures as:

- providing a baseline measure of function
- monitoring progress
- comparison of similar cases
- formulating and altering intervention plans
- prediction: of functional improvement, level of independence, placement on discharge, needs for support or care
- to enhance interprofessional communication
- to establish effectiveness of clinical input.

Whalley Hammell (1994b) adds:

- demonstrating the effectiveness of occupational therapy to funding agencies and other care-givers
- improving the quality of care
- clarifying the role of occupational therapy.

In order to measure something one must first define clearly what is being measured, secondly find a reliable and valid instrument or procedure by which it can be measured, and finally, place a correct interpretation on the results. None of these activities is simple, and all are subject to criticism.

MEASURES OF HEALTH STATUS

What is meant by health? This is a complex question, as measures of personal health and well-being are essentially subjective, and are also culturally determined. The usual approach to this is reductive, 'homing in' on one area of health, perhaps as described by a particular frame of reference, and attempting to define things which can be measured. However, as Cynkin & Robinson (1990) describe, occupational therapists tend to view health holistically, and as expressed by participation in activities.

In the context of an emphasis on human activities health (and its practical correlate function) is manifested in the ability of the individual to participate in socio-culturally regulated activities with satisfaction and comfort.

FUNCTIONAL MEASURES

Since occupational therapy aims to improve function, attention has tended to concentrate on the use of functional outcome measures. Thus ADL indices such as the Barthel index have been proposed; if the patient is assessed at the start of therapy and shows a measurable improvement at the end of it, it can be said that therapy was effective.

But can it? The energetic debate over the Barthel index in the British Journal of Occupational Therapy during 1992–1993 (Murdock 1992a,b, Shah & Cooper 1993, Eakin 1993) indicates the pitfalls. In the first place, how reliable is the tool for measurement? Clearly the Barthel index is one of the better constructed and more standardized of occupational therapy ADL indices, yet it is not without its critics.

It is a narrow checklist, which was designed for use in institutional settings with elderly patients suffering from a limited range of conditions. Can it be generalized? Can the various versions be amalagamated and restandardized? Is improvement of function in a narrow range of PADL alone a sufficient measure? Is the scoring and weighting system subjective or objective? Even the relationship between functional ability and health is unclear. Every question is a research proposal in the making.

If the statistical validity and reliability of even a well-designed test can be questioned, the validity of the 'DIY' tests and indices which are still used by the majority of departments in the UK (McAvoy 1991) is questionable.

Is ADL performance a good outcome measure? This is also disputed. It depends on how one defines ADL, and on whether ADL performance can be seen as predictive of other aspects of recovery or rehabilitation. Again, opinions vary.

Functional improvement measures are often tied to a biomechanical frame of reference, which equates improvement with direct physical treatment of the patient, and often ignores social or environmental factors.

Although function in PADL is a commonly used assessment, therapists certainly deal with many other aspects of life, and outcome measures for, e.g. DADL (IADL), social skills, work skills, cognitive-perceptual skills, would be required to give a wide enough spread to cover all occupational therapy interventions.

Fricke (1993) reviews the whole question of outcome measures and points out the problems and questions with great clarity. There are practical and technical difficulties in every aspect – validity, administration, complexity, reliability, content, interpretation, inter-rater reliability, scoring and weighting. (Some of these issues are discussed in Chapter 13).

It is clear that the profession is faced with a dilemma: unless a way can be found of measuring complex performances which complies in every respect with the strictest criteria for validity, outcome measures using functional tests are bound to remain suspect. Are there, then, alternatives?

McCulloch (1991) examined various measures and concluded that, since occupational therapy aims to improve subjective well-being as well as objective function, the measure should take this into account. Having discarded general health indicators such as the Rosser matrix and the quality-adjusted life year (QALY) as inapplicable to occupational therapy, he proposes that the functional limitations profile (FLP) which considers an individual's subjective view of functional limitations, offers a possible instrument for outcome measurement which might be adapted for use in occupational therapy. This may offer scope, but clearly requires much work and research before it could be widely used.

The Canadian Association of Occupational Therapists Task Force used the occupational performance model as a basis to investigate available outcome measures (Law et al 1990, Pollock et al 1990). They identified a total of 136 assessments, of which, when sifted through to exclude those which were unstandardized, unpublished, or which dealt only with skill components, 41 assessments remained to be evaluated.

The task force concluded that eight measures were compatible with the model, but that all had drawbacks. They proceeded to develop a new measure, the Canadian Occupational Performance Measure (COPM), as a specific outcome measure for occupational therapy.

The criteria used to construct the measure included:

- Clinical utility – easy to administer.
- Responsiveness – specifically able to detect clinically important changes expected from occupational therapy intervention.
- Purpose – to evaluate not simply functional ability, or what a client *can* do, but actual functional performance, or what a client *does* do, in relation to the expectations of the client, his environment and his role.
- Standardization – a standard method of use.
- Reliability – the therapist should be able to use it with confidence.
- Validity – content validity related to the concerns of occupational therapy.

The COPM involves problem definition, in areas of productivity leisure and self-care, problem weighting (in accordance with client's priorities and needs), scoring, re-assessment following intervention and follow-up. This measure is still undergoing development and standardization.

In Appendix 2, a list of functional measures of various types is given, which includes a selection of those standardized tests which have recently been reviewed in published papers, and have been suggested as suitable, to varying degrees, as outcome measures. It should be noted that these are not all developed by, or specifically for, occupational therapists.

The most important points to emerge from this list are that:

- There are now more than enough standardized tests to provide a basis for the development of good outcome measures.
- There is little excuse for using non-standardized tests when so many standardized ones are available. A therapist who has developed and standardized a 'good' test should publish it.
- Many of the most valid and reliable tests do not originate in the UK and may need re-standardization for a UK population.

- The perfect functional outcome measure has yet to be invented.

The development of improved functional outcome measures is clearly an urgent necessity, but given the complexities involved, these measures will take many years to perfect; meanwhile, therapists cannot practice without some means of measuring outcomes.

USING OBJECTIVES AS OUTCOME MEASURES

One possible avenue is to use the achievement of objectives set for therapy or intervention to provide measurable outcomes. This is a problem-based criterion-referenced approach in which the goals are specified in a precise manner which means that attainment can be quantified. COPM is also an example of this approach.

Whalley Hammell (1994) states that:

Identification of the attainment of an objective is a measurement of outcome, which assesses the results of therapy services in promoting effective change in the client's status.

Baseline assessment provides information on the conditions prior to intervention. Whether the goal is that the patient should be able to return to work, or to sustain a conversation for 10 minutes, or to dress with a specified aid, it should be possible to say whether or not, after a given period of time, this has been achieved. The goal therefore becomes an individual criterion for effective therapy.

Although these criteria are relevant only to the individual, it is possible to obtain some measure of overall effectiveness from the percentage of objectives which were achieved. It is a useful measure, for example, to be able to state that 90% of objectives set at the commencement of therapy were attained at the point of discharge; further analysis might point out differences between the types of objectives which were and were not met.

There are objections to this method as, along with other methods, it does depend on the goals being measured. It might, arguably, be possible to set small and trivial objectives in order to show that these were achieved, and the means whereby achievement is judged may be fallible. Austin & Clark (1993) point out that 'patients may lack insight into the severity of their illness. This can impede negotiation of treatment goals and the development of an agreed realistic treatment plan ... the consequent need for sometimes repeated renegotiation of goals seriously complicates the interpretation of measures of outcome.' Nonetheless, this system does offer some scope for outcome measurement.

Medical indicators, such as symptom reduction or relief of pain may be used, but these tend to be less relevant to therapists.

CAN WE PROVE THAT OCCUPATIONAL THERAPY IS EFFECTIVE?

The point of outcome measures is that they should indicate that occupational therapy is effective for any given patient. The major difficulty in this is that, even if accurate measures can be developed, the patient is seldom treated by the therapist in isolation, but rather by a team.

How, then, will it be possible to say that it was occupational therapy intervention which was the major contributor to the improvement? Medical and even social problems resolve spontaneously. Will the improvement last? If the patient is 'back to square one' 3 months later, what was the point of costly intervention?

As with the discussion over assessment methodology, this is not an argument for throwing up our hands and doing nothing, but for a determined effort to undertake applied research, and to develop appropriate outcome measures, related to clearly defined service provision.

DEVELOPING GOOD PRACTICE

The methods which I have just described all contribute to the development of good practice, but they tend to be rigid and structured procedures. An important aspect of practice is capturing

the 'art'. This is difficult to achieve by methods of audit which focus on standards, procedures and protocols, useful though these can be. An important method of developing practice is through personal reflection.

REFLECTION ON PRACTICE

As described by Schon (1983, 1987), professionals typically 'know more than they can say'. It takes time to develop the skill of simultaneous monitoring and adapting of therapy, and only experienced and expert therapists are able to demonstrate it in an advanced form. Even experts (perhaps, especially experts) have trouble in describing the reasons for these apparently intuitive actions.

Novice practitioners are seldom able instantly to be adaptive and often need to stop and withdraw from a situation, and to analyse what is going on and what happens next as a retrospective reflective exercise in order to adapt the session next time.

Reflection following a session is important, even for experienced practitioners. Despite subliminally noticing what was happening one cannot always catch, or react to, all the nuances when one is closely involved. There are, of course, some situations where the therapist must act quickly to prevent a problem or manage a crisis, with no time for reflection until later. No therapist can hope to 'get it right' every time.

Reflection on practice can be described as 'emotion and action recollected in tranquillity'. Reflection should enable the therapist to understand not only what happened, and whether it was effective and why, but also the more subtle and symbolic elements of a situation.

Reflection, although objective in that it deals with a real event, must inevitably be a subjective process, part of which is becoming aware of any biases and assumptions which may have influenced action. Fish et al (1991) proposed that a four strand approach to reflection might be used (Box 12.3):

This is clearly a process which takes time, and it might be impractical to undertake it on every occasion. However, as a means of analysing

Box 12.3 The four strand approach to reflection (Fish et al 1991)

The factual strand	What actually happened and what did you feel, think and do? This should be recorded as soon as possible after the event. It includes setting the scene, telling the story and pinpointing critical incidents. In this it can be related to Mattingly's process of narrative reasoning (1991a, b).
The retrospective strand	This involves looking back over the whole event, seeking patterns and meanings; and reviewing intentions, process, outcomes and personal views.
The substratum strand	This is an exploration of the hidden agenda: what assumptions, beliefs, culture, customs, attitudes or values underlie the event – both your own and those of other participants. Environmental demand might be considered here, or the subtexts of clinical reasoning, or the less obvious effects of an approach.
The connective strand	At this point the implications for future practice are thought through: is there relevance to theory? Are concepts or assumptions challenged? What was learned? What could change? Is a research question suggested?

practice at intervals, or when there is a need to 'unpack' a difficult or complex situation, it offers a practical and useful tool for improving therapy and developing personal mastery and expertise.

Reflections can be shared with others, as a part of professional education, supervision or peer review. As a part of student education it is invaluable, for only by exploring and understanding the dynamics of practice and discussing it with others can a student develop as a competent practitioner.

RESEARCH INTO INTERVENTION

As has been discussed, therapists work increasingly in a market-based environment where managers seek demonstrable outcomes and evidence that money spent on therapy is money well spent. Applied research, testing the efficacy of intervention, is becoming essential. Research is really no more than an extension of the continuum of professional inquiry manifested in all the forms of audit and personal professional development. It is concerned with posing, and trying to answer, some of the numerous questions which are brought to light in the course of everyday practice.

The move from enclosed and self-perpetuating professional training into the academic rigour of mainstream higher education and the development of graduate programmes and post-basic degrees has, finally, meant that both applied research and basic research into the science of occupations and occupational therapy is seen as a necessity.

In the past, therapists have tended to view research as a somewhat arcane process, which was too demanding, impractical or time-consuming to undertake. These attitudes are changing, but the problems remain; it is not easy to conduct research into occupational therapy.

Most of the arguments over research methodology are those which will be re-stated in relation to assessment and the use of outcome measures. Research is merely a more refined and stringent application of similar techniques.

There are two basic forms of research, qualitative and quantitative, and the merits and problems of each are discussed at length. Yerxa (1987) advocates qualitative methods and proposes that quantitative methods, being based in scientific method, are alien to the holistic philosophy and practice of therapy, while others, e.g. Stewart (1990), Carlson & Clark (1991) and Kielhofner (1992) support the use of both methods.

In addition, there is conflict over the legitimate areas for occupational therapy research. Pure research and basic research have been linked to occupational science, which is itself controversial.

To make matters even more complex, the fundamental nature of scientific inquiry is subject to criticism on various philosophical grounds, relating to the theory-dependency of observation, the validity of induction and the problems of falsification (Polgar & Thomas 1991).

Quantitative methods

Quantitative methodology has the advantage of a long and respected scientific pedigree. Deitz (1993) divides types of quantitative research into group research and single system research.

Group research

Group research may be subdivided into experimental research, correlation research and descriptive research. Each of these has different purposes and methods.

Experimental research follows a set procedure. Having defined a specific question or hypothesis in relation to a given population an appropriately sized sample is selected. The sample is divided into groups, either randomly or by a process of matching. An experimental design is then chosen.

The design is crucial in ensuring internal and external validity. Internal validity confirms that the effect on the dependent variable can be attributed to the independent variable, while external validity means that the results can be generalized from the sample to the population.

In pre-test/post-test design, measurements are taken before and after intervention. In post-test design, outcomes only are measured, and the results of the experimental group and control group are compared to measure change. Factorial design enables the investigator to compare the effects of two independent variables on the dependent variable. All of these designs have advantages and disadvantages in terms of internal validity. It is essential that the design controls the dependent and independent variables and eliminates the effects of extraneous circumstances.

Problems of potential observer bias, or the effects on the subjects of being observed, can be reduced by blind and double-blind methods, in which the subjects and/or the person conducting the experiment are unaware of the nature or procedure of the research. This may, however, raise ethical concerns.

The rigorous conditions for experimental research are hard to achieve except in laboratory conditions, and are of questionable use in occupational therapy, where there are too many variables to control. Quasi-experimental methods may therefor be used. Naturalistic studies 'involve the comparison of two naturally occurring groups in relation to one or more measures' (Polgar & Thomas 1991).

Correlation research 'determines the extent to which two or more phenomena tend to occur together' (Deitz 1993). While these methods produce valid results about comparisons between groups they do not necessarily indicate causational links to explain these differences, although hypotheses may be generated. Extraneous variables may intrude and affect results.

Descriptive designs frequently use survey methods, questionnaires or interviews to obtain numerical data. A normative study would be designed to find out what the average state of a given population might be. Such surveys require large samples for validity. Descriptive studies of this kind are relatively simple to undertake (at least when compared to other methods) and are therefore a popular method with therapists.

Single system research

Single subject (or system) design takes an individual or single group and examines the effect of an intervention using the baseline of the pre-test condition with which to compare results following intervention. Alternatively, a multiple baseline design may be used. As with experimental design for groups, there are different single subject designs such as A B, A B C, A B A and A B A B. There are arguments for and against each design. For example, the A B A design, which requires therapy to be withdrawn from an individual for a period, may be ethically unacceptable.

Strengths and weaknesses

Quantitative research depends on statistical analysis of results to indicate amounts, probabilities, and correlations. These days much of this can be done by a computer, which greatly enhances the speed and complexity of calculations and visual presentation of data.

The strengths of the quantitative methodology are also, paradoxically, some of its weaknesses.

Its very precision and the desire, in the search for validity, to control all elements of the research situation, make it potentially inflexible, narrow and artificial. Further problems relate to the technicalities of experimental design, ethical considerations, and possible statistical and sampling errors.

Qualitative methods

Qualitative methods of research have been developed over recent decades by sociologists, anthropologists, educationalists and other professionals who share a phenomenological perspective, emphasizing the interactions of people and environments, and the need to explore complex relationships, meanings and patterns which arise in natural situations. Since occupational therapy has more of the features of a social science than of a pure science, these techniques offer scope for research in areas where experimental or quasi-experimental techniques are inappropriate.

There is a fundamental difference in intention between qualitative and quantitative methods. In quantitative research the aim is to prove or disprove the hypothesis or to quantify and describe the problem: one starts with a specific question. In the qualitative approach the aim is to understand the complexity and subjective meanings of a situation. Whereas quantitative research adopts a 'top-down' approach, starting with a known problem and exploring its nature, qualitative methods are applied 'bottom-up'. By describing processes and the realities of experience, theories are developed; this type of data is called 'grounded theory'. It may serve to identify problems or to create hypotheses for later quantitative research (Glaser & Strauss 1967).

In the course of the research, methodology may be developed and even changed as the situation is explored and understood: this is especially so in the illuminative approach. 'Qualitative research designs range from being loose and emergent to relatively pre-structured' (Deitz 1993). 'Loose' forms involve the researcher immersing herself in and experiencing a situation alongside the participants for an extended period of time, and, in various ways, describing, recording, analysing and explaining it. Techniques include extended interviews, observations, diaries, and video and tape recordings. More structured methods include semi-structured interviews, surveys, open questionnaires and case studies.

Robertson (1988) and Kielhofner (1992) list a number of qualitative approaches. Ethnography seeks to understand a situation from the point of view of the participants, with special reference to their individual beliefs, perception and feelings. Action research is a focused and systematic attempt to evaluate a possible solution to a problem, or the effects of a specific change. A case study involves an in-depth and prolonged study of one individual or environment. The illuminative approach is designed to provide an understanding of complex situations. Since this methodology is still relatively unfamiliar in comparison with the experimental approach, it may be helpful to give examples.

An ethnographic study was conducted by Dyck (1992). The abstract explains that:

This paper addresses the occupational behaviour of mothers of young children, focusing on the relationships between the environment, the women's mothering role, and their daily routines. . . . the use of qualitative methods and a socio-political perspective revealed the meanings the women's mothering role has for them, and the ways in which its content and enactment are shaped within a wider context of social and economic relationships.

Dyck notes that 'Methodologically, it is a considerable challenge to operationalize a socio-political model in empirical research'. This study, conducted on a normal population, represents basic research into occupational science, and Dyck concludes that through it 'we are able to enhance our knowledge of the shaping of occupations and goal directed action essential to the grounding and further development of occupational therapy's theoretical base.'

An applied study was carried out by Hasselkus (1992), entitled 'The meaning of activity: day care for persons with Alzheimer disease'. The researcher used ethnographic interviewing and participant observation to 'gain understanding of the meaning of the daily routines and activities at the day care centre'. The study provided a description of the interventions, and intentions, reactions and emotions of staff. Hasselkus concluded that:

The nature of Alzheimer disease . . . does not lend itself to activity programming which is rehabilitative in scope or emphasis. Instead, the prevention of harm, provision of family respite, and enabling of participation in activities that are meaningful in the present moment are the major source of staff satisfaction.

Qualitative methodology is criticized for its subjective nature, for the effect of the observer on the situation (reflexivity), and for its lack of replicability, experimental rigour and statistical validity. All research is time-consuming, but some qualitative methods require linear studies over periods of months or even years; this is highly impractical for an occupational therapist for whom research is an adjunct to practice, and not a full-time occupation. It may be questioned whether employers view occupational therapy research as an integral part of a therapist's work or as an optional extra for which time and resources can be committed only as a 'luxury'.

Fallacies and biases such as the baserate fallacy, availability heuristic, false consensus effect, vividness effect and illusory correlation may all affect the ability of the observer to draw accurate conclusions. However, researchers who use qualitative methods are well aware of these problems, and use carefully controlled forms of observation.

For example, in reflexive analysis the observer and/or an external supervisor must take account of the observer's personal history, experience, interests and bias. Triangulation involves collection and comparison of data using several methods, or several sources, so that themes can be seen to be consistent. Member checking 'consists of continually testing with informants the researcher's data, analytic categories, interpretations and conclusions' (Krefting 1990). A selection of strategies which minimize such problems is listed by Krefting.

The creativity used in interpreting findings may be criticized as 'unscientific'; however, it may also be argued that it is one of the strengths of the method, leading to new knowledge and fresh thinking. It is undoubtedly more challenging to prove trustworthiness for a quantitative study: issues of credibility, transferability, dependability and confirmability have to be addressed.

It has already been noted that qualitative and quantitative methods serve different purposes and are appropriate in different situations. Much of the critical discussion concerning the best method to use is related to the reliablity and validity of each method. In many respects these methods are mirror images, the strengths of one are the weaknesses of the other. There is, however, no reason why research designs should not incorporate both forms of methodology, this obtaining 'the best of both worlds'. The methods are different, but not necessarily incompatible.

The problem of conducting research in ordinary clinical settings should not be either underestimated or exaggerated. It is a question of selecting a project of manageable scale, which addresses a relevant question, and which can be built into normal practice as far as possible. That being said, research implies time for reading, analysing and documenting results and this must be taken into account. Academics may argue that this should be seen as a normal part of the work of senior practitioners and as essential to the provision of a quality service and to personal and professional development; but managers who are concerned with clinical productivity may have a different view.

SUMMARY OF EVALUATION OF INTERVENTION

Various methods of audit and evaluation have been described: these share features such as the need for standards, structured methodology, and, above all, time. The results validate the process of occupational therapy in terms of its outcomes, lead to improvements in standards of practice, development of therapeutic techniques, and personal and professional development. Findings often lead to research questions, where the therapist may choose to use quantitative or qualitative methodology.

Evaluation works best when it is built into everyday practice, and when it is approached from a variety of angles, so that a cumulative picture can emerge.

13

Assessment and evaluation

ASSESSMENT AND EVALUATION: COMPLEMENTARY PROCESSES

The process of intervention requires the therapist to gather information concerning the patient and all aspects of her situation. Once action has been taken the results must also be evaluated. The therapist uses clinical reasoning to interpret data and to make the necessary judgements and decisions on the basis of it.

In this text the word 'assessment' is used in the sense most common in British practice, to describe actions such as examining, measuring, testing or observing the patient, using structured formats and comparing observed performance to specified criteria, standards or norms. 'Evaluation' indicates the process of determining the value of the results or 'making sense' of them in relation to the individual, and monitoring and judging the success of subsequent interventions as measured by changes in assessment results. These two actions must go together. 'The process of assessment is not confined to the gathering of data but is dependent upon its interpretation and evaluation' (Foster 1992). Because the processes are so closely interrelated, the two words are often used rather loosely as synonyms.

It should be noted, however, that in American texts these meanings are reversed. 'Evaluation refers to data gathered from specific procedures' while 'Assessment yields a composite picture of the patient's functioning' (Smith 1993). The consequent confusion is regrettable, but seems unavoidable until a standard terminology can be accepted on a worldwide basis.

Assessment has become a misused and abused term, 'Doing an assessment' is in danger of becoming an end in itself, whereas it only has use and meaning when assessing for a purpose, in order to gain very precise information on the basis of which intervention may be planned, adapted or ended.

Occupational therapy assessment is concerned with identifying the abilities or dysfunctions of an individual. It looks at the individual as an actor engaged in activity (Cynkin & Robinson 1990). It focuses on the nature of individual performance in all its complexity, 'What the person does, what he needs to do, and what he wants to do' (COPM). The activity has demands and the environment has demands; each can be analysed; the important part is how far the individual is able to meet these demands, and what help she will require to do so. If there is a problem, what must be adapted – the nature of the performance demand, the nature of the physical or social environment, or the skills, knowledge or attitudes of the individual?

Assessment may be:

Descriptive: Stating an objective view of a person at present usually in comparison to some predetermined norm, scale or standard.

Evaluative: Noting changes in the individual over time.

Predictive: Making a statement about how, in consequence, the individual will be in a given situation at some future point in time.

Description is, relatively, the most simple of these forms of assessment, since it requires accurate observation, measurement and recording on only one occasion, without implications for the past or future. Norms, scales or standards must still be precise, accurate and relevant.

Evaluation becomes more complex, for sequential assessment implies a high degree of reliability and validity if results are to be meaningfully compared.

Prediction is the most difficult of the three, since predictions are based on probabilities, which in the area of human performance are fraught with complexity, and with a whole set of problems concerning the validity of the assessment procedure or instrument.

Assessment may be:

Informal: Observations made in natural settings in the course of other contact with the patient which are noted by the therapist as significant. Such observations are mainly descriptive, but may be evaluative.

or

Formal: Happening at a particular time, in predetermined circumstances, for a specific purpose, and recorded in a precise and structured manner. These assessments may be descriptive, evaluative or predictive.

The fact that much valuable information can be gained by informal methods has augmented the confusion concerning assessment. When, for example, is a dressing practice a therapeutic exercise for the patient, and when does it become an assessment? The two are not the same, although the means may be similar and the processes simultaneous. That something was done and ticked off on a checklist does not make it the subject of an assessment; it becomes something which has been assessed when it has been observed critically and compared to some target criterion or standard.

Standardized assessments have a set procedure and results which can be compared with and rated against normative scores obtained by testing a sufficient, selected sample of people. If validated the procedure has been tested to ensure results are consistent in use.

Unstandardized assessments are not related to normative scores, or tested for, e.g. validity or inter-rated reliability. A criterion – a referenced assessment in which some individual performance or goal is used as a baseline – is the most useful form of unstandardized assessment.

STANDARDIZED ASSESSMENT METHODS

Assessment frequently involves the use of an assessment instrument – a form, usually with a rating scale – by means of which performance of some carefully structured task or normal activity can be recorded and measured by a trained observer.

The format of the assessment instrument and situation is crucial if the results of the assessment are to be depended on. The problem is that one starts with the premise that assessment construction is difficult, and that the perfect assessment has yet to be developed.

There has been considerable debate in the professional literature concerning the utility, or lack of it, of various assessments. In considering this, Law et al (1990) propose the tests which an assessment should pass before use. A similar set of headings is used by Murdock (1992) in evaluating the Barthel index, and by Fricke (1993) in discussing outcome measures. Smith R (1992) also discusses design in relation to purpose.

The issues may be summarized as:

Utility: aim: clinical applicability practicality
Construction: validity, reliability, sensitivity, scoring
Administration: instructions, training, procedure.

UTILITY
Aim

What is the intention of the therapist in conducting the assessment, and is it suitable for this purpose? Judging suitability is a matter of looking critically at the proposed assessment instrument or method and confirming that it provides the required information.

Assessment is not normally an end in itself, except where a report has been requested by the referring agent and is the sole object of the intervention.

An assessment should add some specific information which is not otherwise available and which will serve as a basis for action. There is little point in spending time defining in general terms a problem which is already obvious, or in exploring a situation when no further intervention is planned.

Aims of assessment include those given in Box 13.1.

Smith R (1992) explores the conflicts which can arise between these purposes, and points out how the reductive approach necessary to obtain quantifiable 'hard data' giving valid results may be at variance with the holistic and more phenomenological view required to give a meaningful picture of individual function.

Clinical applicability

Some tests are generic while others are designed to be relevant to a specific condition, age group or situation (see population-specific reliability, p. 201). In the latter case the therapist must beware of using it in circumstances other than those for which it was designed, since results may be invalid unless re-standardized.

Practicality

The most important considerations are the complexity or simplicity of the test procedure, the need for special equipment or environmental conditions, and the time required to administer the test or undertake the observation. The degree of expertise required may also be a consideration.

CONSTRUCTION
Validity

Validity is concerned with determining the extent to which a test measures what it states it is measuring. The evaluation of valdity is a complex and technical matter. There are different kinds of validity and interpretations of these in relation to occupational therapy assessments vary between authors. It should be noted that much of this language is derived from psychology or research, and the applicability of these concepts to occupational therapy tests should be viewed critically. A valid test should:

Box 13.1 Aims of assessment

Description

To diagnose	To discover the nature of a problem, condition or situation from an occupational perspective
To identify dysfunction	Noting specific instances of dysfunction in roles, relationships or activities, and relating the level of dysfunction to some criterion
To explore subjective responses	Patient's perceptions and concerns responses

Evaluation

To set a base line	In order to plan therapy or intervention or to quantify change
To measure	Specific physical capacity, level of skill or ability
To chart progress	To measure by objective means whether improvement has been made or deterioration has occurred
To quantify learning	To see if learning has taken place effectively
To reassure concerning progress	Patient, carer (or therapist)
To provide outcome data	Assessment results may be used for managerial purposes when evaluating service efficacy

Prediction

To plan future action by therapist	Need for further therapy or intervention
To enable patient to take decisions	Concerning personal future and actions
To inform co-professionals	So they may include this information in their own decision-making

---

- predict a criterion accurately
- correlate with current behaviour
- sample a representative array of the content in question
- be related to a consistent network of constructs.

(Baraon & Byrne 1987)

Face validity is the superficial relevance of the test in relation to the purpose of the test.

Content validity is a more careful examination of relevance and comprehensive coverage of the area to be assessed, as judged by usual standards of professional knowledge and expertise. Would other competent therapists agree that this is what should be assessed, in their circumstances?

Construct validity means that the test does measure the changes which the designer predicted that it would measure.

Criterion validity is the most complex of the validity concepts. A criterion is a measure whereby the success of a predictive test is verified (Atkinson 1993). For example, suppose a person scored well on an assessment designed to predict recovery of functional power grip, and subsequently was able to undertake a predetermined task requiring the use of such a grip for which

there was another validated test with known standards. The successful completion of the task would be a measure of the value of the test and could act as a criterion.

Criterion (or empirical) validity therefore concerns the predictive validity of the test. It is possible to work out a coeffiicent of correlation between the early test scores and later performance. If this relationship – the validity coefficient – is high, the predictive value of the test is good.

However, in many situations, and commonly in occupational therapy, there may be no one criterion which the investigator is willing to accept as a true measure of the concept being evaluated. This is known as 'the criterion problem'.

In this case, research must take place to confirm construct validity; first, to support a theory that predictive links can be made between a performance or test score and subsequent events, and secondly, to establish that the test in question does seem to produce results in line with such theoretical expectations. In general, the therapist must beware of making predictions where such inferences cannot be substantiated.

To confuse matters further, the word 'criterion' is also used more loosely to indicate a form of measurement where individual standards or goals are used as the reference points rather than 'norms' for a whole population. This is called criterion-referenced (as opposed to norm-referenced) assessment. For example, if a person could, before an injury, lift an object of a certain weight, then the ability to lift that object at the end of therapy might be used as a criterion for measuring whether therapy had achieved its aim.

Concurrent validity confirms that the test results relate well with other measures of the same thing. It may take as a 'gold standard' a well-estalished test and evaluate the results of the test in question in relation to this one; this of course implies retesting the patient using the same test, which may be possible in a research and development setting, but seems unlikely in a clinical situation. The comparison of other tests with the Barthel index (Murdock 1992a, b) is an example of this, but indicates how even a well-established test may be subject to criticism.

Reliability

If a test is to be regarded as reliable it must produce consistent results whenever it is used, provided the situations are comparable.

Inter-rater reliability (also known as inter-tester reliability, interscorer agreement and inter-judge reliability) means that different people using the same assessment on the same person or event, either at the same time, or at different times, produce identical, or at least very similar, logical and consistent results.

Intra-rater (intra-tester) reliability means that the same person can get consistent results when using the measure on successive occasions.

Parallel reliability is the extent to which tests of the same thing produce similar results.

Temporal stability. If a test is given to a person or group on two occasions without either any intervention between the two tests, or any other circumstances which might legitimately change the situation, the results should be the same. The test is then described as having temporal stability or test–retest reliability.

Population-specific reliability relates to tests which are designed for a particular population; the results are reliable for that population, but the test may not be generalized for use with others, and may require re-standardization. Fisher et al (1992), for example, describe testing the assessment of motor and process skills (AMPS) on a Taiwanese population to confirm validity and reliability for that population.

Tests of reliability may be built into the assessment. Internal consistency is the degree to which various parts of the test are all measuring the same thing, and the results are agreeing with each other. Anomalies would indicate poor reliability, but if internal consistency is usually good, they might also reflect a deliberate attempt by the subject to falsify results.

Sensitivity

The most valuable assessments are those which are able to discriminate to a high degree between types or levels of performance, and which consequently give information which may be used diagnostically to differentiate between types of problems, levels of performance and predictive outcomes.

Sensitivity is a combination of appropriate and specific test content and accurate methods of scoring or measuring. However, the more sensitive the test, the more difficult it may be to achieve inter-rater reliability.

Scoring

Scoring is a technical matter which requires well-developed numeracy if all its intricacies are to be understood. It is doubtful whether occupational therapists in general, unless conducting research, are equipped to make or use such scales effectively. The defence of the Barthel index by Shah & Cooper (1993) and the critical review of ADL scales (Law & Letts 1989) illustrate well the degree of numerical fluency required to provide a critical evaluation of a scoring system and consequent test validity.

To have a score it is necessary to define expected standards of performance. If the test is standardized this should have been done by careful research into performance norms, using a sufficient sample of subjects, and ensuring that scores can be related to these norms.

However, if the assessment is unstandardized, which is common in occupational therapy, scoring is often designed on the basis of assumptions about 'normal performance' or the likely effects of dysfunction. Scoring systems must be very clearly explained and the definition of each level in a score given unambiguously so that there is minimal risk of varying interpretations.

Scores may be totalled and may be expressed as a percentage, or as a mean score (average) or, in more sophisticated tests, as standard deviations. To design such scoring systems one requires a knowledge of statistics, and if this is lacking or inadequate the result may easily be misinterpreted.

Some scoring systems are weighted to take account of factors not directly included in the scoring system; e.g. in an ADL index it may be decided that ability to do some tasks is more significant in predicting readiness for discharge than other abilities. Again, this raises questions of the basis for the initial distribution of weighting.

Rating scales are full of pitfalls for unwary assessors. A rating scale for a standardized, validated test should be reliable, provided that the test procedure is followed. Unstandardized rating scales, however, can give a spurious appearance of validity, and may encourage subjectivity.

While recognizing that standardization is a slow and cumbersome process which may be impractical for the therapist, it is nonetheless essential that when a rating scale is used all users should have the same understanding of it. A user's handbook, or a set of very precise definitions, can save considerable confusion, and small-scale pilot studies with the user group can be revealing.

Value-laden words such as 'good' or 'poor' should be avoided, but even apparently clear scales can be confusing. For example, the following instruction may at first sight seem straightforward:

Rate performance using the 4-point scale provided:
0 is unable, 1 requires assistance, 2 needs supervision, 4 is independent.

However, what is meant by 'independent', and what is the difference between assistance and supervision? Unless definitions are given it is quite likely that different observers might enter different ratings.

Such scales often imply a norm, and the basis for establishing this should be questioned. Is it based on research or on assumption? To whose expectations does it relate – those of a society or culture, those of the therapist or those of the patient?

A 'one-off' assessment has minimal value, since it records only a performance or condition during a small slice of time which may or may not be representative. It is more usual for assessment to be sequential. The first assessment of the patient can be used to set a baseline against which future, similar, assessments of the same individual may be compared.

Factors such as previous performance, performance of unaffected skills of functions, and individual aspects such as age, roles and occupational requirements can contribute to the evaluation of the results, and the setting of realistic targets. However, the results of such an individual assessment are relevant only to that individual, and can be compared with those of other individuals only with caution and in very general terms.

As Smith R (1992) points out, occupational therapists are not alone in encountering the problem of ensuring accurate measurement. Given all the problems and arguments over validity and reliability, are we even using the appropriate methodology, and if not, what ought we to do to develop more appropriate, yet still valid, assessments?

ADMINISTRATION

Instructions

Any assessment which is to be reliable and valid must have a fixed format and instructions for users. These must include interpretation of terminology, scoring systems and, where relevant, specific test organization and procedure.

Training

Training is essential for some standardized tests (usually psychometric tests), and their use is prohibited unless suitable training has been given. However, most assessment procedures can be improved if the people using them have received training aimed at ensuring that assessment is conducted competently, in a similar fashion, on each occasion using a common understanding of terms, scoring and procedure, and with a similar interpretation of results. This not only improve skills in using the tests, but can show up difficulties in design, administration, inter-rater reliability or other issues which can be resolved by improving the assessment format. New users should practise under supervision until competent.

Procedure

The procedure should state the conditions under which the assessment is to be carried out, and specify the need for special equipment, sequence, and special verbal cues or instructions (or whether these are to be avoided). A defined procedure for a standardized test must be followed if results are to be reliable and valid.

In informal assessments, especially ecologically based observations (those conducted in natural surroundings), arrangements will be more flexible, but since performance is situational the environmental demand, social factors and other relevant influences need to be noted and explained.

PROBLEMS IN CONDUCTING ASSESSMENTS

In the preceding section it will have become apparent that the process of assessment is complex and filled with difficulties.

These difficulties relate to:

- technical problems of assessment design and administration
- problems derived from the nature of occupational therapy and the types of assessments required by therapists
- problems affecting the objectivity of the assessor
- problems affecting the person being assessed.

Technical problems and the nature of assessment in occupational therapy

Concerns over reliability and validity, as measured against the standards required for psychometric or specific performance tests, have been discussed earlier in this chapter. It is clear that even well-constructed, standardized tests have their problems. Since many of the assessment procedures used by therapists are not standardized, they must be even more subject to criticism, on these grounds.

Norm-referenced assessments depend on the use of well-researched data, and are applicable only in defined circumstances. There is still a dearth of information on norms and standards of occupational performance which would be relevant to occupational therapy assessments.

Criterion-referenced assessments also require careful research and development, and in the case of functional performance it may be difficult to find an appropriate single criterion which can be used for all patients.

However, it may be possible to develop a set of criteria for an individual against which the predictive value of assessment results might be measured. Indeed, this is what tends to happen in practice: a set of specific objectives are defined for the individual, and the degree to which these are achieved is measured. The therapist is therefore concerned less with whether the patient has attained some ideal level of competence, or with comparing patient A with patient B, than with whether she has reached a personal target, related to a personal criterion of ability with reference to past or desired performance. This is the basis of the Canadian occupational performance measure (Law et al 1990a, b).

Assessment results can be used evaluatively

to measure progress towards these targets, or predictively to measure whether these targets are likely to be reached. If, over time, the assessment shows consistent predictive value for many patients, its construct validity and reliability become more trustworthy.

It is necessary for the therapist to guard against making predictions on insufficient evidence about performance in very different circumstances. Such predictions, if made, are best expressed as probabilities. It is perhaps preferable to report assessment results as true for the day of assessment, but without prediction, where there is any degree of uncertainty.

As discussed in Chapter 12, the use of assessment results as outcome measures to test the effectiveness of therapy is equally problematic. If a baseline assessment was performed before therapy commenced and testable objectives were set, it is relatively simple to decide whether or not improvement has taken place; but is improvement due to the occupational therapy intervention, or to any one of a number of other interventions or causes?

The methodology of formal, standardized assessment was developed largely by psychologists, kinesiologists and other researchers who are concerned with isolating and measuring, e.g. tiny performance components, traits and the effects of interventions. The higher one travels up the levels of occupational performance, the harder it is to design assessments which are, in precise scientific terms, valid and reliable.

It is relatively easy to design a test to measure a specific skill component; the main problem is isolating the skill. It is possible to make very specific observations of measurable physical or cognitive functions. It is also possible to observe performance of task components or simple tasks in isolation from each other with a reasonable degree of accuracy. The environmental and performance demands can be controlled and restricted. In all of these areas, the therapist is concerned only with the proto-occupational, developmental level of function.

As soon as the therapist seeks to explore complex and integrated function, the performance of whole activities or chains of activities in normal environments, where the situational and existential elements of performance, motivation and meaning become significant, the use of scientific assessments becomes difficult. There are too many variables, no precise criteria, and there is simply too much occurring at once.

A QUESTION OF METHODOLOGY – WHICH FRAME OF REFERENCE?

These problems are not an argument for giving up on the development of better assessment methodology, but for the selection of appropriate models for such development. The psychometric or biomechanical frames of reference may be appropriate for certain specific skill components, but if such tests become inappropriate higher up the occupational scale, then the therapist must seek alternative models.

Discussion of these problems can be related directly to similar discussion concerning quantitative or qualitative research methodology. Quantitative methods can be appropriate when there is something capable of being quantified in a valid statistical form, but when there is not, other methods must be used. Just as the therapist may feel pressurized into using quantitative experimental methods inappropriately because of the need for scientific respectability and credibility, so he may similarly be pressed into producing quantitative assessments with numerical scores because this is what the recipient expects, or seems to respect, rather than because it is the best method of obtaining and explaining assessment data.

AN EDUCATIONAL MODEL

It is often instructive to seek parallels between professions to see if these can illuminate a problem. The discussion of assessment in education, especially higher education, provides a good example. The similarities are interesting, bearing in mind that the role of the therapist is frequently that of 'teacher' as much as, or even more than, that of 'treater'.

Assessment produces volumes of anxious educational analysis, which often revolves around issues of reliability and validity. Rowntree (1981) makes some pragmatic comments which can be translated into therapeutic terms.

He begins by distinguishing between assessment and evaluation, as follows: 'You assess your students (patients), but you evaluate your course (the methods and results of your therapy).' He points out that the student may well be a participant in her own assessment, since she is trying to find out about her own learning. Several occupational therapy authors make a similar point concerning the patient's involvement with and interest in her own situation. This active view of the nature of assessment is important: psychologists or researchers tend to talk of 'subjects' – relatively passive objects of study; this is not the way in which therapists view their patients, nor the way in which educationalists view learners.

Rowntree proposes six reasons for educational assessment; occupational therapy equivalents are suggested in brackets:

- to aid in selection (placement, allocation)
- to maintain standards (as a part of outcome evaluation and quality control)
- to motivate students (patients/clients)
- to give feedback to students (patients/clients)
- to give feedback to teachers (therapists/others)
- to prepare students (patients/clients) for real life.

He condenses these into two main purposes: to teach the student and/or to report on her. The objectives seem relevant to much of the practice of occupational therapy, especially those regarding the use of assessment as a means of motivation and feedback, and as an integral part of the therapeutic/learning process.

The question of reports is of interest: despite presentation of detailed assessment instruments, how often do recipients simply wish to read the report summary? Given that this is the case, what purpose is the assessment, e.g. the functional index, serving? It is fine if it genuinely informs the therapist, but if completion of the assessment becomes a ritual confirmation of what the therapist already knows, its utility should be questioned.

Educationalists, like occupational therapists, speak of skill, knowledge and attitudes. Activities require the integration of cognitive and attitudinal as well as performance components; assessment often needs to consider all three elements.

Bloom's (1956) hierarchy of five cognitive levels: knowledge, comprehension, application, analysis, synthesis and evaluation, is still a valuable reminder that integrated performance occurs at the higher levels. (This is recognized in the design of the assessment of motor and process skills). Rowntree comments: 'The essence of a skill is that it can be used to create something or to change the state of something. So in order to assess a skill we must ask our student (patient) to create something or change something.' There are many more recent texts which extend Rowntree's discussion.

The point is that educationalists, being concerned with assessment and faced with the need to involve their students in the process, also find the question of reliability and validity a major problem, and have taken various routes to overcome the difficulties, all of which have advantages and disadvantages.

Options vary from controlled 'examination' type tests, through open tests which the student may complete in her own time, to self-assessment. Further discussion centres on whether assessment should be intermittent, sequential or continuous. There is also a large body of information on competence-based assessment which is highly relevant to therapists.

It is suggested that the educational model is likely to be relevant in providing assessment methodology for performance at effective level, and that there is a great need for research into the applicability of these methods in occupational therapy.

SOCIOLOGICAL MODELS

Sociologists, like therapists, take a phenomenological perspective, and in consequence have adopted qualitative methods of research, and would probably speak of investigation and observation rather than assessment. Yet they are happy to make evaluations and judgements on the basis of the collected data.

They, again like occupational therapists, are concerned with complex situations which fail to resolve themselves neatly into comparable sets of statistics. As far as I can discover, occupational therapists in Britain have not yet explored sociological methods for relevance to assessment to any great extent, although their value as research tools is becoming acknowledged. While accepting that sociological methods are usually developed to look at groups, it may be possible to adapt these for use with individuals.

The correlation method involves structured observation in natural surroundings to detect relationships between two or more variables. For example, one might observe a patient in a number of different locations and situations in order to observe when outbursts of aggression occur, and by looking at the features of the situations in which they occur detect similarities and draw conclusions about possible triggers.

Most of this methodology relies on highly skilled observation. The forms of observation are well-defined, and can be classified as proposed in Box 13.2 (Polgar & Thomas 1991).

In observation of natural environments, the observer notes and reports acts and activities, meanings, participation, relationships and settings. The observer will attempt to detect themes and meanings and may record large amounts of information, both objective and subjective, using diaries, notes, recordings and other methods, while endeavouring to remain detached and objective. In order to increase reliability the observer may use triangulation – taking data in several different ways, on different occasions, or from different people to compare results.

Predictably, each of these methods has advantages and disadvantages. One of the acknowledged difficulties is the effect of the observer on the subject. The knowledge of being assessed, and the resultant extra attention from the assessor, may itself improve performance (the Hawthorne effect), or may, conversely, provoke anxiety or 'problem' behaviours. The complete observer may be viewed as a threatening presence. The complete participant is likely to become subjectively involved in the situation.

The expectations of the assessor concerning whether the patient may succeed or fail can alter the manner of observing and the interpretation of results in both positive and negative directions (the Rosenthal effect). The more naturalistic the environment and form of assessment, the more difficult it may be to prevent such effects.

The therapist may also be influenced by his desire to see the patient improve, not only for the sake of the patient, but also to meet his own needs; therapists report lack of progress in patients as a significant cause of stress (Sweeney et al 1993).

BASIC SKILLS OF ASSESSMENT

There are many types of assessment procedures and a full explanation of all those available to therapists would fill a large book. Most occupa-

---

Box 13.2 Forms of observation (Polgar & Thomas 1991)

Non-participant observation	The observer as 'fly on the wall'
The complete observer	One who neither interacts with participants nor discloses his purpose.
Participant observation	The observer takes part in the situation being studied, using ethnographic or illuminative approaches to understand the situation.
The complete participator	One who is totally immersed and becomes part of the situation.
The participant as observer	One who participates fully but discloses his identity as an observer.

tional therapy texts contain descriptions of them. Smith (1993) provides a useful summary of frequently used assessments and a list is given in Appendix 2. There are many procedures which derive from specific frames of reference, and others which are functionally-referenced. The purpose of this section is to discuss the basic skills of assessment, rather than the use of particular methods in relation to specific conditions or problems, for the latter, the reader should refer to specialist texts.

If this section seems to be a statement of the obvious, that is perhaps because basic skills are just that – very basic. To a senior practitioner this is 'old hat'; for this reason they may be taken for granted, and therefore a brief recapitulation seems justified, especially to assist the novice practitioner.

OBTAINING INFORMATION

The precursor to assessment is obtaining information. This may come from case notes, resource files, or interviewing the patient, relatives, or other professionals. Simply obtaining information is not in itself assessment, but evaluation of information should indicate whether assessment is necessary and suggest what assessments should be undertaken.

The therapist uses basic clinical knowledge to discriminate between relevant and irrelevant items when collecting information, usually on the basis of some preliminary hypotheses made as a result of the information on the referral. Where such information is inconclusive, a wider examination of information must be made before it is possible to say what is currently relevant.

OBJECTIVE ASSESSMENT

Much assessment is objective; the therapist attempts to be as accurate as possible in obtaining and recording data concerning the observable actions and interactions or condition of the patient. This is not always a simple matter. The problems of observer bias or expectations and the effects on performance of being observed need consideration, as do the observation procedure and

system of recording observations. It may be questioned whether an observer can ever be truly objective, but it is possible, at least, to become aware of, and reduce, tendencies towards subjectivity.

The different forms of observation have been described. Observation is an integral part of therapy. The therapist continually makes observations, conducts small tests, and makes consequent evaluations and adjustments. This type of assessment relies on awareness of the salient isues, directed attention, and a mind like a video camera, capable of both 'freeze frame' and 'action replay'. Indeed, the therapist may no longer have to rely on the 'mental camera' – video-recording a therapy session, with the consent of the patient, can be of great benefit.

Objective observation is a skill which must be learned, developed and practised. Simply being a therapist does not necessarily make one instantly observant. Since the locations and situations of therapy are so variable it is not easy to give specific guidance on techniques.

The principles of objective assessment are:

- accurate observation
- precision
- clear recording
- replicability.

Accurate observation

Observation is the skill of being able to 'tune in' to things which are significant, and to retain that information for analysis. The first difficulty is deciding what is significant.

If you go for a walk along a pebble-strewn beach, an overall impression is gained. You may be able to say if the pebbles were many, or few, if they were large or small, and what was the main colour, but the detail is lost in the mass of information. In assessment terms this kind of general impression is useful as a quick scanning exercise, but it is relatively imprecise.

If you are asked to go and look for green pebbles of a certain size, your information about them is likely to be more accurate, and you will be able to pick them out from the background.

Similarly, if you know that you are trying to assess a patient's ability to lift an object, or to initiate a conversation, it becomes simpler to set up a situation and structure precise observations.

Precision

The statement 'there were quite a lot of large green pebbles on the beach' is not very helpful. A statement that 'in a survey of 10 square metres of beach, the average number of green pebbles per metre was 10, and of these an average of three were more than 12 cm in diameter; 29 such pebbles were counted' is considerably more useful.

Observation should provide precise answers to questions such as:

- how often?
- for how long?
- when?
- was it consistent?
- how effective was it?
- why did it happen then?
- what happened next?
- how did the person react?

There are many more questions than these few examples; the task of the therapist is to frame the right questions in such a way that pertinent and useful information can be obtained, and checked against future results. A frame of reference may therefore be useful in narrowing the field of inquiry and suggesting appropriate investigations and techniques.

Clear recording

Assessment data cannot be carried for long in one's head; it needs to be written up as soon as possible, preferably at the time of the observation, although that is not always desirable or practical, and the experienced therapist must carry much of the data collected informally during a session in his head until it is convenient to document it. It is not wise to attempt to carry too much information in this way, especially when it concerns several patients. In some circumstances, flow diagrams or action charts can be used to record events or interactions.

Each assessment record should be dated and signed by the assessor. Only actual observations should form part of the record. It is also useful to separate judgements made as a result of the observation from the observation itself.

Although the value of a checklist can be overstated, it does help to make the record clear and to speed up the process of recording. However, it should always be possible to compromise on a form that is both of manageable length and sufficiently comprehensive to cover all eventualities.

Replicability

'One-off' assessments have their place, but the data obtained must be compared only cautiously with that obtained in dissimilar circumstances. If such comparisons do indicate patterns of performance, dysfunction or relationships this can be revealing, but it is easy to impose patterns where they do not exist.

If the data is required in order to carry out a sequential study of progress or deterioration, it is important that the circumstances of the assessment can be repeated. This may mean not only the same test or task, under similar circumstances, but also at the same time of day, and with the same assessor. In some performance tests, however, the patient may simply learn to do the test, without necessarily generalizing the performance into other activities.

It may be necessary to repeat an assessment at different times and in different environments if the purpose is to test whether abilities are consistent and generalized. The therapist, by using activity analysis, can provide assessment situations which, although apparently different, actually test the same skills. This may be useful in assessing actual or potential ability as opposed to the lower level of ability that the patient may expect of herself in a specific situation which she finds difficult or stressful.

Despite an understanding of environmental demand on performance it can still surprise a novice therapist when the performance of a patient changes in differing situations – hence, for example, the exasperation of a nurse when faced with an occupational therapy report stating that the patient can dress and undress herself when the nurse's assessment is that she cannot. In fact, the patient may be able to do so at 9.30 a.m. in the homely occupational therapy bedroom, where the therapist has provided suitable equipment and cues, but not at 7.00 p.m. on the ward, when the items she needs are not readily accessible, and when she is tired and becoming confused, and the cues are absent.

SUBJECTIVE ASSESSMENT

Self-assessment by a patient may be the only method of investigating her personal perceptions and concerns. Although such data is 'soft' and difficult to test, it is nevertheless revealing, especially if there is a discrepancy between self-assessment and objective assessment. Adult learners typically underrate their own performance. This kind of data can form the basis of discussion or goal-setting. Some subjective tests are standardized, such as those which require the subject to select a statement with which she agrees.

Involvement of the patient in any assessment procedure is another matter of debate and differing frames of reference. Is the assessment to be seen as a kind of 'unseen examination' where the patient is the subject of 'tests', or is the patient to be closely involved in the process of monitoring and evaluating her own progress and condition? Is the patient even to be made aware of being assessed – ethical considerations notwithstanding, there may be reasons why this is undesirable.

CONDUCTING THE ASSESSMENT

Explanation

Unless the patient is to be unaware of being assessed, some form of explanation of the purpose of assessment and the nature of it needs to be given.

Any assessment situation is liable to provoke memories of examinations, appraisals or tests in which success or failure were at stake, and consequent anxiety and stress. Even if it is indeed a test of this kind, it is important for the therapist to spend some time in gaining a rapport with the patient, and in presenting the assessment situation in a positive manner.

It is useful for the therapist to practise some appropriate introductory phrases until they become automatic, for it is very easy to use the wrong words. For example, 'I want to see if you are safe to go home' may be correct, but may also indicate to the patient that safety is in doubt, and that failure may jeopardize the chance of going home, both of which feelings are likely to create anxiety and reduce competence. It is obviously preferable for the patient to feel involved in the assessment process, and to see it as dealing with her own concerns in a sympathetic and practical manner, with a view to solving the problems. If the patient can set her own agenda for assessment, so much the better.

However, some patients deny having any problems, even in the face of obvious difficulties, some may be too confused to understand the situation and others simply refuse to cooperate with any overt form of assessment. Also, the Hawthorne effect can create problems, and it is sometimes necessary to observe a patient without her being aware of this. This really does need to be subtle and occasional, otherwise the patient will feel continually 'watched'.

When the patient is involved in the assessment situation it is natural for her to want to know 'how did I do?'. This needs careful handling. In many cases a sympathetic explanation in accessible or lay terminology helps the patient to make informed choices and decisions. Feeding back information to the patient can be therapeutic. For example, it may be possible for the therapist to describe observations, asking a patient to give a subjective response – 'I noticed that you were more at ease in the group today; you made several useful points in the discussion. How did you feel about this?'

Assessment which is sequential and shows clear improvement – 'look, this is much better than when you started treatment' – can boost morale, improve motivation and build confidence. Conversely, results which indicate a steady deterioration may have a demoralizing effect unless handled very sensitively.

The patient has a right to be given information about herself but does not have an automatic right to see reports of everything which the therapist may have observed, or the conclusions to which he may have come.

Rehearsal

The need for rehearsal should be considered, and the fact that it has occurred should be recognized. Occupational therapy assessment often takes place after a period of practice during which learning can occur. When the objective is to improve performance this creates no problem. In this kind of developing situation an assessment might take an average of a series of performances, or a 'best effort' as the test result. Bearing in mind educational models of assessment, if one of the aims is to provide the person with feedback and motivation then it is important that success is built into the situation. Some techniques of 'errorless learning' provide ideas for how this may be done.

There is sometimes the need to present a patient with a test 'cold' to find out what abilities are present at this moment in time. Some tests allow a period of familiarization with equivalent tasks and then use different ones for the actual test.

Over-rehearsal can be counter productive. It may actually decrease skill, or may result in 'learning to do the test' but not a functional performance.

Performance

During assessment both patient and therapist need to concentrate and be undistracted; quiet and privacy are important. The exception is when assessment is undertaken in a group, or in a normal environment where distractions abound, since part of the assessment is likely to be concerned with whether the patient can cope with the task in a distracting or stressful environment.

While recording an event or performance the therapist has to strike a balance between the necessity of recording things as they happen, and the necessity of giving attention to the patient, the event, or the test procedure.

Where the therapist is simultaneously conducting some kind of therapy and attempting an assessment, accurate observation is difficult. In these cases it is useful to have a co-therapist acting as observer and assessor, although it has to be remembered that a non-participating observer is often regarded as a threat. One solution is to have the observer permanently present until he becomes accepted, but many therapy areas do not have the luxury of allocating staff in this way.

In informal situations and during practice the therapist may cue or prompt the patient, provide aids or assistance, or otherwise shape performance, but if such facilitatory devices are used in an assessment this must be recorded.

In standardized assessments the therapist must ensure that the conditions of the assessment, the equipment and the procedure are as specified for the test.

Recording

Once again, there is a need for explanation: the therapist should normally tell the patient what kind of recording is being used, what is being recorded, the purpose of this, who will see the results and where the information is to be kept. It should also be made clear whether or not the patient will have access to the information.

The most frequently used form of recording is an itemized form, but other types of recording may be used, e.g. tape-recording, video-recording, visual representations, graphs and diagrams.

It is essential that all records contain the name or other identifying details of the person assessed, the date (and perhaps time and duration) of the assessment and the name of the assessor.

EVALUATING THE RESULTS

Interpretation

Data is of little value unless it leads to some form of action, decision or additional knowledge. Following evaluation, information should be used to shape further intervention. Therapy may need to be changed, advanced or discontinued; some action may be needed, resources obtained or discharge plans commenced. When action is consequent upon assessment data the links should be clearly noted, and the action recorded.

The problem for the therapist is to make sense of the data in respect of the unique situation of the individual. This requires experience and the use of clinical reasoning.

Providing that a baseline was obtained at the outset, it is relatively easy to decide whether or not an individual is making progress. Sequential assessment should show a steady curve. If, however, the results show a 'zigzag' pattern in which performance seems to fluctuate unpredictably the therapist recognizes an anomaly in the pattern and is challenged to find a reason for this: it may be the patient's condition, an environmental factor or an effect of therapy – but equally it may cast doubt on the validity of the assessment procedure.

The difficulty of using assessment data predictively has already been noted, yet predictions are often what the originator of the request for information seems to want. The therapist must avoid being pressurized into the role of 'clairvoyant', and should remember that written predictions which prove inaccurate could expose the therapist to litigation.

If the assessment is being used to decide whether a particular therapy is effective, it may be necessary to adopt a more structured research approach to evaluation.

Communication of assessment results to others

Assessment data is of primary interest to the therapist as a means of making clinical decisions and monitoring the process of intervention. The therapist needs far more information, in more detail, than other professionals or, usually, the patient.

In communicating information to others the therapist has to consider the person who needs the information, how much is needed, whether it is appropriate to communicate it, any legal considerations, and how best to present it. The people who most frequently need the information are other professionals, or the patient's relative or carer.

When communicating with other professionals it is usual to summarize the information in a written report, or to report it verbally, adding a written confirmation later. Reports are the visible part of professional practice, by means of which others may form impressions and opinions of the therapist's competence and efficiency, and they must be given due attention.

It can also be difficult to know how much information to disclose to a relative or carer. 'Talking about a patient behind his back' may raise ethical problems. It is good practice to ask the patient if she is willing for the therapist to talk to the person concerned.

In situations where the patient is likely to impart confidential information which the therapist wishes to convey to others, it is wise to make the ground rules for such disclosure quite clear to the patient at the start of therapy. The therapist must avoid being placed in a position where disclosure looks like a breach of confidentiality, even if it is in the patient's best interests. Material which indicates risk to the patient, in the form of, e.g. self-harm, suicide, or abuse by others, must be disclosed and recorded in line with local policies, and the patient must be told from the outset that this will be the case.

ASSESSMENT AS A FORM OF RESEARCH

It should by now be apparent that in many ways the process of assessment – e.g. pose question concerning subject, test, intervene, test, evaluate – is similar to research, and therefore an awareness of the pitfalls of research methodology are helpful in improving accuracy and validity. Indeed, a structured approach to assessment can provide data for research without imposing added work for the therapist. The occupational therapy art and practice can become a research laboratory; a series of single subject studies could provide valuable data if systematically recorded and evaluated.

As has been discussed, many of the techniques of performance analysis are related to qualitative methods where a quantified description or comparison is produced. During an assessment the therapist often regards the patient as a research subject. A question is formulated, e.g. 'Compare the right hand grip to that of the left; does this show deficit?', 'How does it relate to norms for age and sex?', 'Has therapy improved the ability to grip?', 'Does this lady initiate conversation?' 'Does environment affect her ability to do so?', 'What critical incident provokes an anxiety attack?' 'How often do these occur?' Deitz (1993) illustrates how single subject research designs can be used to answer such clinical questions, and points out the advantages and disadvantages of various forms of design.

The therapist, like a researcher, must structure a test situation, observe and record data, and evaluate results. The importance of accurate observation is a recurring theme.

Assessment checklists or indices, and specific tests of performance benefit from a 'research approach' to design and validation. Basic research provides norms, standards and criteria. Applied research assists in testing and validating assessments. Research literature contains much helpful advice about the design of questionnaires and observation record forms.

Qualitative research may both illuminate the treatment process and provide further information on which to build theory and evaluate assessments or observations, especially in more complex, subjective and experiential areas.

FUNCTIONAL ANALYSIS

Occupational therapists are primarily concerned with functional assessment, i.e. with determining whether a person is able to do the things she needs to do in order to carry on with her daily life, hence the adoption in this text of the term 'functional analysis' as a generic description of this type of assessment.

Most therapists would assume that they have a clear idea of the concept of function so it may come as a surprise that even such a well-used term is open to interpretation. If, as Unsworth

(1993) suggests, therapists do not have a well-defined concept of function, they are certainly going to have difficulty in assessing it.

She points out that 'definitions do not convert the theoretical idea of function into a defined statement regarding the way in which it should be measured. Therefore functional assessments appear poorly linked to theory.' Her review of 22 ADL indices 'highlighted inconsistencies in what ought to be measured, confusion between measuring skills and tasks, and different approaches to scale construction.'

The Concise Oxford Dictionary (COD) defines function in two ways relevant to this discussion: 'activity proper to person or institution; mode of action or activity by which thing fulfils its purpose'.

Function is therefore the ability of a person to perform activities in a manner which achieves the desired purpose. It then becomes necessary to define ways in which the performance of such activity can be described.

The concept of function has become closely associated with that of personal independence in ADL, but this is a narrow view. A person requires levels of function in all areas of life, including work and leisure; these aspects are often relegated to second place in the belief that ADL, having 'survival value', is the most important area. In this therapists may be in danger of imposing their own values on the patient.

FUNCTIONAL ANALYSIS IN RELATION TO THEORETICAL STRUCTURES

Integrative models of practice developed by therapists typically suggest headings under which assessment should be conducted, or provide assessment instruments or checklists. The main effect of using a model is to indicate where to start and where to put the emphasis of the assessment.

For example, the model of human occupation places importance on the volition subsystem as the head of the hierarchy, and indicates exploration of this system as a priority, including subjective rating by the individual. The habituation and performance subsystems also have assessment procedures.

Much research has been undertaken on a standardized performance assessment measuring specific skills, the assessment of motor and process skills (AMPS), which consists of 35 motor and process (cognitive) skill items used in the performance of activities. Therapists can be trained and accredited in the use of AMPS. The rating system allows for adjustment for personal idiosyncrasies in scoring (Fisher 1994).

Adaptation through occupation (Reed & Sanderson) proposes assessment of three performance areas: sensorimotor, cognitive and psychosocial; and three environmental areas; physical, biopsychological and sociocultural. In a later presentation of the model, Reed adds other elements specific to occupational therapy including orientation, order and activation, and suggests a skill assessment derived from the work of Gagné significantly, an educational theorist.

The Canadian occupational performance measure (COPM) (Law et al 1990a, b) is a criterion-referenced outcome measure within the model of occupational performance (which was derived from the work of Reed). While paying strict attention to reliability and validity, this takes a more holistic approach 'based on the belief that the individual is a fundamental part of the therapeutic process' and describes an individual's occupational performance as:

A balance between three areas: self-care, productivity and leisure. Factors which interact with these three areas include the individual's mental, physical, sociocultural and spiritual characteristics . . . this model involves the assessment of abilities and disabilities of the individual client within his/her environmental and role expectations. Together the client and therapist determine therapeutic goals, implement treatment and assess the outcomes of treatment.

The assessment 'incorporates roles and role expectations within the client's own environment. It considers the importance of the skill or activity to the client using a semi-structured, individualized interview approach.' The client is asked if she needs to, wants to or is expected to perform activities within various categories, and if the reply is positive, is then asked if she can

perform, does perform and is satisfied with her performance. 'When the client identifies a need as well as an inability to perform ... this performance area is identified as a problem.'

The COPM is described as having several advantages in terms of applicability to occupational therapy: relevance to the client, and improving responsibility for, and motivation to engage in, therapy. An interesting comment is that 'the true priorities of the client became evident and these priorities were often different from the therapists' initial ideas.' This is an example of a highly integrated approach where outcome measures are built into the process and where assessment automatically contributes to client-centred evaluation.

Frames of reference direct the therapist towards particular areas of function, e.g. cognition, movement, relationships and effective responses. Particular areas of practice, e.g. paediatrics, orthopaedics and mental health, require differing focuses for assessment.

Despite the ways in which such theoretical structures may direct assessment, the actions of the therapist tend, in the end, to relate back to the core concerns of assessment in relation to occupations, as modified by the chosen approach.

UNRAVELLING COMPLEXITY IN FUNCTIONAL ANALYSIS

Taking as an example the assessment of a person's ability to eat a meal, the therapist wants to know if the meal was eaten, from start to finish, with no problems. If so, the person is a 'competent eater'.

However, in terms of an ADL assessment, what does one mean by 'eating a meal'? Is it a real meal or a pretend one? Is it something the patient likes and would normally eat? Did she want to eat the meal at all? Does it provide enough nourishment or meet dietary requirements? Was help provided or were adaptations made to tools or environment, and does this affect the judgement of competence? Because human actions are complex, variable, social and symbolic as well as functional, assessment becomes a difficult matter, except insofar as the norms, goals and wishes of an individual can be identified.

Eating a meal is only one activity in a long chain which, for an independent person in the community, would include planning, shopping, preparing, cooking, serving, eating and clearing up afterwards. How many of these activities are required by the individual who is being assessed?

A distinction is often made between PADL, personal activities of daily living, which are those required for health and physical survival, and DADL, the domestic activities which support these basic activities or which are socially necessary. The latter are sometimes referred to as instrumental activities. Attempts have been made to view these as arranged in some kind of hierarchy where some activities are more essential than others, but this may be misleading. There are few activities of this kind which need not be performed at all. The first question is not whether they are done, but who should do them, the patient, or someone else, and how much assistance may be required.

The second question is, 'how far does the quality of performance at PADL predict performance at DADL?' Although, logically, there is a negative link, in that marked inability in PADL would make it highly unlikely that DADL could be attempted, the fact that PADL can be managed does not necessarily predict that DADL will be also.

If the person is unable to perform an activity it becomes important, by means of task analysis, to identify the point at which performance broke down and the reason for this. Incompetent performance may or may not relate to a deficit in skill. There may indeed be a lack of skill, or even of the potential to acquire it; equally, however, the skill may be there, but another factor – psychological, emotional, social or environmental – intrudes.

A STRUCTURE FOR FUNCTIONAL ANALYSIS

The structure for functional analysis described in the following section mirrors that for occupa-

tional analysis, occurring at the same levels, and from both objective and subjective viewpoints. The chief difference is that whereas in occupational analysis it is the occupation, activity, or task which is studied, in functional analysis it is the nature of the performance of an individual. (The reader may find it helpful to refer to the section on occupational analysis in Chapter 5 where the forms of analysis are explained.)

When studying performance, the therapist is concerned with skills and competencies. In the same way that it is possible to arrange occupational performance in a hierarchy, it is also possible to see skill acquisition in a similar way. The two continua can then be related to each other, which helps to clarify the methods and objectives of assessment at each stage; however, the relationship should not be seen as rigid.

Levels of skill

Skill components have been described as the 'building blocks of performance' (Ch. 4, p. 62). These components – sensorimotor, cognitive and psychosocial – are combined and coordinated through mastering task components and then task stages and tasks, into smoothly integrated, skilled performance of activities.

Skill components build into skills, and skills into competencies. Once competencies are acquired the person may, in some occupations, go on to develop mastery and expertise. The levels of skill in relation to occupational levels are illustrated in Table 13.1.

Skill acquisition typically follows an upward path, flattening towards the end, which is described as a learning curve. Sometimes it may proceed in a more step-like fashion with plateaux between phases of learning, during which consolidation takes place. The early stages are characterized by experiments and mistakes which gradually reduce until, finally, performance is smooth and automated. Only when the stage of automation is reached is performance likely to become reliably competent.

In physiological terms, for complex motor skill, this stage signals a transfer of control from 'conscious' use of the motor cortex to achieve parts of the action – where the person is aware

Table 13.1   Levels of skill in relation to occupational levels

Level of skill	Definition	Occupational level
		Developmental (proto-occupational)
Skill components	Linked specific skill components	Task segments (smallest part of a task) e.g. grasp spoon, more spoon to pudding, get pudding onto spoon
Skill	Smoothly integrated skills	Task stages (integrated task components) e.g. take spoonful of pudding and place in mouth, return spoon to plate
Competence	Skilled and adequately successful completion of a task	Task (completed section of activity) e.g. eat pudding
		Effective and organizational (productive and occupational)
Competence	Skilled, automated, adequate performance	
Mastery	Fluent and faultless performance	Activities and processes
Expertise	Consistently exceptional performance	

of each stage of the task and struggles to combine the elements of performance, to unconscious control by patterns located in the cerebellum – where the whole action is smoothed and 'polished'. Once action reaches this point it is quite difficult to make further adjustments, and to do so requires feedback from an outsider who can observe the performance and locate the problem.

It may be hypothesized that other habitual and automated actions involving process skills, once learned, are similarly stored at a deeper level of cerebral control where they are less susceptible to change.

At the proto-occupational level, the therapist is concerned with the development of skills, but the more complex performance becomes, the more difficult it is to distinguish individual skills, and the more important it becomes to look at the effects of performance as an integrated whole. Once the effective level has been reached, it becomes increasingly hard to describe skills other than in terms of the quality and results of performance. For this reason, the term 'skill analysis' will be used at developmental level and 'performance analysis' at the higher levels.

Types of functional analysis

Assessment always starts with an appreciation of the unique needs, concerns and occupational requirements of the individual, in view of her past medical, social, psychological and environmental history, current situation, and future needs and aspirations. This focus frequently eliminates many assessments as irrelevant or unnecessary, although in more complex situations, more global assessment may be required.

The following description of types of functional analysis is a representation of all the possible investigations which may be carried out; however, it would be unlikely that all those described would be used with one individual, except over a very extended timescale.

The distinction between objective assessment data – that obtained by the therapist based on tests or observations, and subjective assessment data – where the patient's memories, thoughts and feelings influence the information, needs to be retained in the therapist's mind, although in practice the two types of information may merge.

Table 13.2 demonstrates the types of analysis in relation to occupational levels. Since assessment often follows a development sequence, the developmental level will be presented first.

DEVELOPMENTAL LEVEL
Skill analysis

In assessing skill the therapist is concerned with both process and product. He needs to know how

Table 13.2 Functional analysis in relation to occupational levels

Level	Type of analysis	Aims
Developmental	Skill analysis	To investigate in a clinical setting the performance of skill components or skills in relation to task segments or tests of function.
Effective	Performance analysis	To analyse the effectiveness of an individual's engagement in an activity, and the level of competence achieved.
	Participation analysis	To describe the individual's pattern of participation in activities over a short timespan.
	Existential analysis	To describe subjective reactions, values and personal meanings which an individual attributes to activities, and subjective purposes and motivations.
Organizational	Role analysis	To describe the occupational and sociocultural roles held by the individual, and her subjective view of these.
	Participation analysis	To describe the pattern of occupational participation for an individual over an extended timespan.
	Existential analysis	To describe subjective reactions, values and personal meanings which an individual attributes to occupations.

well the objective of the task has been achieved, but also to evaluate the method by which it was carried out and the skills used to perform it.

Both applied skill (skill as actually used) and potential skill (signs that performance could improve because ability is there but as yet undeveloped) can be relevant.

Functionally, the therapist, and the patient, need to see the results of the effort in terms of task completion – that the patient put on a shoe, filled a kettle, drank tea, got out of bed, wrote a message, answered the phone. At earlier developmenal stages this assessment might focus on performance of task stages or even single task components.

From the point of view of skill analysis, the therapist needs to decide whether the task was completed competently (using standards relevant to the individual), and whether there were any observable skill deficits. If there were, subsequent analysis will reveal which of the many skill components were lacking, and what may be required to improve performance.

Analysis of skill components

Skill components are assessed by using task analysis to identify the task stages and segments, and the skill components required to perform these. The performance of the patient can then be observed to check whether the required skills are present, and to establish how efficiently they are used.

It is sometimes necessary to assess very specific skill components in a purely clinical manner, divorced from any context of functional performance. Examples of such skill components include; perception, attention, memory, vision, range of movement, righting reflexes and muscle tone (see list of skill components, p. 62). The purpose of such testing may be diagnostic, or to provide a precise baseline for measuring improvement.

This can be useful, but it is essentially an artificial process. Functional performance is always integrated, and it can be hard to construct a test which isolates a specfic skill without 'contamination' by another. This is particularly true in relation to the 'unscrambling' of cognitive, perceptual and sensory deficits.

There is a particular danger in designing 'DIY' test procedures. The test which appears to test one thing may in fact be testing several things, or even something quite different, e.g. if the spatial perception test relies on comprehension of verbal instructions, or visual acuity, or even basic literacy, results could be distorted. There is much less likelihood of such problems occurring if the test has been correctly standardized and validated. A number of suitable psychological tests are available.

Specific skill assessment is time-consuming, and may not always be justified by the value of the results. If the therapist find that a specific test only confirms observations already made during functional performance, without adding further information concerning differential diagnosis or guidance for therapy, it may be worth questioning if such testing should be repeated.

EFFECTIVE LEVEL

Performance analysis

This is concerned with the individual's ability to perform activities. It is most frequently related to work or personal care (perhaps because many of the procedures originated within the medical rehabilitation model), but leisure and social activities may be included.

This is an objective analysis of what a person actually does, and how effectively she does it. The aim is to identify areas of dysfunction with a view to intervention or therapy, or to monitor the results of such intervention.

There are three different facets to performance analysis, emphasizing the product, the skills and the environment.

Product-related assessment

This looks at the performance of an activity or activity sequence as a gestalt, and defines the level to which the product or purpose of it is, or is not, satisfactorily and competently completed. The questions relate to the whole activity, e.g. 'Can he get dressed?', 'Can she cook a meal?', 'Can she drive to work?', 'Can he ask friends in for coffee?'

Assessment of performance skills

This analyses the means whereby the activity is achieved and the performance skills required, and looks for areas of achievement or deficit. Broad classifications of skills, e.g. sensorimotor, cognitive and psychosocial, may be used as headings to direct attention to specific performance areas.

The main use of this type of analytical assessment is to identify problem areas and to direct therapy. For example, an ADL assessment indicates that the patient is unable to dress. A performance assessment will discriminate between a cognitive or motor skill deficit as the origin of the difficulty. Having identified a skill deficit, this form of assessment is conducted more practically at the development level, focusing on the problem tasks or task stages.

Performance-related assessment is frequently secondary to product-related assessment.

Assessment of the environment in relation to function

This is important in identifying barriers or providing means to facilitate performance. Differing environments, both human and physical, can have distinct effects on performance. To consider the participant in isolation from the environment is relatively meaningless in functional terms. It is therefore necessary to record not only the nature of the performance, but also the location and time, the presence or absence of others and their contribution to the situation, and the tools, furniture or equipment used (see Ch. 15).

Participation analysis

Information about actual use of time is very helpful in providing objective evidence of what the patient really does in daily life. For this a diary may be kept by the patient for a week (or some other finite period), charting which activities are engaged in and how long is spent on each. Periods of inactivity, rest and sleep should also be noted. This is a fairly demanding activity which may be beyond the scope of some clients.

This type of assessment can indicate the extent of occupational dysfunction, or areas of imbalance, and may suggest areas which would benefit from more detailed assessment and evaluation. Participation analysis is commonly used in models related to occupational performance or adaptation and several checklists and procedures are available (see Appendix 2).

In evaluating such information, the things which are not done are of as much significance as those which are, since these exclusions may reveal the nature of the patient's difficulties. Reality is sometimes different from personal perceptions, and this too can be significant.

This information can also be usefully linked to a record of the extent to which the person perceives the things he does as pleasant and meaningful.

Existential analysis

The term 'existential analysis' has been coined to describe the highly subjective impressions which individuals have of their lives and choices. This is frequently linked with participation analysis and is concerned with the individual's perceptions of purposes, products and processes, and the feelings these engender. The individual is best able to give meaningful answers in reponse to specific questions such as 'do you like doing that?' or 'why do you do that so often (or seldom)?', in relation to each activity.

Subjectively, it may be difficult to disentangle purposes, products and processes, as one can objectively, since the purpose of participating in an occupation or activity may well be related to personal perceptions of the product, or participation in a process. Participation may even be for reasons only tangential to the actual activity. This is best illustrated by some examples.

If you analyse gardening as an occupation, you can define some of its general purposes, products and processes. However, gardening has many processes, and most gardeners have preferences. The individual gardener is likely to give different responses to the question 'What sort of gardening do you undertake?' – it may be vegetable growing, flowers or patio planters, or all three.

When you know what kind of gardening is engaged in, it is possible to explore the exis-

tential background to such participation. Individuals are likely to give varied answers, depending on their values, likes, dislikes, prejudices and experiences, and sociocultural setting. For example:

- 'I like to grow fresh vegetables, and I don't want any chemicals sprayed on them. It saves money too.'
  (Valuing the product, economy, and an organic style of production)
- 'I don't much like gardening, but my wife (or husband) drives me mad if the grass isn't cut, and I don't want the neighbours to complain.'
  (Social pressure unconnected with personal liking of process or product)
- 'I like getting out onto the allotment because I meet friends and we can have a good chat. I've won prizes too.'
  (Valuing social contact and affiliation, and experience of personal achievement).
- 'I love roses, all the colours and scents; I am always buying new ones. Being in the garden brings me peace.'
  (Valuing product and a quality of experience)
- 'I don't know much about flowers, but I like pottering in the garden because it gives me the chance to get some fresh air and exercise. I like seeing the birds and insects, too.'
  (Valuing the process more than the product)
- 'I don't much like gardening, but I do like having somewhere nice to sit in the summer.'
  (Valuing a consequence, and therefore tolerating the process.)

These subjective views give personal meaning to participation and are often much stronger motivators (or de-motivators) than the objectively identified purposes or products of the activity.

Likes and dislikes may have rational origins, or may have unconscious sources: the origins of the latter may be disregarded unless one is using an analytical frame of reference; it is the effect on participation that matters.

Negative experiences feed back into negative attitudes to an activity, e.g. 'I never keep houseplants, they always die on me.' Kielhofner speaks of beneficial and vicious cycles in which successful or unsuccessful participation reinforces and builds either positive or negative self-image and perception of competence.

In fact, the attitudes of the participant can be double-edged tools when it comes to assessing a patient: a familiar activity may have too much meaning, being associated with too many past experiences; this may be helpful, but equally, it may be counterproductive.

An activity previously valued, at which competence is no longer possible, may simply provide new experiences of frustration and failure. Perhaps this is where the novelty and challenge of mastering a new technique can be used to advantage, since there are no preconceptions, and where the skill of the therapist lies in engineering success.

The point is that individual perceptions of purpose, standards, associations and meaning are just that – *individual*. Even though it may be possible to predict a likely range of reactions or meanings within a given culture, the precise reactions of an individual cannot be taken for granted. The more the therapist can explore the personal values and perceptions of a patient during the assessment process, the more likely it is that a deeper understanding of that patient's needs will be obtained, and that therapy will be effective.

It should equally be recognized that within some frames of reference, exploration of meaning is irrelevant, and a more utilitarian approach to activity is used. It is arguable, however, that meanings are so ingrained in human experience that it may be impossible to disregard them.

ORGANIZATIONAL LEVEL

At this level the therapist seeks to obtain an overview of occupational participation for the individual. What roles are taken? What occupations and activities are performed? What is the spread of occupations in areas of work, lesiure and personal activities (or other classifications relevant to age and culture)? The purpose of such assessment is primarily descriptive, although it may become evaluative where the assessment is repeated at some point following therapy to determine changes due to intervention. Predictive value is limited, although obvious trends may suggest or confirm assumptions.

Role analysis

As discussed in Chapter 5, occupational roles 'come with the job'; they are derived from a title associated with the occupation, and such titles are always regarded as highly significant definitions of who, and what, that person is. Social roles define a relationship or other social function.

The first concern of the therapist is to identify which occupational and social roles the person possesses. The spread of roles, like occupations, changes with age, and is subject to strong cultural influences. Social roles tend to lead to the requirement to adopt occupational roles. In some cultures roles are gender-linked and it would be highly inappropriate to ask a person to cross the gender boundary. In Britain such attitudes are changing, but are persistent in some areas, while in other countries, e.g. Africa or India, these distinctions are still clear. Roles are linked to status; this is also culturally determined. It is essential for the therapist to use the appropriate cultural norms when evaluating roles.

There are a number of secondary questions to ask once a pattern of roles has been established:

- How does this pattern compare with that expected of a person of similar age, sex, culture and social status (e.g. is it richer, impoverished, atypical)? Is there the expected balance (allowing for individual variation)?
- What does the pattern reveal about the individual (e.g. relationships, responsibilities, interests, abilities)?
- Is the person coping satisfactorily with these roles? (If not, in what way is she dysfunctional?)
- Does the person acknowledge ownership of her roles?

A limited repertoire of roles, inability to perform a significant role, or rejection of a role, may be signals for intervention.

Participation analysis

Occupations are conducted over a length of time: it is therefore useful to review what the spread of occupations was at some previous point, what it is like now, and how the individual thinks it will be in the future.

Most of this information can be obtained by means of a semi-structured interview, or by asking the patient to complete a self-rating checklist.

At organizational level it is difficult to obtain more than a general indication of where problems or difficulties in occupational performance occur; this is best done at effective level in relation to specific activities. As part of participation analysis, however, it is useful to identify which occupations present difficulties, and whether these relate to only one area of function or to several.

Existential analysis

The person's view of the sociocultural nature of her occupations, e.g. whether they are viewed as work, leisure or self-care, is useful in indicating general themes and whether a lifestyle has the expected balance for that individual. However, notions of balance must be treated with caution; in addition, it should be recognized that occupational designations are affected by changes in situational elements.

Similarly, questions concerning subjective reactions to occupations can only produce general indications, since occupations include many processes, some of which may be liked, while others are not enjoyed. Reactions to these questions are highly individual. For example, the person who says, 'I like being a secretary' may really mean, 'I like my boss and the contact with people, and I quite enjoy word-processing, but I hate filing.'

CONCLUSION

The process of assessment is instrumental in setting the aims of intervention and monitoring its effectiveness. The therapist needs a range of basic assessment skills and procedures.

Therapists have attempted to use reductive and analytical methods to produce valid assessment data, but have found it difficult to confine the rich and highly individual patterns of human activity within a methodology that was developed originally for research.

It has been suggested in this chapter that educational and sociological models may offer alternative methodology. It is further suggested that, while improved methodology is being developed, it may be helpful to adopt a more structured approach to functional analysis – one which recognizes that different occupational levels raise different concerns and require different forms of investigation.

14

Occupational analysis and adaptation

OCCUPATIONAL ANALYSIS

Of all the processes of occupational therapy, this is the one which differentiates it most from other professions with shared concerns.

The term 'occupational analysis' is used as a convenient generic description, but there are several different forms of analysis. Macroanalysis is concerned with understanding the nature and performance demand of occupations. In a similar way, activity analysis provides a description of activities, and microanalysis describes tasks. These three forms of analysis are 'pure'; they are concerned with the nature of what is done, not with the performance of an individual 'doer'.

Applied activity analysis or task analysis is the means whereby the therapist uses activities or tasks as therapy to enable, enhance or empower performance.

Occupational analysis and applied analysis are linked to functional analysis, which is concerned with the level of competence of individual performance (see Ch. 13), and also to environmental analysis (see Ch. 15).

Table 14.1 shows how these different forms of analysis are related to each core element – environment, person occupation and therapist, and to differing timeframes – past, present and future.

MACROANALYSIS

Macroanalysis takes place at the organizational level and involves description of an occupation

Table 14.1 Forms of analysis in relation to occupational levels

Area of core concern	Environment	Person	Occupation	Therapist	Time frame
Type of analysis	Environmental analysis	Functional analysis	Occupational analysis	Applied analysis	
Organizational level	General analysis	Participation analysis	Macroanalysis		Extended (past, present, future)
Effective level	Demand analysis	Participation analysis	Activity analysis	Applied activity analysis	
		Existential analysis			Extended or current
	Adaptive analysis	Performance analysis			
Developmental level	Demand analysis	Performance analysis	Microanalysis	Applied task analysis	Current (duration of task)
	Adaptive analysis				

using the '10P' analysis headings. (Readers who need to remind themselves of the occupational taxonomy and '10P' headings should refer to Chapter 5, page 85, Box 5.5.

Attributes are divided into two groups: sociocultural and observable. Sociocultural attributes are subjective phenomena which may be difficult to observe, while observable attributes relate to aspects of the occupation which are overt and can readily be studied by an observer.

Using this 10-point structure it would be possible (but very time-consuming) to produce a detailed and comprehensive analysis of an occupation at all levels. A more far-reaching, indicative approach would enable a general understanding of the occupation to be obtained. It is comparatively simple to make precise statements about attributes which are readily observable. It is far more difficult and time-consuming to make precise statements about sociocultural attributes, which are often implicit.

THE PARTICIPANT

An occupation is merely an abstract concept unless it has a participant. The participant is given a title derived from, or related to, the title of the occupation. However, it is important to

recognize that in macroanalysis one is concerned not with the individual participant but with the characteristics of the 'typical' participant.

This might include consideration of age, physical and psychological abilities, education, training, and any other relevant factor, so that a profile of an average participant may be obtained.

This is akin to the kind of profiling carried out for recruitment or educational purposes (but should not be restricted to occupations which are obviously 'jobs', since the therapist has a much wider definition of occupation). Some occupations are open to a wide range of participants having differing abilities and characteristics, others require the participant to possess a narrow range of skills and abilities.

SOCIOCULTURAL ATTRIBUTES

These attributes are difficult to analyse, which may be therapists have not, so far, tended to pay much attention to such analysis, accepting sociocultural features as part of a set of general, background assumptions. However, in terms of understanding occupations as sociological or cultural entities they become important.

Sociocultural attributes are based on the beliefs, attitudes and opinions of the participants in the occupation, and of those who are external to it in a specific culture. These attributes change only slowly, and may sometimes lag behind external events, causing a mismatch between the occupation and the reality of the world in which it now operates.

A description of such attributes can be obtained only by ethnographic or illuminative studies over an extended period of time. This area of qualitative investigation may well be one with which occupational scientists will in future concern themselves. The tools to do this require development, and the following summary indicates the breadth and potential difficulty of the area of study.

Principles

These are the intellectual foundations of the occupation which may include concepts, ideas, assumptions, values or ethics. All occupations, however simple, have some implicit guiding principles, but some complex occupations have many, and it would take a great deal of careful analysis to tease these out.

Position

This relates to the sociocultural position of the occupation. Is it generally regarded as work, as leisure, or as self-care, or perhaps as all three, under differing circumstances? What social status does the occupation have? Is there a hierarchy within it? Are there any cultural aspects affecting or limiting participation?

Possessions

These are the territories claimed by participants in the occupation and recognized by others as owned by the occupation. This may relate to intellectual territory, a sphere of action or a place in which the action takes place.

Purposes

These are the reasons for the occupation to exist. They include a summary of the practical inten-

tions, and socio-economic or cultural benefits – but not the subjective purposes of a particular individual, which are a different matter.

OBSERVABLE ATTRIBUTES

These are attributes which the therapist might identify by observing the occupation in practice.

Products

A product may be tangible or abstract. Between the commencement and ending of a process or activity some result must have been achieved: something can be observed to have changed, a thing has been made, a service provided, an idea transmitted, some new knowledge found or some experience gained. It should therefore be possible to make a list of what, in total, is made, achieved or changed.

It is important to try to separate purpose – the reason why something is done, from product – the result of action, although the two things may be very similar in some cases, where the purpose is 'to produce the product'.

By the time the products are viewed at organizational level they are usually visible and readily identifiable. However, at lower performance levels, products may be less tangible, e.g. in the forms of ideas, plans or mental calculations. These are just as important (sometimes more so since they form the foundation for performance) as tangible, observable products, and must not be excluded.

Processes

Processes are the means whereby the purposes and products of an occupation are accomplished. Metaprocesses organize a chain of processes, generic processes describe a typical type of performance, and integrative processes link a series of activities in sequence.

A process usually has a descriptive title, and can be analysed as having several typical actions, purpose(s) and products(s). Processes may be independent of each other, or linked as stages in the production of a complex final product to form a metaprocess. (Refer back to Figure 11.1 on page 158 for an illustration of process analysis).

To understand a process in detail, further analysis would be required to identify its component activities. Activity analysis and microanalysis would provide further detail so that it would, theoretically, be possible to describe the processes of an occupation through chains of activities, into task sequences, tasks and task stages down to the smallest task segment.

This would, however, be an exercise of impractical size and complexity, and it would result in a reductive list which might not contribute to the understanding of the occupation as a whole. It has been found useful to analyse a sample process as an academic exercise for students in making the complexity of an occupation apparent.

A process may be an occasional, frequent or continual component of an occupation. It may have a fixed timescale or a very loose and flexible one. Nonetheless, a process remains a generalized, organizing and descriptive concept, and is not tied to a specific time and place. For example, gardening is an occupation; growing herbaceous plants is a metaprocess; tending the herbaceous border is an integrative process; staking is a generic process or action, but as soon as the gardener speaks of going out after lunch to stake the delphiniums, it becomes an activity.

Integrative processes which are organizational or preparatory, involving the use of skills within the cognitive – affective domain such as planning, problem-solving, inventing, imaging or other creative actions within the potent sector, are harder or observe, but are essential to competent performance. In some occupations, inability to undertake such processes would be seriously detrimental, and even simple occupations involve some planning or preparation. It is frequently at this stage that personal emotions, values and preferences intrude to affect internal processing and subsequent actions.

Patterns

At this level, patterns refer mainly to organizational temporal elements and sequences. Occupational patterns may change in relation to the age of the participant. The patterns of an occupation are typically extended over a long period of time. They include, for example the times when the occupation is performed, seasonally, or over a week or day: the duration of processes within the occupation; the repetition of processes and the sequences in which these are commonly arranged.

Practical requirements

At the occupational level it is useful to restrict analysis to a broad approach, giving a general list of the types of human resources, tools, equipment, machines, transport, materials and environmental factors required for performance. At this level, taking carpentry as an example, it is practical to list, e.g. workshop, timber, materials for fixing and finishing, hand tools and machine tools.

However, it would be quite possible to provide a complete list of everything which might conceivably be required for an occupation to be carried out: the DHSS Building notes and equipment schedules which give detailed specifications for building and equipping various hospital departments are examples of this.

Performance demand

At organizational level, identification of performance demand is best restricted to generalities, describing the types of knowledge, skills, attitudes and abilities required for effective engagement in the occupation.

A detailed analysis could, of course, be undertaken; this is the type of analysis required when planning a competency-based educational programme for a vocation, e.g. National Vocational Qualifications. Analysis of performance demand, like that of practical requirements, is more easily achieved at effective level.

ACTIVITY ANALYSIS

Activity analysis provides the therapist with a tool whereby the nature and performance of an

activity may be understood, its demands described and its therapeutic usefulness evaluated. This form of analysis is context-free, in that it is not related to the needs of any specialty or individual patient, although is a useful precursor to applied analysis.

In practice, one is seldom required to undertake an exhaustive activity analysis, except as an academic exercise, although this does greatly improve the understanding of the nature of activities and their place in human life.

It is more common to concentrate on particular aspects – social, physical and cognitive – which are currently relevant. For the therapist in a hurry, Johnson's (1992) 'How, what, why, where, when and who' checklist is a practical alternative, but it should not replace thorough activity analysis.

Activity analysis involves the consideration of stable and situational elements, and of a number of factors. Such analysis can be conducted as and when there is time or need, and could readily be used to build a portfolio of basic analysis for a specific clinical area or typical client needs, which could subsequently serve as a time-saving resource for applied analysis(Table 14.2).

It should be immediately apparent from Table 14.2 why the bulk of the practice of occupational therapy is focused at the effective level, rather than the organizational level. An activity is capable

of analysis and control, and acknowledges individual responses to, and the meanings of, a unique episode, whereas an occupation, while providing an organizing framework or a useful overview, is too generalized and complex for specific therapeutic application.

STABLE ELEMENTS

Stable elements are those which can be observed objectively and are relatively consistent features of the activity.

Purpose and product

These elements are usually readily identified. They are implied in the activity title and simply need re-stating or expanding.

Procedure and practical requirements

Components tasks are listed in sequence. The usual requirements for, e.g. tools, materials, space, time and environment are listed in relation to each task.

Performance demand

This is an analysis of all the performance skills which are utilized during the activity. At the

Table 14.2 Activity analysis

	Stable elements	Situational elements
Purpose	General intention and sociocultural classification	Potential variations in intentions and motivations
Product	General description and possibilities; accepted standards or values	Potential for variations in product or outcome, design options, personal choices, personal standards or values
Procedure	The usual sequence of routines and task	Potential for alterations to sequence
Practical requirements	The need for time, space, tools, equipment, furniture, materials and environment	Alterations to these factors
Performance demand	The knowledge, skills and attitudes generally required for competent performance	The potential for altering performance demand
Participant	General person specification	Potential for altering general person specification

simplest level, it may be sufficient to make a superficial analysis of general performance demand, such as simplicity or complexity, need to follow instruction and whether physical action requires strength or dexterity, and to make a generalized list of skills in each domain. This will provide an activity performance profile which will indicate the main features.

A detailed analysis of performance demand, such as is described by Mosey (1986) as 'the generic approach to activity analysis', can be extremely lengthy. Mosey lists 10 considerations, each of which have many subsections. Johnson's (1992) list of demands is similar but more generalized. Simon (1993) gives further examples. A version of the lists given by Mosey and Johnson is included for comparison (Table 14.3).

Participant

Once performance demand is understood a profile of the 'ideal' participant can be formed, stating the general abilities, knowledge and skills which will be needed to complete the activity effectively.

SITUATIONAL ELEMENTS

Situational elements can be identified in general terms, as a list of things which may potentially alter from one occasion to another. This listing process is a useful tool in pointing out areas where therapeutic adaptation may be possible, but it has to remain generalized.

Purpose and product

The potential personal purposes or motivations for undertaking the activity (as opposed to the objective purposes) are listed in general terms.

The potentials for individual variations connected with the product can be listed, e.g. size, shape, colour, quantity; there may be either a great deal of scope for choice, or little scope.

Procedure and practical requirements

Taking the previously described task sequence, the points are identified where variation in

sequence, additions or omissions is possible. Opportunities to vary, e.g. environments, performance conditions, tools, materials and number of personnel can be noted. Again, some activities have rigid procedures which are hard to change, and permit little variation in practical requirements, while others are very flexible. Flexibility is an asset when therapeutic adaptation is required.

Participant

It is quite apparent that the individual participant will affect the activity, but in the absence of a real person further analysis is difficult. It may be possible to make some general comments about changes likely to result from more or fewer people being involved, or from differences in age or culture.

When an activity is actually to be performed by a particular person it becomes possible to analyse the stable and situational elements in relation to that person, on a given occasion, in relation to needs (see applied analysis, p. 229).

MICROANALYSIS

Microanalysis, as its name implies, involves the detailed examination of tasks and their constituents. Task analysis uses structured observation, and/or written analysis or flowcharts, to break the task down into task stages and, if necessary, task stages into task segments.

It is often difficult to determine the level of performance – is it a task, or a task stage? There is no definitive way of deciding this, since tasks vary greatly in complexity, but in general it should be possible to divide a task into a manageable series of stages, and these into chains of task segments which are not too long.

If sequences become long and seem involved, or descriptive terminology seems to have been exhausted before the task has been analysed to its smallest segments, then it is probable that analysis has been commenced too high up the hierarchy of performance. Further examination will usually reveal that what was thought to be a

Table 14.3 Headings for activity analysis (Mosey 1986, Johnson 1992)

Mosey (psychosocial dysfunction)	Johnson (physical dysfunction)

I Sensory integration
    Sensory input
    Opportunity for integration
	I Motor/physical
	    Position
	    Movement
	    Grading
	    Sensory

II Motor function
    Functional capacity required
    Types of motions	

III Cognitive functions
    Attention
    Memory
    Orientation
    Though processes
    Abstract vs concrete thinking
    Intelligence
    Factual information
    Problem-solving
    Symbolic potential
	II Sensory
	    Visual
	    Auditory (including language)
	    Olfactory
	    Gustatory
	    Tactile/kinaesthetic

IV Psychological function
    Dynamic states
    Intrapsychic dynamics
    Reality testing
    Insight
    Object relations
    Self-concept
    Self-discipline
    Concept of others
	III Cognitive
	    Motivation
	    Learning (including memory)
	    Problem-solving
	    Logical thinking
	    Communication
	    Organizational ability

V Social interaction
    Interpretation of situation
    Social skills (dyads, groups, communication)
    Structured social display
	IV Perceptual
	    Agnosia
	    Apraxia
	    Spatial relationship disorders
	    Self-awareness disorders

VI Occupational performances
    Relevance to social roles (family, ADL, work, leisure)
    Temporal adaptation
	V Emotional
	    Activity demands/offers

	VI Social Activity demands/offers

VII Age
    Age specific?
    Relevance to developmental tasks
    Adaptation to loss
	VII Independence
	    Activity demands/offers

VIII Cultural implications (meaning, relevance)
    Ethnic groups
    Socioeconomic group
	VIII Cultural
	    Activity demands/offers

IX Social implications
    Involve social network?
    Involve family members?
    Implications for sick role
    Community resources
    Physical environment	

X Other considerations Includes: time, task sequence and breakdown, equipment, materials, space, noise, dirt, cost	

Note: Further subdivisions and subsections have been omitted from both lists.

task was in fact an activity, or perhaps that a task stage was really a task, and microanalysis needs to be taken further down the chain. It is important that sequences do not become too long and involved as this makes it difficult to teach or apply the task.

At developmental level, subjective considerations become less relevant since a small portion of an activity is regarded as part of the activity, and therefore is viewed subjectively in that context (see Ch. 5). Task analysis is an exercise in objective observation. Similarly, a single task has low sociocultural significance. Interpersonal aspects, other than basic communication skills, are better considered at the level of activity.

Microanalysis is used for several purposes, including: facilitating teaching; identifying the point at which performance may become difficult for an individual, and offering a solution to this; eliminating stages, or re-designing task sequence to make performance simpler or to save energy. Considerations are:

- sequence of stages (or segments)
- performance requirements – tools, materials, etc
- environmental considerations – human and non-human
- skills required

SKILL ANALYSIS

Linked to task analysis is skill analysis, which is used to identify which of the basic skills are employed in task performance. The results of skill analysis indicate performance demand at developmental level. This can provide information for skill development, or for therapeutic application.

A general skill analysis can be useful in screening for probable causes of dysfunction and to identify therapeutic application in broad terms. Skills can be described in three domains: sensorimotor, interactive and cognitive–affective. The headings given in Chapter 4, page 62 are also convenient for use in microanalysis.

Once again, a clear distinction must be made between skills analysis, to find out what skills are required to do the job, and performance analysis, in which the ability of the person to use his personal skills to perform the task competently is assessed.

FRAMES OF REFERENCE FOR TASK ANALYSIS

Task analysis may be conducted within a frame of reference which narrows the scope of inquiry to a specific area of performance. This is normally done in association with applied analysis; some commonly-used frames of reference are briefly described below.

BIOMECHANICAL ANALYSIS

The itemizes the muscles used, the type of muscle and the types and ranges of movement during task performance. It may also take note of sensory requirements such as type of touch, or sensitivity to heat or cold. It is used especially in relation to the function of the hand and upper limb, where analysis of praxis and different types of grip becomes important. This requires detailed use of kinesiology, in relation to a specific task.

NEURODEVELOPMENTAL ANALYSIS

This considers implications for positioning, reflex activity, balance, posture, the effects of gravity, the potential for sensory stimulation or sensory integration, and other elements related to neurodevelopmental frames of reference. It may include consideration of the degree to which particular agnosias or apraxias may affect, or be influenced by, task performance.

COGNITIVE–PERCEPTUAL ANALYSIS

This examines the perceptual content of the task and/or the need for cognitive skills, especially attention, memory, recall, planning, sequencing, problem-solving, and concrete and abstract reasoning.

INTERACTIVE ANALYSIS

As previously noted, single tasks provide little scope for interaction, but at developmental level it may be necessary to conduct a microanalysis considering the components of communication between therapist and patient during the task, e.g. eye contact, expression, body language, verbalization, listening, and following demonstration or instruction.

BEHAVIOURAL ANALYSIS

This is concerned with defining the sequence of task stages and components and framing these precisely. It is linked to applied analysis in which behaviours may be cued, prompted, and reinforced in specified ways. Environmental cues may be considered as well as those provided by the therapist.

APPLIED ANALYSIS

Applied analysis is what enables a therapist to turn participation in an activity into therapy. There will be some specific objective or objectives; in general terms the aim of participation in a therapeutic activity will be to provide therapist and patient with more information concerning his present condition, or, where a need has already been recognized, to enable or enhance performance, or provide opportunities through which the patient can be empowered to learn, change, or experience something.

A therapist's preliminary assessment of an individual and the preliminary stages of the case management process will have provided some understanding of the patient's abilities, needs or dysfunctions, social and environmental circumstances, personal interests, wishes and aspirations. This will lead to a number of decisions about the case, such as:

- the significant clinical features
- the significant sociocultural features
- the priority problems or needs of the patient
- the patient's interests, attitudes, concerns or wishes
- whether the information is sufficient
- whether further assessment needs to be done
- whether occupational therapy is appropriate
- the general purpose of treatment or intervention (to enable, enhance or empower by means of rehabilitation, development, education or other processes)
- aims and objectives to be achieved
- possible approach.

Each of these issues generates many ideas, connections, speculations and decisions which affect the purpose and process of analysis.

In general terms there are four main purposes:

- to enable the therapist to select a suitable activity (or options) which meet treatment needs and offer appropriate choices to a patient or group of patients
- to assist the therapist is setting up, organizing and sequencing the activity
- to facilitate teaching and learning
- to enable appropriate adaptation of the activity.

Applied analysis takes as its starting point the general information obtained by activity analysis and/or microanalysis. This provides an outline understanding of the activity or task. The objective of applied analysis is to relate this information to the specific individual on a particular occasion for a defined therapeutic purpose.

In theory, the therapist starts with an infinite array of potential activities. In practice, the needs and interests of the patient, environment of therapy, practical considerations and performance demands will reduce this to a few, potentially relevant activities. Which should be chosen? How do the aims of therapy affect this choice? Who makes the decision, therapist, patient, or both? A screening or filtering process needs to take place before an activity, or several activities, can be considered for a treatment programme, for the process of analysis is time-consuming.

The therapist, therefore, has to exercise considerable skill in clinical reasoning before making a shortlist of activities or a final selection. The clinical reasoning process provides a rapid 'elimination scan' which may result in a definite decision, but results more often in a shortlist, or 'let us try that and observe what happens ...'. No therapist will always select the right activity first time, but the expert practitioner will make the right decision fairly consistently, and will rapidly be able to make modifications to programmes as they progress.

Applied activity analysis must consider both objective and subjective elements of the activity. Objective considerations are those related to the stable elements in a basic activity analysis. Subjective considerations relate more to the situational elements. The degree to which each of these elements is of importance will again vary with the chosen approach and the needs of the individual.

The most useful information is that provided by the summary of performance demand and the analysis of situational elements, which indicate how adaptable the activity may be. This must be related to the needs and interests of the patient and to the aims and objectives of the intervention. These factors may place some limitations on the available options.

OBJECTIVE AND SUBJECTIVE CONSIDERATIONS

Objective considerations

The following factors need to be considered:

• The demand for performance: what general characteristics is the participant required to possess to succeed in this activity? Is there a match between these and either the existing or the desired abilities of the patient?
• The specific performance requirements: cognitive, sensorimotor and interactive. Do these match the therapeutic objectives? Is there potential for therapeutic adaptation? This is usually achieved by analysing the activity into tasks and analysing the performance requirements of the tasks.
• The degree of complexity of the activity – if too complex, can it be simplified?
• The degree of structure – a continuum of rigidity to flexibility. What is needed?
• Duration of activity; opportunities for rests and changes in routines.
• The practical requirements: tools, equipment and environment.
• Risks, hazards and precautions.

Subjective considerations

The following factors should be taken into consideration:

• Patient's needs and wishes, likes and dislikes. Opportunities for choices.
• Sociocultural considerations: positive/negative, appropriateness for age, sex and status.
• Potential for engagement of patient interest and participation.

• Familiarity versus novelty; safe exploration versus challenge.
• Potential for exploration of affective responses.
• Potential for exploration of roles and relationships.
• Potential for providing positive experiences: enjoyment, exploration, mastery, competence and control.
• Temporal focus – does the activity facilitate exploration of the past, experience of the present or projections about the future?

It should be evident from the above description of the process of selection that this is no way a matter of using a formula. Each patient requires an individual programme, and while similar problems may result in similar prescriptions, this can not be taken for granted.

To reassure the reader who by now feels that this implies an overly directive and prescriptive approach on the part of the therapist, of course this process should be conducted in collaboration with the patient. However, the expertise of the therapist lies in eliminating some activities and suggesting others, and in making specific adaptations. The processes of activity analysis and applied analysis are not ones in which the patient is equipped, or very probably even motivated, to engage. An interested person can always be given a suitably condensed explanation of what has been involved and its relevance to his situation.

Occupational therapy is quite often compared to an iceberg, in which the visible tip represents only a small part of the whole. There is nothing wrong with this. However, the therapist should be prepared to explain and justify the 'unseen' parts of therapy, if the patient wishes this.

STAGES IN APPLIED ANALYSIS

The first stage is a clinical reasoning process, whereby the therapist reviews the needs of the patient and the therapeutic goals or objectives, and provides a shortlist of compatible activities.

The second stage is to rewrite the basic activity analysis of one (or more) potential activities in terms of the precise event which is being considered (or to undertake a new analysis if required.)

The process of applied analysis involves looking at the activity analysis of the event or situation thich the therapist proposes to set up, and asking a number of questions related to the following considerations.

In the third stage the potential therapeutic activity can be analysed and evaluated to see if the match is good, and if it could be improved by some alteration of the situational elements. At this stage, applied environmental analysis may also be needed.

This sounds complex – and can be – but it becomes much simpler given a real patient and a real situation.

FACTORS TO BE CONSIDERED IN APPLIED ANALYSIS

Therapeutic relevance

The whole point of using an activity as therapy is to produce a desired result for the patient. An activity which lacks therapeutic relevance may be relaxing, enjoyable and 'therapeutic', but it is not occupational therapy.

The therapist must be able to justify, to colleagues, patient and referring agent, that the chosen activity does have therapeutic relevance. It is also necessary to be able to discriminate between the potential relevance of different activities. However, therapeutic relevance is not the only factor, and the other factors must also be considered. It would be of no use, for example, to select an activity which satisfied therapeutic aims as a 'paper exercise', if it was something which was considered unpleasant or irrelevant by the patient, or which took up far too much time in preparation.

Practicalities

The commonsense consideration of feasibility needs to be remembered. In order for an activity to be performed effectively all the necessary tools and materials must be available. The environment must be capable of producing the right demand. The cost may need to be considered.

The preparation of, and clearing up or disposal following, the activity and any antecedent, contiguous or consequent activities must be identified. It is important to note whether preparation will be undertaken by the patient (or another), in which case further analysis of the antecedent activities may be required, or by a member of staff, in which case the effective use of time must be considered.

It is of little use to involve the patient in a task, however relevant, if it takes a therapist or assistant half an hour to set it up and another to finish it off or clear up afterwards. Another common problem is caused by initiating an activity which is part of an extended process which must, once started, be completed. For example, sowing seeds implies pricking out, potting up and either selling or planting: it would lose meaning if the planted seeds are simply to be thrown away.

Elimination of undesirable features

Undesirable features are those situational elements which are not relevant to the treatment aims, or which may impede the performance of an individual. Sometimes these can easily be altered, but sometimes they cannot. Examples include: a stage in an activity which is irrelevant – perhaps someone else can do it; a risk factor, e.g. heat, dirt or a particular movement which is contraindicated; too much, or too little, choice; a difficult working position; or an anxiety provoking situation.

Enabling or empowering

The purpose of therapy is often to enable or empower an individual in a particular way. The activity may contain opportunities which can be adapted or exaggerated in order to achieve this.

Enhancement

Where the therapist seeks to enhance the quality of performance or experience, the situational elements of the activity can be reviewed to see where there may be scope to achieve this by emphasizing or altering certain features, providing aids or cues, or changing methods.

Grading

Grading is 'The measurable increasing or decreasing of activity. Measurable changes may be graded by length of time, size, degree of strength required or amount of energy expended' (Reed & Sanderson 1983).

This definition stems from the biomechanical frame of reference. Although grading is often used in the context of physical performance components, it should also be applied to grading of cognitive or perceptual complexity and the intricacies of sequencing and organizing the activity.

At this stage the therapist is concerned with evaluating the potential for grading in relation to specific treatment objectives. Methods used to provide grading are describe later (Box 14.2).

Readiness to meet performance demand

This refers to the readiness of the patient to participate in the activity, in terms of current knowledge, skills and attitudes. It may well be that a patient may need a period of training, education or practice before he is ready to attempt the activity.

This may be a simple matter of a few minutes' explanation and demonstration, or it might take several weeks of planned training and development. The activity may be too difficult for a particular stage of recovery or development. Unless the activity is being used as a deliberate challenge or as an assessment of the level of function, it is generally unhelpful to expect a patient to tackle an activity for which he is not ready.

Individual relevance

An activity may be theoretically relevant to the treatment of a condition and able to meet defined aims, but inappropriate to the individual. Judgements about individual relevance must consider a range of sociocultural and personal factors. These may include: age appropriateness, gender implications, cultural attitudes and prohibitions, personal likes and dislikes, personal interests and personal goals.

There are many therapeutic situations where the subjective elements of performance are far more important than the objective ones. In such cases, the therapist is concerned less identifying the skills needed to perform than with involvement the patient in the performance. This is especially common in the mental health setting, where aims relate to psychosocial responses or self-esteem and confidence-building. This is where patient choice and involvement in the selection of activities is an essential part of the therapeutic process.

Preservation of meaning

The experience of an activity as meaningful is a complex phenomenon which is difficult to predict. At this stage, it is important to ensure that the meaning which is normally attributed to an activity within the relevant culture is retained during the therapeutic experience.

In simple terms, fun activities must stay fun, work should feel like work, problems to be solved should be seen as real relevant, purposes – whether objective or subjective – should be genuine, not contrived, and creativity should remain stimulating. Meaning can be changed by over-adaptation, by the artificiality of a clinical area, by incorrect environmental demand, and by the manner of presentation.

Individual choice

The therapist must have a clear view of the degree to which the choice of the patient is to be promoted or constrained during therapy. It must be recognized that in some cases patients are unable to cope with choice, or at least with too much choice, due to cognitive or affective dysfunction, hence free choice from many options, instead of being pleasant, becomes bewildering and stressful. Patients who have become institutionalized often need much guidance and re-education in making choices and accepting responsibility for them.

There are, equally, patients for whom it is necessary and desirable to offer real choices and options as part of the process of personal direction of therapy.

The points in the course of the activity where choices can be made should be identified, and consideration given to whether these choices should be exaggerated or diminished.

CHECKLIST FOR APPLIED ANALYSIS

The points listed in Box 14.1 may be used as a checklist.

A list similar to that given in Box 14.1 would be used to evaluate an activity for use with a group, with the addition of questions about the ways in which the activity involves, and is appropriate to, all the group members. This process is illustrated in Figure 14.1.

THERAPEUTIC ADAPTATION

Applied analysis may indicate that adaptation of the activity is needed in order to meet the aims of therapy. Each aim will provide a reason for selecting an activity. How far will the individual be involved in the choices? What kind of activity analysis is needed? These elements will be decided in relation to a model or frame of reference.

In many cases the activity contains the therapeutic elements with little or no need for adaptation. In Chapter 5 I made the proposition that the activities most suited for use as therapy are those which have low performance demand, i.e. those which can be engaged in by the majority of patients, or which can be presented

---

Box 14.1   Checklist for applied analysis

1. What elements in the performance demand, purposes and products of this activity relate to the roles/needs/abilities/interests of this person, as stated in the treatment goals or objectives? Do these relevant elements form the major part of the activity? If the purpose is assessment of the individual, how does the activity provide opportunities for this? (*Therapeutic relevance*)
2. Is it realistic to engage in this activity in terms of its practical requirements and procedures? (Available time for preparation, completion and clearing up, tools and materials available, cost, enough space, appropriate environment, etc.) (*Practicalities*)
3. Are there elements which do not relate to needs/abilities/interests?
    Are these a major or minor part of the activity? If a minor part, can the situational elements be adapted to minimize the irrelevant aspects? How can this be done? (*Elimination of undesirable features*)
4. Which features of the activity contribute to enabling or empowering the patient? Are there elements which will make the activity difficult for this individual? Can these be eliminated or adapted to facilitate performance? How can this be done? (*Enabling/empowering*)
5. Do the situational elements enable these relevant performances or experiences to be emphasized? How can this best be done? (*Enhancement*)
6. Is the activity to be performed on a single occasion, or repeated?
    Is there a need to grade the activity – if so, how might this be done? (*Grading*)
7. Does the individual need instruction/information, or any other form of preparation before engaging in this activity? If so, a teaching programme will be needed, based on activity and task analysis. (*Readiness to meet performance demand*)
8. Does this activity have relevance to this individual (age-appropriate, culturally appropriate, meaningful purpose, product or outcome, etc. (*Individual relevance*)
9. Do therapeutic adaptations to the activity of the environment intrude on the gestalt of the activity and affect meaning or relevance? (*Preservation of meaning*)
10. How does engagement in this activity relate to any expressed choice or preference of the individual? Can the individual be given a choice of activities, or opportunities for choice within this activity? Must choices be constrained? (*Individual choice*)

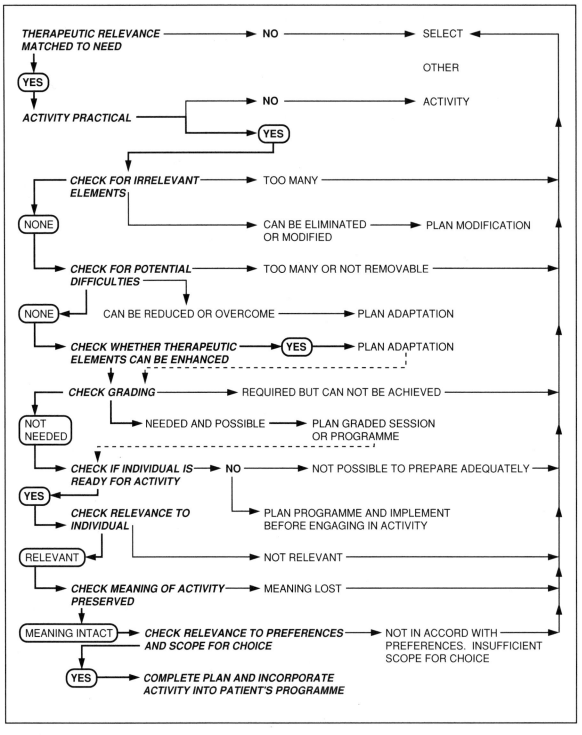

Figure 14.1 Flowchart illustrating applied analysis.

in a 'user friendly' manner. However, in the context of therapy, one or more of the 'normal' elements of the activity may require alteration.

The general purpose of adaptation is either to make participation more specifically therapeutic, by emphasizing the desirable features and reducing those which are undesirable or have no therapeutic value, or to enhance and enable performance by removing barriers or providing aids.

The question of therapeutic adaptation is one which requires careful consideration; an activity has its own gestalt. Many familiar activities become personalized in their performance. If the activity is heavily adapted, presented in an obviously artificial manner, or minimalized in order to achieve some specific therapeutic objective, it can be difficult to retain its coherence, normality, and the parapherhalia of subjective responses which would usually be associated with it.

It has been said that the art of fine cooking is to take the best ingredients and to do as little as possible to them. This seems to me to be very appropriate advice on the use of activities. Therapists are concerned with normal, purposeful activities. Once an activity is perceived by its participant as abnormal, or if it loses its purpose, then the dynamics of occupational therapy are altered.

In general, such adaptation requires divergent thinking, problem-solving, and a predisposition to look for alternative ways of tackling a task, rather than accepting a given format. It is difficult to adapt an activity with which the therapist is unfamiliar. Activity analysis provides information concerning the potential for adaptation. Where the activity is unfamiliar the therapist may need to observe it being performed by a number of people, and also, where possible, perform it herself, in order to appreciate the nature of performance and the consequences of adaptation.

An activity is adapted in order to make it different in some useful way, e.g. longer, shorter, more complex, more simple or more sociable; the list of potential adaptations is as long as the list of potential therapeutic objectives. The skill of the therapist lies in making such alterations as

unobtrusive to the participant as possible, or where unavoidably obtrusive, in ensuring by explanation that the reason for the adaptation is understood.

The point has already been made that therapists can view an activity in a variety of ways when providing therapy, alternatively emphasizing the process, the product, the purpose and the meaning. Different frames of reference have differing perspectives on this. A more client-centred response may consider any adaptation irrelevant and may value the product or successful outcome more than any specific therapeutic by-product of the process.

FEATURES OF AN ACTIVITY WHICH MAY BE ADAPTED

Features of an activity which may be adapted include:

- environment; location, setting, milieu, demand
- equipment: quantity, availability and presentation of tools and materials; adaptations to tools and equipment, e.g. size and shape of handles
- technique: the way in which an activity is performed
- sequence: the order of tasks, omission of non-essential tasks, rests, rigidity or flexibility of sequences
- temporal features: duration and repetition; focus on past, present or future
- performance demand: sensorimotor domain; cognitive–affective domain; interactive domain (grading)
- standards: sociocultural norms; achievable goals or products; use of design to enhance simple products
- cultural meanings: generally accepted sociocultural symbols and attributes.

Adaptations to equipment and materials

Physical alterations to, e.g. shape, size and length, using biomechanical principles such as leverage or torque, are usually those which come to mind first. Colour and texture may also be altered. Many such adaptations are described in current texts on physical rehabilitation, but the elaborate paraphernalia of adaptations to, e.g. looms and printing presses with pulley circuits, weights, slings and springs, which were formerly used have now passed into history.

Useful though these forms of adaptation may be, adaptations to positioning of tools or materials, and of the patient in relation to these, can be equally important, and sometimes render physical adaptation unnecessary.

For example, in the sensorimotor domain, positioning extends or reduces range of movement, requires work to be done with the resistance or assistance of gravity, and alters the amount of strength and endurance required.

In the cognitive domain, positioning materials to be used can bring things within the scope of the patient's attention, or require him to seek it. It may indicate a pre-planned task sequence, or may be haphazard, requiring the patient to impose his own sequence. In the interactive domain, having to ask another person where something is, or to pass things or share things will promote communication.

Adaptations to technique

In physical rehabilitation, techniques may be adapted so that a different movement is required; this may also be useful in overcoming a dysfunction, e.g. joint protection techniques used with rheumatoid patients.

Imaginative adaptations are sometimes needed so that a severely disabled person can participate in a version of an activity, e.g. playing a game on computer, or from a wheelchair. However, this alters the nature of the activity so considerably that it is often equivalent to the invention of a new one, and it may be better presented as such.

Adaptations to sequence

In order for the sequence of a technique or method to be adapted, the standard task sequence must first be understood. It may then be possible to condense stages, remove a stage, or alter the order of stages, in order to reduce effort or complexity. Breaking the activity into stages and introducing rests between these is a frequently used adaptation.

A cognitive approach may be concerned with how information is presented or sequenced, or whether decisions which have to be made in the course of the activity are offered to the participant as problems or solutions.

Temporal adaptation

The length of time which an activity session takes may be adapted, and an activity may be condensed or, more often, stretched over several sessions.

The time elements in an activity which relate to the present may be emphasized, typically those which serve to orient to time of day and associated activities, or to a season. It is also possible to emphasize the retrospective elements, e.g. nostalgia or reminiscence, or those which call attention to the prospective elements – the need for planning and the effect which current actions will have on future actions.

A somewhat different temporal adaptation, which needs to be recognized as an artifice, is the undertaking of an activity with a strong temporal connection, e.g. undressing and going to bed, at an unusual time of day, for practice purposes. This may be quite acceptable to some patients, but to others it can be confusing, or may alter the nature of performance.

Adaptation to performance demand

Grading of the performance demand of an activity, implies a sequence of increasing (or, in some cases, decreasing,) challenges in one or more domains of skill. This is usually in the context of repeated performance where the 'goalposts' are moved progressively as the patient meets each level of challenge and becomes more able. It may also be used to get the demand right on one occasion, or to set an appropriate level for a person whose abilities are unlikely to change.

The performance components which may be

Box 14.2 Performance components which may be graded

Sensorimotor domain	*Interactive domain*	*Cognitive–affective domain*
Range of movement	Proximity to others	Attention
Power/effort	Need for verbal communication	Memory
Stamina/endurance	Need for non-verbal communication	Planning
Repetition of movement	Expression of emotions	Sequencing/organizing
Speed of movement	Listening to others	Problem-solving
Precision of movement	Sharing/turn-taking	Literacy
Coordination	Cooperating	Numeracy
Balance	Showing regard for others	Perceptual skills
Tactile discrimination, e.g.	Taking a leadership role	Following instructions
texture, temperature, pressure	Being assertive	Seeking information
		Making choices
		Taking decisions
		Control of emotions
		Self-confidence
		Self-motivation
		Responsibility for self/others
		Initiative

---

graded are numerous. Box 14.2 indicates some of those which are most commonly adapted.

Adaptation to standards

A standard is an expectation concerning the quality or quantity of performance whereby competence may be judged. The standard may be set by the therapist, by society, by an employer or by the individual. The important point is recognition of who has set the standard and what purpose it serves in the process of therapy.

Personal standards are closely connected with personal culture and values, and it is easy to impose an inappropriate standard on an individual. This is an area where close involvement of the patient in describing the standards he wishes to meet is important.

In a rehabilitation setting, standards may be set and altered as part of grading; the therapist has to face the possibility that the patient may perceive the standard differently from the therapist, especially if insight into the current level of ability is lacking. Striving for an 'unattainable' standard is discouraging and frustrating, but so is being asked to do something at a standard which is perceptibly much lower than the patient would previously have been capable of attaining. Unless this is handled carefully, it may have the effect of 'rubbing the patient's nose' in his dysfunction.

Adaptation to meanings

As meanings are so intensely subjective and personal, adaptation may be viewed as irrelevant or impossible. Meanings may be experienced as positive or negative: positive meanings need to be reinforced and built upon, whereas negative meanings may serve to develop insight or coping skills. Perhaps all that the therapist can hope to do is to try to structure experiences which have positive meaning, as opposed to those which do not, and to use negative meanings constructively.

15

Environmental analysis and adaptation

THE CONTENT AND INFLUENCE OF ENVIRONMENT

As described in Chapter 6, any environment is composed of physical and sociocultural elements. Physical elements are those which are, more or less, stable and capable of perception by the senses, including human constructs and natural features. These may serve practical or aesthetic functions. Sociocultural elements are subjective, mutable and may have a symbolic content. They reflect, and are perceived as a result of, learned cultural and social norms, rules, values and expectations; these, however, become less significant at the lower end of the hierarchy of performance.

In the western world the majority of environments in which humans live and work have been created by people to serve various purposes. This is especially true in a small country such as Britain. Even the apparently 'natural' landscape in the countryside has been created by generations – sometimes dating back several thousand years – of cultivation and exploitation. True wilderness is becoming rare where humans live, even in the less developed parts of the world. People affect environments and environments reciprocally affect people.

Environment influences human responses in both subtle and obvious ways. In the course of normal living an individual seldom stops to analyse these responses unless awareness of the environment becomes conscious, usually because some pleasant or unpleasant feature has intruded.

Too much noise, crowds, or someone else's rowdy or unsettling behaviour will make the individual decide that this is not a comfortable place to be and she will leave. The glorious summer weather and breathtaking view may grasp attention and demand that the person stops to experience and enjoy it. Far more often, the environment is subliminally noted, analysed and accepted, and the individual either rapidly ceases to observe, or remains largely unaware of why she is hurrying and anxious, or quiet and restful, or feeling sociable and relaxed.

Conscious awareness of environment varies considerably from one person to another; some people are acutely sensitive and responsive, while some seem virtually unaware.

In ergonomic terms, the design of an environment can aid or impede functional use. Again, many people are aware only of the results of this – they know that in some environments the task seems easy, or tiring, or that it is hard to maintain concentration, but often find it very difficult to say why. Because people differ in shape, size and strength the 'perfect' environment for one person may well present problems for another.

As individual responses are so varied, it may be questioned whether it is practical for a therapist to attempt environmental analysis or adaptation for therapeutic reasons. If such manipulation was, in fact, ineffective, a legion of designers, marketing consultants, ergonomists, architects and others would be forced out of business. Responses may be individual, but some things tend to work, in any given culture. If the superstore can influence the rate at which shoppers move and the amount of an item which they buy, by changing the piped music or pumping tiny quantities of scents through the air-conditioning, and finds it worthwhile to spend money on such things, then there is surely scope for the therapist!

The occupational therapist is not normally dealing with complex and sophisticated elements of the environment, but with very simple adjustments to basic features. He is concerned with the adaptation and exploitation of the environment in order to facilitate human performance and interactions. In this he seeks to provide a setting in which all or a selection of the following can take place:

- activities can be performed effectively
- interactions can take place
- information may be obtained
- learning may occur
- the patient can explore or practise
- assessment can take place
- therapy can happen.

These aims are achieved by the use of environmental analysis and adaptation, which are closely linked, but distinct, processes. The environment may be that encountered in the client's home, in everyday surroundings, indoors or outside, or in clinical settings.

In order to alter an environment one must first understand it. From an ecological standpoint, environment, users and performances interact, so all these factors must be considered. Alterations need to be made for clear reasons.

From an occupational therapy perspective, therefore, consideration of an environment cannot easily be separated from considerations of the purposes that environment was created to serve, the nature of the users, and the activities or occupations which may take place within it. Such consideration may be purely utilitarian, but must frequently take account of the symbolic function of environmental features, or their special meanings to individuals.

This is particularly important when considering the personal environment created by an individual for her own use. The majority of people, given the opportunity and resources, do like to make some personal alterations and adaptations to their homes. This is a reflection of complex psychological, cognitive and emotional needs, including the need to impose control and ownership on a personal portion of space. It also mirrors the individual's interests, lifestyle and personal history. Indeed, the lack of opportunity to influence one's personal environment, as a result of poverty, homelessness or institutional controls, can be very damaging.

The purpose of environmental analysis is to determine the content of an environment in order to assess the nature of its demand and the potential for adaptation, in relation to therapeutic requirements, or the occupations, activities or roles of an individual.

Environmental adaptation is a secondary process which may or may not be required. During this process, the therapist deliberately manipulates some aspect of the environment in order to enable or enhance performance or to provide more specific therapy.

The foundation of environmental analysis is proficient, structured observation and accurate recording. These skills can be acquired only by repeated practice and experience.

ENVIRONMENTAL ANALYSIS

There are three forms of environmental analysis:

Content analysis: Objective observation of who and what is there.

Demand analysis: Appraisal of the subjective effects on people and their behaviours.

Adaptive analysis: Identification of elements which need to be altered, and of how this may be done.

CONTENT ANALYSIS

Content analysis may be conducted at any occupational level. The technique is similar at each level, but the scale and detail of the analysis differ. The aim is either to record the total content of the environment, or to focus on an aspect of it.

At organizational level content analysis, like macroanalysis, takes a broad-ranging approach, and is aimed at providing an objective summary of the main features and uses of an environment. The location will be somewhere large, e.g. a factory workshop, office, shop, precinct or playground, or a set of rooms; this is related to general occupational uses. It is important in this type of analysis not to become preoccupied with details, which are best dealt with at effective level.

Content analysis can be conducted in relation to a smaller area, e.g. a single room, and in this case it is usually related to one or more of the activities performed within that area. In this kind of analysis, much more detail can be included. For example, a content analysis at organizational level might state 'modern office furniture' with a brief note of colour, style, size or quantity. At effective level it would be necessary to list all the items, and to describe in detail those which have particular uses in connection with the activity being performed.

At developmental level content analysis relates to a small, circumscribed area where a task is being carried out, e.g. a table top. Clearly the content of such an area will be very limited, but the position of objects and their relationship to each other and to a user will become significant.

A 'who, what, where, when, how' approach is needed for content analysis. A checklist may be constructed using some or all of the following headings. However, it is not necessary to ask questions about purposes, meanings or the effects of the environment on the user: this is done in demand analysis.

Natural elements

A general description of non-human features – e.g. climate, geography or natural resources, and organisms – plants, trees or animals, is useful in setting the context of the environmental observation.

Human elements

- *People:* the users of the environment. A description of age-range, gender, and any noticeable sociocultural features, e.g. class, ethnic grouping or cultural subgroups, may be helpful.
- *Constructs:* things which are built to serve human needs, e.g. buildings, roads, bridges and railways. Rural constructs such as farmland, hedges or woodland could be included.
- *Utilitarian artefacts:* things which are made to

be used in occupations, activities and tasks, e.g. tools, equipment, vehicles and furniture.

- *Aesthetic artefacts:* things which exist in order to fulfil decorative functions.
- *Cultural or symbolic features:* things which serve to express cultural identity, or to symbolize cultural, religious, political or other attitudes, values and practices relating to either the users of, or providers of, the environment.

Occupational uses

A description of the occupations or activities for which the environment is used, such as the following:

- work
- leisure
- self-care
- play
- social activity
- cultural affirmation
- religious observance
- education
- social organization/control.

Pattern of use

In some environments the general patterns of use in terms of timing, frequency and duration may need to be noted, together with the number of users at any one time, and whether the pattern is stable or fluctuating.

ANALYSIS OF ENVIRONMENTAL DEMAND

The concept of demand and its importance in occupational therapy have been explained in Chapter 6. Demand is the effect which environment has on shaping human behaviour. It is generated by the combined effects of people, plants and animals, design, objects, tools and materials, uses, activities, rules, expectations and meanings within a given environment at a given moment in time.

These effects predispose the users of the environment to behave in certain ways, to refrain from other behaviours and to have certain subjective responses. People have to learn to recognize environmental signals, to interpret contexts, and to make the links between these and expected behaviours. Most of the signals, once learned, become subliminal triggers which the person no longer consciously recognizes or analyses.

By creating the appropriate demand the therapist may be able to enhance the quality of performance. If the demand is in some way inappropriate, or if the individual, because of deficits in perceptual, social or learning skills, has failed to recognized the demand, performance may be impaired.

The production of demand is often linked to a process of conscious environmental design. Architecture, decor and furniture, contribute to the desired effect. Design is equally important in the utilitarian aspects of demand. The fitness of tools or equipment, storage and handling of materials for their purpose contributes to create demand which facilitates performance. If design is inappropriate for the occupations and activities which will be carried out in an environment, then performance will be impaired.

There is some overlap in this area with the work of ergonomists who are also concerned with occupational and environmental demand – fitting the task to the man' (Grandjean 1988) – but this tends to be in relation to groups of people, such as factory or office workers, rather than to individuals and 'normal' (in the sense of average) populations. Environmental psychologists are also concerned with identifying the relationships between environment and behaviour.

The occupational therapist is concerned with matching the task, the environment and the skills of an individual in order to facilitate occupational performance, often for a person with special needs. The therapist is also concerned with adapting environments for therapeutic purposes, which is beyond the remit of the other professions.

Some of the analytical techniques used by ergonomists and psychologists can, however, be useful to the therapist, and a general awareness of the principles of ergonomics is necessary when designing an efficient and effective environment for a specific purpose.

The analysis of demand identifies the features which contribute to subjective reactions to the environment, and the nature of the reactions which are observed, or which it is hoped to promote. This is best conducted in relation to one activity (or a linked series) within a defined area such as a room or a limited outdoor space, and taking account of the abilities and needs of a known user or user group.

This is for purely practical reasons: a thorough environmental analysis can produce a substantial amount of information, which becomes overwhelming or over-generalized if too large an environment or too many users, processes or activities are considered. Content analysis may be used as a precursor to provide an objective summary of the area. Adaptive analysis may follow if alterations are thought to be necessary.

ADAPTIVE ANALYSIS

In the context of therapy, analysis of content describes what is there, and demand analysis describes whether it is suitable for the activity and the therapeutic objectives of the user. Adaptive analysis is used similarly, in relation to a known user and her activities, in a particular area, and describes the potential for adaptation and suggests what features might be changed to improve therapy. Adaptive analysis can also be used in domestic or work environments to define the alterations needed.

Headings used are similar to those for content analysis, but are more specific and include more detail. Since both demand and adaptive analysis use the same headings it is useful to consider them together (Table 15.1).

Potential for adaptation

The following information is required before the analysis can be conducted.

Occupational use of environment

The purpose(s) and activity (or activities) for which the area will be used need to be defined.

User(s) profile

The main features of the user should be described, and any special needs, risks, precautions or contraindications should be noted.

Aims of therapy or intervention

The aims and objectives, and any relevance to environmental features should be noted.

ADAPTING ENVIRONMENTS

GENERAL CONSIDERATIONS WHEN PLANNING ENVIRONMENTS

Therapists may be involved in planning a person's own environment, in cooperation with that person, or in developing residential or clinical environments.

Except in the case of minor modifications it is useful to prepare a design brief to ensure that the environment meets the user's requirements. Such a brief is especially useful when communicating with architects, builders or designers. The brief is concerned with definition of uses and users, consequent architectural and design considerations, specials needs and cost limits.

The headings used for content analysis and demand analysis can be combined (deleting any which are inapplicable in the circumstances) and used to provide a planning guide. However, in this situation, the questions become, not 'What is there, and is it suitable?' but 'What ought to be there? What are we trying to achieve? How can we best achieve it?'

If designing a multipurpose area, it must be taken into account the potential number of users and activities can be large. It can be a time-consuming and complex process to analyse all possible uses and requirements and to ensure that they are all met.

Table 15.1 Headings for environmental analysis in demand and adaptive analysis

Heading	Demand analysis	Adaptive analysis
Architectural features and services	The shape, size and design of the room, position of doors and windows, access and services, e.g. heating, lighting, ventilation, water. Relationship to other rooms if relevant.	Suitability for activity/user? What may need to be altered? How? Define options.
Furnishings	Furniture and fittings; flooring, curtains or blinds. In an external area note also landscaping and planting.	
Decoration	Colour schemes, aesthetic artefacts, plants, patterns, textures, etc.	
Cultural or symbolic features	Hangings, pictures, artefacts and objects with special meaning. Cultural associations linked to usage or location of area.	Suitability for activity/user? Consider ethnic/social/cultural implications. Can meanings be emphasized if needed?
Stress production	Is there an appropriate degree of stimulation or challenge? What features contribute to this?	Suitability for activity/user? Can engagement be increased by adding to stimulation? How? Does stressful stimulation need to be reduced? How?
Stress reduction	Does the environment press to reduce stress? What features contribute to this?	If a relaxed atmosphere is needed, how can this be promoted?
User control	Does the environment permit and encourage, or inhibit, user control? How?	If user control is to be promoted, how may this be done?
Utility	Is the environment designed and equipped to promote effective and efficient use in relation to user needs and activity performance?	If not satisfactory, can it be altered? How? Define options.
Tools/equipment	Is everything required available? Is it suitable for user abilities and activity? (Check activity analysis.)	What may need to be altered? How? Define options.
Materials	Is everything required available? (Check activity analysis.)	Alteration required? Consider quantity, choice, etc.
Positioning	Are all objects for use located in the optimum position?	Is alteration to position needed? How? Define options.
Distractions	Will the environment distract user from activity? Will other users distract or be distracted?	Can distraction be removed or reduced?
Other considerations	Any other relevant factors?	Any other adaptations?
Promotion of interaction*	Is interaction promoted or inhibited? Describe the features which contribute to this.	Suitability for activity/user? What may need to be altered? How? Define options.
Promotion of movement*	Does the environment require, encourage or inhibit movement? What type of movement? What features affect this?	Need to increase or decrease demand for movement? How?
Sensory stimulation*	What sensory stimulation does the area provide? What provides it?	Can this be enhanced or decreased?
Cognitive information*	Does the environment provide any kind of information, by means of words, sounds, visual cues or instructions? Is this sufficient?	Need to increase or draw attention to information content? How?
Therapeutic aspects*	Does the environment contribute to the aims of the intervention/therapy? Have risks, precautions and contraindications been considered and are special needs met? (Check aims and patient profile.)	Is adaptation required? How? Define options.

Note: Headings marked * are relevant in clinical situations, but are not always needed in normal domestic or work situations.

DESIGNING AND USING CLINICAL ENVIRONMENTS

In new developments it is necessary to draw up 'room loading' schedules which contain literally everything. The Department of Health produces design briefs, technical information and equipment schedules of hospital departments. These can be an invaluable starting point, but they do need to be revised with care since they are generic and are not always up-to-date. Although the time required may seem daunting, and the minutia tedious, personal experience has convinced me that it is always time well spent.

The chance to participate in planning where one starts with a 'blank sheet' is relatively rare. The need to adapt an existing area is more usual. Much therapy still takes place in hospitals, clinics and similar formal settings. In these clinical areas the therapist's ability to manipulate the environment may be limited, because much of it is formed by needs and purposes other than his own. The therapist must therefore be able to exploit given environments. The exception is the occupational therapy department, where the therapist can arrange things, within some limitations, to meet his own requirements. Although all aspects of demand require consideration, the following points need extra attention.

Occupational uses

The primary consideration is the identification of the purposes and activities for which the area is to be used, and whether there is one purpose or many. Multipurpose areas may be unavoidable, but if there are to be activities requiring specific equipment or facilities, they may be impractical. List the activities or purposes, note the essential requirements, and check if the area will provide these, or can be adapted to do so.

Therapeutic uses

Therapy areas often have primary and secondary uses. What is the primary use – is it patient treatment or some other form of intervention such as confidential discussion, or is it physical examination, social interaction, participation in an activity or assessment? Whatever it may be, does the environment contribute positively to this objective, and could it be improved so that it better enables or enhances performance?

Secondary uses may complement or conflict with the primary one. Even non-therapeutic areas may be used by clients at times, and if such use is at all likely, it should be taken into consideration.

Sociocultural factors

These factors relate to the numbers of people using the area at one time, the roles these people will take, and the associated cultural norms and values.

The need for privacy, so often in short supply in clinical settings, is a very important consideration. Real privacy – not the substitute provided by token drawing of screens or curtains, and lowering of voices – must be guarded. It is especially important in interviews, one-to-one sessions, assessments requiring silence and concentration, and physical examination of the client.

Open plan office areas and wards present extra difficulties; it is easy for the therapist to become over-familiar with these, so that the noise, distractions and intrusions are no longer registered – although they are by the patient.

By contrast, the need to promote social interaction may be considered. Positioning of chairs, tables, tools and materials can contribute substantially to facilitating conversation, sharing, and cooperation.

It is surely a matter of commonsense that if someone is to work, she needs a light, bright, functional area which communicates activity, efficiency and productivity. By the same token, for relaxation, dimmer light, quiet, soft colours and soft furnishings facilitate the desired response. Therapy groups are likely to interact better in informal, comfortable settings with neutral soft furnishings.

Most therapists will take account of such factors as a matter of course, but in the real world compromises do have to be made. It is necessary to recognize, however, if an environment is too incompatible with the activity for it to be used for the intended purpose.

Special considerations concerning users

This involves being aware of any precautions, contraindications or special needs of users, and ensuring that the environment takes account of these. This might include, for example, risk of self-harm, absconding, fits, falls, confusion, impaired sight or hearing, need for ready access to a toilet, or mobility problems. However, it is important to balance such considerations with the need to provide normal experiences, and to avoid 'nanny mentality'. The importance of thinking through potential problems during the planning stages cannot be over-emphasized, as it is often difficult to remedy problems at a later stage.

Architectural factors

Unless one is planning from scratch, structures, e.g. walls, doors, windows and ceilings, are fixed features, which were present before the arrival of the therapist. This does not mean that they cannot be adapted, but conversions are often complex, and are usually expensive and time-consuming.

The most frequent structural problem with which the therapist must cope – even, at times, in purpose-built buildings – is access. There may be, for example, too many stairs, no ramps, doors which are too heavy or which open the wrong way, or inconvenient or distant toilets. It may or may not be possible to adapt these, but the therapist needs to scan the environment and observe such problems before deciding to use the area.

Space – usually too little, but sometimes, in institutional settings, too much – is another important consideration.

Less obvious is the question of services – heat, light, ventilation, water, power and drainage. It is easy to overlook these, so a checklist, mental or actual, can help to ensure that the positive aspects and requirements are present, and that negative aspects, e.g. cold, glare, draughts and excessive noise, are not.

Furnishings

Appropriate furnishings contribute to both ambience and function. It really can make a difference which colour scheme is chosen, or whether there is a carpet, or pictures on the walls. The difference made by ergonomically-designed seating and work surfaces, and pleasing designs should need no further explanation.

In evaluating furnishings, a basic consideration to be borne in mind is whether the use of the area is productive or social (or both), and whether the atmosphere is to be, for example, formal or informal, functional, relaxing or stimulating.

In a familiar area it is again easy to become habituated to the accepted features of a room, especially accumulated clutter or professional paraphernalia, and to forget that these may have a different impact on a patient to whom they are unfamilar. There is a world of difference between an area which looks interestingly cluttered, inviting informal exploration, and one which is simply a chaotic mess, or which contains an intimidating array of incomprehensible equipment.

It can be an instructive exercise to take someone with reasonable powers of observation who is unfamiliar with the profession into an occupational therapy area, and to ask for 'first impressions' – these may not be in the least what the therapist expects.

Materials, tools and equipment

The practical questions are what is needed, and for how many people? This will lead to the consideration of location, access and storage.

In planning for a specific activity, it is not difficult to list the requirements; it is worth having checklists for commonly-used activities, as this saves time and frustration, especially if equipment has to be taken to an area for use. This is where an activity can be useful.

Temporal factors

Temporal factors have a peripheral influence on environment, but are worth considering. The most relevant factor is how frequently the room is used, over what period and in relation to how many people. This may affect some basic spatial and furnishing considerations, and can have implications for services such as heating and ventilation. People passing through for short sessions may have different needs to users who occupy a room for extended periods. Use at night will affect lighting provision.

Ownership

The question of who owns an environment is of fundamental importance. Objectively, the legal owner (landlord, freeholder, company, council, trust) has rights and responsibilities which will affect and limit the use of an environment, and may affect what the therapist is able to do with it.

While this is of practical and legal importance, the more subtle matter of subjective ownership needs careful consideration. Territorial instincts are primitive and deep-rooted, and the symbolic and cultural nuances of whether one is on one's own territory, 'neutral ground', or someone else's 'patch' are complex and important, and will affect all the actions and interactions within the environment.

In clinical settings, areas are either neutral, or are 'owned' by a profession. The etiquette of negotiating the use of someone else's area can be intricate, but must not be disregarded.

The loser in these territorial politics is usually the patient, who may have little or no territory of her own. A bed-space, or a chair in a dayroom, may become the personal space of an individual, and needs to be respected as such.

The psychological 'balance of power' rests with the owner of the territory. The therapist may use this to advantage on occasions, but in developing a partnership with the patient in a clinical setting it is important that the environment reflects an egalitarian approach, and does not subliminally promote the authority of the therapist.

A therapist wishing to provide an area of which patients can feel ownership, has to consider both social and physical aspects of the environment. Involvement of the patient in decisions concerning her environment is essential if ownership is to be experienced, for ownership is linked with control. The therapist must be especially sensitive to the matter of ownership when intervening in a client's own home.

ENVIRONMENTS FOR INTERVIEWS

Formal interviews typically take place in an office or interview room which is designed for the purpose. An appropriate design should provide privacy, security, tidiness, and a degree of comfort relative to the length of the interview. Therapists should beware of cluttering up an office which is also used as an interview area. It may provide them with a comfortable and informal working environment, but is unlikely to provide the client with a first impression of efficiency and professionalism. On the other hand, starkly clinical rooms are intimidating, and should be avoided unless needed for physical examinations.

There are various options for the arrangement of desk/table and chairs in interview areas (Fig. 15.1). Of these, the arrangement shown in Figure 15.1B is commonly used, since it permits use of the desk, without separating the therapist from the patient.

Informal interviews can take place almost anywhere, and are sometimes unplanned. There may be little that a therapist can do to avoid this, other than to retain an acute sensitivity to the nature of the environment and the appropriateness of what is being said or done within it. It is wise to terminate any interview or discussion which is out of place – or indeed, to avoid starting one. In personal experience, busy senior professional staff and managers are notorious for 'seizing the moment' and wishing to discuss sensitive matters in public places. This should be courteously refused.

An interview area of informal design is

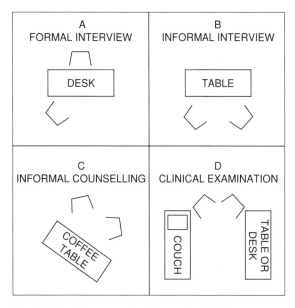

Figure 15.1 Arrangement of desk and chairs for an interview.

normally used where the interview is likely to be prolonged or of a more probing and sensitive nature, and should be designed for comfort and a feeling of security. Since such sessions may move unpredictably into counselling, the arrangement in Figure 15.1C is more appropriate, although the chairs would be softly upholstered, and the table may be a coffee table. A light-coloured carpet, curtains, pictures and potted plants all help to produce a relaxed atmosphere.

ENVIRONMENTS FOR ASSESSMENT

Therapists assess people for many reasons and in many different ways, from clinical evaluation of physical or psychological condition to practical tests of competencies in occupations, activities and roles. Interviews may be a precursor to assessment and the same environment may be used.

CLINICAL ASSESSMENT

Clinical forms of assessment, in which the physical and/or psychological state of the patient is examined, usually require privacy, a neutral area without distractions in the form of noise, people or telephones, and the necessary assessment equipment or instruments, which should be neatly stored and readily accessible. If physical examination is necessary, the therapist must be able to wash his hands and maintain hygiene.

On the subject of physical examination, it is worth noting that even when screened or private, very informal areas or work areas, as well as being of potentially doubtful hygiene, may make some people feel uncomfortable during a physical examination which requires undressing, especially if they are culturally educated to associate this with doctors' surgeries or similar environments. The demand is wrong; intimate touching which is 'safe' in the clinical area (which the patient may associate with that of a doctor) is much less 'safe' in the dayroom (which feels like a hotel reception area), even though screens are provided.

ASSESSMENT OF PERFORMANCE OF ACTIVITIES OF DAILY LIVING

The problem encountered when creating an environment for use in assessment of occupational competence is that of achieving the balance between risk and reality.

This is true in all areas of assessment, but especially in ADL. In occupational therapy departments, assessment areas such as bedrooms, kitchens or bathrooms, while designed to be 'domestic', are in fact safe and protected areas which may be far removed in both design and equipment from those in a person's own home. In addition, the increasingly stringent requirements of hygiene and safety in public buildings may add constraints and increase the non-domestic appearance of the area.

Practice and assessment of ADL in a safe environment is often an essential stage in therapy. The therapist can remove hazards, facilitate performance and provide aids, while observing, charting and monitoring progress. It is essential for the therapist to remain conscious of the artificiality of such an environment when making an assessment, and to note when aids, equipment or cues are used, since performance may be less functional if these are not available.

Normal living involves taking normal risks; human beings do not and cannot exist in a totally safe environment. No therapist would deliberately put a patient 'at risk', but it is a matter of professional judgement when and whether the patient should be allowed to cope with the normal hazards of daily life. There must come a time when the patient is to be allowed to pour boiling water into the teapot, deal with a hot oven, walk unaided across the room, or be left alone to get out of bed and cope with dressing or toileting.

Skills must eventually be generalized into other situations and less safe places. It is one thing to be able to cope with the necessary activities and occupations of daily life in the safety of the occupational therapy area. It may be quite another when it comes to dealing with the same things at home, especially when alone. This can work both ways; a familiar, comfortable home environment can enable the patient to produce more competent performance – but it may equally show up problems which had been masked in hospital. A difficult, stressful environment can produce immediate dysfunction in a patient who appeared to cope well in a protected area. Such problems may lie in the performance of the patient, or in the environment itself.

Where an in-patient is taken from hospital for an assessment home visit, great care must be taken in making appropriate arrangements; there are both practical and legal considerations. Clear guidance on these visits is given in the COT standards document (   ) and there should be written policies and procedures, of which all staff are aware.

It is impossible to simulate some aspects of daily life satisfactorily in a clinical setting: shopping, busy streets, public transport and driving are part of life for many people and can only be assessed properly in the community. Again, for an in-patient, such arrangements must be made with care following local policies.

Since such realistic community-based assessment is not always practical, the therapist must often make judgements based on an evaluation of observed competencies in the clinical environment. It is possible to make an accurate assessment under these circumstances; however, it is wise to avoid over-extrapolating conclusions about individual abilities derived from limited evidence in restricted environments. Most therapists become skilled in seeing opportunities in the grounds or public areas of a hospital or clinic where more realistic assessment can take place. An external assessment area, such as a garden, can be valuable, for both work and ADL assessment.

ENVIRONMENTS FOR WORK ASSESSMENT

Since jobs are becoming ever more varied, demanding, and dependent on technology, it is usually very difficult within the confines of an occupational therapy department to do more than assess simple versions of skills which may be required as part of a job. These can be useful indicators, but have limited predictive value.

Except in specialized work assessment or training units, it is simply impractical to have a sufficient range of equipment and options available. Work assessment should ultimately be conducted in the workplace if it is to have any real validity, and may need to be conducted over an extended period. Employers are frequently cooperative, but the therapist should check the need for special permissions and insurance cover. It may well be necessary for the therapist to make one or more visits to a working environment in order to observe, analyse and understand job requirements before attempting to assess the individual.

THERAPEUTIC ADAPTATIONS TO THE ENVIRONMENT

ROOM MANAGEMENT AND PREPARATION

The term 'room management' is used here in much the same sense as one might use the theatrical term 'stage management' (not in the more specific sense of the behavioural management system which has the same name). Like stage management, room management is concerned with 'setting a scene': arranging furniture, decorations, tools, materials and even 'props' to create the desired environmental demand. It takes place consciously, and much of it happens before the 'audience' – the users of the room – arrive; however, the 'scene' may also be changed, or adjusted, during use.

A therapy room, like a stage set, may be managed and arranged in many ways, changing the reactions and expectations of the users, facilitating in turn, group work, social interactions, individual concentration, problem-solving or relaxation. As an example of the occupational therapy approach to this, the selection and use of chairs and tables is explored next, but this is only one aspect of room management.

CHAIRS AND TABLES

Considering how essential to many activities these items of furniture are, it is surprising to find little formal attention given in occupational therapy texts to description of some of the basic principles of selecting and arranging chairs and tables. It is probably one of those aspects of therapy which is assumed, incorrectly, to be simply commonsense.

Although there can be no rigid formula for selecting arrangements, it is necessary for a therapist to experiment with and understand the uses of, different patterns of arrangement, both of the chairs and tables, and also of the objects, materials or tools with the use of which they are to be associated. (The following description does not take account of specific physical disabilities which may require special seating and positioning.)

Selection of seating and tables

The variation of human size and shape means that it is impossible to make a chair which suits everyone equally. Designers and manufacturers are obliged to work towards suiting the larger percentile of the population. Old people and children do not fit within this general grouping and need different sizes and proportions of seating.

While it is clearly impractical to have a range of seating to suit all possible shapes and sizes of user in a small department, benefit is to be gained by choosing chairs constructed on sound anthropometric principles and having a selection of suitable cushions and footrests with which to adapt these. Good back support and foot support are essential in order to avoid fatigue and to maintain healthy sitting posture.

The therapist has to make several clinical decisions when choosing a suitable chair for an individual, e.g. seat height, width and depth, type of backrest, arms or no arms, upholstered, or not, and by what means. The practicalities of chairs which have to be moved or stacked have to be considered and weighed against user needs. The activity for which the chair is required is also important: chairs for relaxation and informal social use are not the same as those for work. To the therapist, a chair is no simple object, it can have therapeutic, functional, symbolic, social and cultural implications.

If the chair is required for the user to work at a table, the height should enable the user to place forearms comfortably on the table with the elbows at right angles, without pushing shoulders into elevation, or obliging the person to bend over to reach the table.

Tables also have pitfalls in size, space, portability, surface characteristics and utility. These notes are not intended to be comprehensive, merely to alert the novice therapist to the necessity of taking as much conscious care over the selection of basic furniture as he would over the selection of specialist equipment.

ARRANGEMENTS FOR TABLE ACTIVITIES AND SMALL GROUP WORK

Figure 15.2 shows a number of different arrangements of a basic room setting. It should be apparent that these arrangements have advantages and disadvantages in relation to differing forms of activities.

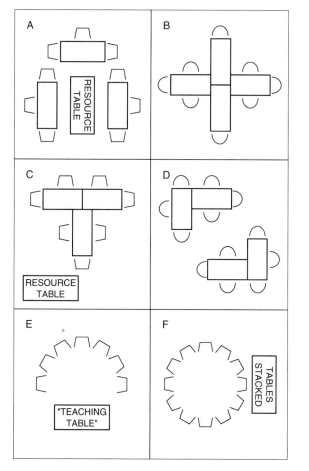

Figure 15.2 Various arrangements of a basic room setting.

Box 15.1 Types of group used in psychosocial settings (adapted from Mosey 1986)	
Evaluative groups	In which the therapist may observe the client's performance and/or interactions with others.
Task-orientated groups	In which completion of the task by the group is the primary purpose; the therapist leads and assists.
Parallel group	Where a client (or clients) not yet able to work as a group member works individually but in a group setting, with some minimal interaction with others. Activities are led, prompted and cued by the therapist.
Project group	The therapist leads and runs the group. The joint project is used to enable group members to work in twos or threes, to cooperate, share and interact.
Egocentric–cooperative group	The group is encouraged to select and achieve its own activity with the therapist acting as facilitator and problem-solver when required.
Cooperative group	The group is relatively autonomous, self-directive and self-sustaining. The members work together to achieve a common goal.
Mature group	In which all members, including the therapist, are peers: activities may serve as a focus for exploring current issues and concerns within the group.
Thematic group	The group 'focuses on gaining knowledge, skills and attitudes necessary for mastery of performance components and occupational performances.' The activity might be work, leisure or ADL. The emphasis is on structured participation and learning; the therapist acts as a 'teacher' using a more or less directive model as required.

TYPES OF ACTIVITY GROUPS

Mosey (1986) lists a number of types of activity group used in psychosocial settings. Some of those listed are summarized in Box 15.1, not from the point of view of exploring the psychosocial construction and aims of each group (for which the reader should refer to the original text, which describes this in detail), but in order to consider how room management, by the selection of different arrangements of tables and chairs (Fig. 15.2) might contribute to each group.

It would further be necessary, as part of room management, to consider where each individual should sit in relation to each other, to features of the room such as tools or the door, and in relation to staff.

PHYSICAL AND COGNITIVE LIMITATIONS IN RELATION TO THE ENVIRONMENT

Some of the group structures just described may be used in a physical setting, where cognitive or physical skills are to be used, rather than psychosocial skills. Where there is physical or sensory limitation, the environment can be used to facilitate performance by provision of the correct furniture, equipment and sensory cues, whether for groups or for individuals.

BIOMECHANICAL ADAPTATIONS TO THE ENVIRONMENT

In physical rehabilitation, the biomechanical approach uses the principle of extending physical ability, by providing environmental and performance demand which requires the patient to stretch and extend his current ability in order to meet the challenges.

Environmental factors may require alteration in a graded manner to achieve this, with a change in features such as type of seating, position of user in relation to height of work or distance of work from user, and location of tools and materials.

These adaptations involve the understanding of kinesiology and basic mechanical principles such as leverage, pulley systems, torque, equilibrium and the effect of gravity. These effects can be calculated mathematically, but in practice, adaptations are often achieved by trial and error, since what works may depend on human factors as much as on mechanics.

Positioning of the patient in relation to work-surface, tools and materials may enhance performance, or require the patient to perform in a particular way, as may adaptation is the tools themselves.

Typical adaptations to tools include: extending handle length, changing the shape or size of a handle and fitting some adaptation to change the direction of a movement, e.g. to change a rotary movement into a linear one or the reverse.

Alterations to the positions of tools and materials also use biomechanical principles. An activity may be positioned higher or lower to alter the range of movement, or so as to use gravity to assist or resist its performance.

Texts on physical occupational therapy provide many examples of such adaptations. It is worth noting, however, that environmental adaptation is not always necessary; alterations may be made to working methods and procedures rather than to the equipment used. Sometimes both kinds of adaptation are needed.

Conversely, deteriorating physical conditions will require incrementally increased assistance and reduced demand.

ADAPTATIONS TO MEET COGNITIVE NEEDS OF PATIENTS

Allen (1985) draws attention to the importance of the placement of materials and tools in relation to the cognitive level of the patient. In the context of psychiatric illness she describes how patients with impaired cognitive (levels 3, 4, 5) are variously unable, depending on the level of cognitive function, to cope with the demands of hunting for things outside their present field of vision, making connections between objects, or between personal actions and their effects on objects or people, making choices about elements in the environment, or sequencing the use of successive tools or materials.

On the other hand, patients with more intact cognition can make choices, problem-solve, use logic, and make correct connections between objects – spatially, temporally and symbolically.

Allen suggests that tasks should be selected to match the cognitive level and that the environment should be prepared in advance of the activity to provide precisely the right level of cognitive demand. Alterations can be made to the quantity of objects presented to the patient, to their location, and to their general characteristics – size, shape, colour, spatial relationships and necessity for choice.

It is interesting to note that she challenges the view of the traditional rehabilitation approach of 'stretching' cognitive abilities by providing an environment which has a demand above the capacity of the current skills of the patient, and argues that, until the patient has, by whatever means, (e.g. chemotherapy, remission of symptoms, improved physical health) attained a higher cognitive level, such challenge is ineffective or counterproductive.

Allen has developed this concept into a system of assessment and placement of patients by observation of their abilities and reactions during tasks and in relation to environmental features, including people, objects, location and time.

Personal experience of working with individuals who have severe brain damage following a cerebral vascular event or head injury, suggests that function at these different cognitive levels can also be observed in these patients.

The process of cognition requires input, throughput and output. When input is reduced or inaccurate, resultant cognition can be impaired or reduced. Patients with sensory or perceptual difficulties may be disadvantaged both by environments which give insufficient information, and by those which provide too much.

Lighting levels and surface colours are often overlooked, but are especially important for people with visual impairment, who benefit from bright light and well-constrasted differentiation of surfaces and objects. Hearing loss may be improved by an induction loop system, and by removal of extraneous noises.

Reliance on information provided by notices or signs is now so much part of our culture as to be overlooked, yet this can cause problems to people who cannot read, or who use a different language.

Sensory loss may require that textural features are exaggerated, or that a soft environment is provided. Adaptations may remove or enhance appreciation of certain perceptual stimuli or cues.

General environmental content can be important when dealing with clients or patients who are confused or disorientated. For example, in a day hospital for people suffering from dementia, cues to usage and location can be provided by consistent colour coding of doors, clear signing backed up by symbols, and differentiation in the colour schemes of rooms. Handles to 'no-go' areas can be made hard to operate, whereas those to accessible areas or toilets are easily managed. Equipment and furniture may be deliberately domestic in style. In some units 'old-fashioned' furnishings, household goods or other items have been used as environmental cues to provoke reminiscence, although the usefulness of this can be overestimated.

It requires great imagination to view an environment as a confused elderly person may perhaps perceive it. In one example, it was complained that elderly male residents in a home were using the lavatory washbasins inappropriately as urinals. On visiting the home it was found that the small white porcelain washbasins did indeed bear a remarkable resemblance to mini-urinals – it was not surprising that the men were responding incorrectly to this cue.

AREAS WHICH PROVIDE SPECIAL COGNITIVE–PERCEPTUAL INPUT AND SENSORIMOTOR STIMULATION

Snoezelan

Snoezelan is a composite of two words of Dutch origin, roughly translating as 'sniffing and dozing', but meaning sensations which promote relaxation. This is an example of an environment which is designed to produce very specific demands. All external stimuli are excluded and the content of the environment can be varied by the therapist to produce the required degree of stimulation.

These areas vary in size and complexity, and range from a room fitted with a totally soft environment, in which general lighting can be dimmed to emphasize the effects of coloured light displays, vibrations, sounds and mobiles, to quite complex, large rooms which can be walked through and explored, featuring a great variety of exciting or restful visual, tactile olfactory and auditory stimuli.

Snoezelan has been used successfully with profoundly handicapped individuals, and with a range of other clients, either for sensory stimulation or, more usually, for relaxation. Marked positive changes in behaviour and awareness have been reported when clients use such areas, although much more structured research is needed to quantify these (Long & Haig 1992).

Soft play areas

Equipment such as a ball pool, foam blocks

covered in brightly-coloured plastic, tunnels, swings or trampolines may be used for 'soft play', and physical activity and exploration with handicapped children.

These are used also for adults with severe learning difficulties; but although this equipment is developmentally appropriate and often gives much pleasure, the age-appropriateness is highly questionable and may be considered unacceptable. The dilemma is whether to respond to the physical and cognitive developmental age, and needs, of the individual, or to the chronological age and adult social needs. This is a matter in which doctrinal and philosophical issues have to be weighed against therapeutic advantages.

ADAPTING AND USING EXTERNAL ENVIRONMENTS

A great deal of human activity takes place out of doors. The demand produced by an open space is very different from that of a room, and promotes a different range of reactions and performances.

Attention tends to be directed towards adapting indoor environments, yet use of, and adaptation to, outdoor areas is equally important.

External environments are at least as rich and varied as interior ones, and indeed, in terms of sensory stimulation, are often more so. Bustling, noisy cityscapes, quiet suburbia, small villages, parks, gardens or rural landscapes have obviously different characteristics, but some differences are far more subtle, and depend on social and cultural perceptions. There can be, for instance, distinctly different demands in a park and in a domestic garden, despite the fact that the actual content – trees, lawns, flowers – is the same. There are even differences between acceptable and unacceptable behaviour in back and front gardens in some neighbourhoods.

Open air environments permit a wider range of behaviours than indoor environments. It is more permissible to run, shout, swear, sit on the ground, eat with fingers, and dress minimally in various outdoor areas than it would be indoors. A wide range of work and leisure occupations take place out of doors, as do many domestic activities. Mobility within open air environments is important.

There is some evidence to indicate that green landscape, especially when it contains water, engages the attention, and produces relaxation more effectively than urban scenes. In one study, it was demonstrated that levels of discomfort and recovery time following operation were improved when the patient had a view of greenery through the window as opposed to a view of a brick wall.

The therapist may need to make a conscious effort to include open air environments in assessment and therapy, but to ignore these is to reject a large part of normal experience, and also valuable therapeutic potential.

THERAPEUTIC USE OF LANDSCAPE

The landscape nearest to a building – its curtilage – is that likely to be most accessible to therapists. Landscape is describe as 'hard' – walls, paving, paths and structures, and 'soft' – plants. Uses may be described as active – directly related to the care and cultivation of plants, or reactive – for recreational, social, or other uses.

Active uses include:

- therapeutic gardening
- reality orientation through plant material
- sensory stimulation through plant material.

Reactive uses include:

- relaxation
- socialization
- games and exercises
- observation of wildlife
- assessment and practice of mobility
- assessment and practice of daily living/work skills.

External areas requires as much attention to analysis, design and adaptation as do indoor areas.

Designing therapeutic gardening areas

Gardening offers much potential as therapy, both physical and psychosocial. On a smaller scale, it may be used for single tasks, sequential tasks and long-term projects (Hagedorn 1987). On a larger scale, commercial horticulture and market gardening can be used for education and rehabilitation. Adaptations are mainly to promote access and to provide the right opportunities for project work. Raised beds may be useful for people with a physical disability, but must be designed with care since the requirements of therapy and skilful horticulture are to some extent opposed. Ground-level beds worked with long-handled tools are often overlooked as an alternative.

Reality orientation and sensory stimulation

Plant material is rich in symbolism and is closely associated with the passage of time. It can therefore be used in reality orientation to trigger memories and responses, as well as to provide material for project work.

Carefully chosen plant material can stimulate all the senses, and may be used to provide pleasurable stimulation. Plants must, however, be chosen with knowledge and care as many are toxic to a greater or lesser degree. In one project, a garden for profoundly handicapped children was designed with plants which could be touched, smelled, tasted and rolled upon.

Reactive uses

In most cases, little special adaptation is required for reactive use of external environments, the most essential requirements being ready access to a suitable environment. In some cases, however, attention must be paid to special needs, security, supervision and protection from the extremes of weather.

OUTDOOR RECREATIONAL ENVIRONMENTS

As a result of the move towards care in the community and the closure of large institutions with their own private recreation areas, therapists have made increasing use of community facilities, such as swimming pools, bowling centres, riding centres or places of entertainment, and outings to park, seaside or country, for purposes of assessment, training and therapy.

This may be desirable, but it does raise considerable managerial problems in terms of organization, number and skill-mix of accompanying staff, insurance cover, special qualification for instructors, first aid arrangements, funding, and a host of other practicalities. It is wise to ensure that carefully written policies and procedures and checklists exist to cover all eventualities, and that all staff involved are appropriately trained, particularly if clients have special needs.

From a therapeutic perspective, the therapist has very limited control over such public areas. It is helpful for an exploratory visit to be undertaken before the visit to ensure that the facilities meet therapeutic and practical requirements, that the management is prepared to accept the visit, and that there are no unforeseen hazards. A mobile 'phone is a recommended accessory, in case of emergencies.

ADAPTING THE HOME ENVIRONMENT

DOMESTIC ADAPTATIONS

Enabling a disabled person to remain in, and cope better in, her own home is a central role of occupational therapists, especially those based in the community. This has always been important, but is increasingly so in view of the conscious shift in the philosophy of care towards community living.

Minor adaptations are those which involve provision of easily fitted equipment and small alterations such as rails and ramps. Major adaptations range from removing a partition wall, installing a lift, or fitting a toilet, to building or 'attaching' customized home extensions.

This is a complex and challenging area of work which can require the combined skills of therapist, technician, tradesman, architect and builder. Often the therapist must be at least a little of each of these in order to assess the problem, solve it, and communicate with the client and those who will do the work.

As well as the technical complexity of the task, home adaptations raise many other considerations concerning individual preferences, choices and modes of living. The therapist must be especially sensitive to the matter of ownership when intervening in a client's own home. There, the therapist is a visitor and guest – perhaps not always a welcome one – and must comply with all the local cultural expectations and rules of visiting. He needs to use quantities of tact and empathy to avoid being seen as an invader, who, with whatever good intentions, is about to disrupt a settled way of life and impose solutions.

Proposals for altering something as personal as a home environment have to be made cautiously, allowing the client to express ideas, anxieties and preferences, and to contribute as much as possible to the process. Some clients are imaginative and adaptive and solve their own problems with a little facilitation from the therapist. Others may be stressed, overwhelmed, and find it almost impossible to translate plans from paper into reality, and are happy to rely on the therapist as an intermediary. As with any other intervention, the client has the ultimate right to reject proposed alterations or assistance, however much the therapist may feel these would be in her best interests.

There is a quantity of information about ways of adapting homes and the equipment available to do so. This information, and the regulations which apply to home adaptations and the systems of provision are constantly being updated, and there is little point in attempting a summary. Therapists must acquaint themselves with the current information and must keep abreast of new ideas and local policies.

The following notes indicate some of the basic considerations for major adaptations.

On-site assessment

It is essential to take detailed notes and accurate measurements (using a metric rule), and advis-able to make sketch plans, however crude, at the same time.

User brief

As previously described, it is helpful to begin by working with the user to produce a simple design brief, identifying what is wanted and any special needs. As well as providing the therapist with information about what is required, the discussion and negotiation will help to firm up the design brief and iron out misunderstandings about what is and is not practical. It is essential that the complexities of funding the scheme are explained at the outset, and that no promises or

Box 15.2	Headings in the preparation of a user brief
Users	Who? Describe and list user(s), main and occasional Special needs? Precautions or contraindications? User preferences – likes, dislikes, wishes, ideas and cultural implications (include all main users)
Uses	What? Describe and list uses and purposes When? How often?
Practical requirements (related to use and user)	
Structures	Built features – walls, doors, windows, access, space, etc
Services	Heating, lighting, power, water, drainage and ventilation
Furniture and fittings	Furniture, domestic appliances, tools, storage, materials, decor, etc
Advantages and constraints	How does the existing environment enhance or impede occupational performance and meet needs of user?
Adaptations	Minor adaptations – equipment, rails, etc Major adaptations
Cost	Details of who will fund project, cost limits, need for grant, etc
Options	Note any alternatives in general terms

commitments are made by the therapist unless these can be fulfilled. All discussion and correspondence needs to be recorded or copied.

The headings listed in Box 15.2 are useful in preparing a user brief.

Plans

Initially, the therapist will need to produce simple metric scale plans of the existing structures and those which are proposed, as these will help to clarify the design process and involve the client, as well as assisting when discussing options with an architect or builder.

Proposals must take into account local site features and structures. The therapist has to be aware of basic practicalities such as the location of drains, load-bearing or partition walls, access, light, ventilation and the restrictions imposed by conservation or building regulations.

The builder or architect will provide advice, and will produce the final design and professional plans. It is usually necessary to seek planning permission for a major adaptation, and to go out to tender for building work, so professional plans are essential. Ownership can affect what can be done and the need for permission.

The therapist must develop a facility for reading architectural plans and spotting potential problems, errors or omissions at the design stage.

Funding

The formulae for funding adaptations for a disabled person's home are complex and subject to alteration. There is normally a means-tested element which the client must pay. The therapist must be fully briefed on national and local policies and procedures. The most important point is to ensure that the client really understands the position, and has agreed to it, and that no work is started until all the necessary formalities are completed, which may take some time. Meticulous recording of progress and agreements is essential.

RESIDENTIAL CARE IN THE COMMUNITY

A therapist may be called upon to contribute to the deisgn of a group home, hostel, or other setting providing supervised care in the community. The principles for this are the same as for any other exercise in environmental planning and adaptation, but there is an added dimension, that of the philosophy under which the home will be run.

This may lead to conflict between 'political correctnesss' and practicality. The term 'normalization', for example, was devised to describe the deliberate de-institutionalization of residential care settings, especially for people with special needs and severe learning disabilities (mental handicap), with a view to preventing discrimination and increasing personal choice and participation.

In creating such areas, everything from the size and type of food packaging, to furnishings and decoration, has to be considered to ensure that they are domestic in character, and in all respects equivalent to those used by the 'normal' population.

This is an admirable philosophy, but is not always easy to put into practice. It can be difficult to meet the restrictions imposed by planning and other regulations affecting residential care or group homes and hostels, while retaining a normal domestic environment. Fire precautions and hygiene regulations are necessarily stringent but can create an institutional impression unless handled with flexibility and imagination by planners. In my experience, these complications have sometimes created such serious delays and difficulties that the opportunity to acquire suitable property for adaptation has been lost in a maze of bureaucracy.

There is also sometimes a tension between the philosophy of 'hard-line normalizers' and the practicalities of care. Assessment of residents' needs must be realistic; it is of little use to place upon residents optimistic demands for maintenance of self, house and garden, simply because this is 'normal', even though they will in fact be unable to cope.

Advocates of normalization tend to emphasize the beneficial effects on clients. In many cases these do exist, but personal experience indicates that, where clients are profoundly handicapped, to an extent that awareness of environment is very limited, the primary effect is, in fact, to de-institutionalize *staff* and to promote in them attitudes and values related to normal patterns of living; it is these which are of benefit to clients.

16

Therapeutic use of self

INTRODUCTION

The development of a therapeutic relationship is the most delicate and nebulous of processes – difficult to pin down and hard to communicate. Reduction of it to a list of basic skills makes it seem artificial or mechanistic; capturing the complex interplay of dynamics which are different for each relationship, and change during a relationship, is more easily achieved by a novelist than by the author of a textbook. The general considerations have been discussed in Chapter 4. If, therefore, this seems a short chapter in comparison with others, this should not be taken as a comment on the importance of the topic, but on the difficulty of communicating it without either being reductive or covering overly well-trodden ground.

I define therapeutic use of self as the artful, selective or intuitive use of personal attributes to enhance therapy. 'Artful' should not be interpreted as artificial or deceitful, but as use of the art of therapy to select aspects of one's own personality, attitudes, values or responses which will be relevant or helpful in a given situation, and equally to supress those which may be less appropriate. The therapist is not expected to be 'perfect'; honesty, integrity and authenticity are the keys to therapeutic use of self.

Much personal interaction is spontaneous, and it would be disastrous if this were not so, but the expert therapist learns to identify and retain techniques which are helpful, and responses which appear intuitive may in reality be based on rapid professional judgements of which the therapist may be, at least at the time, unaware.

SELF-AWARENESS

In order to employ oneself effectively in a therapeutic relationship one must be both aware of oneself, in the sense of having a well-defined concept of who one is and what one has to offer as a therapist, and sensitively aware of the other person.

It is also necessary to judge the situation in order to know what kind of relationship may be required. Some therapeutic contacts are brief, formal and business-like. Others may be long-term, and may require interaction at a deeper level.

Self-awareness relates to the therapist's conscious monitoring and control of her own inner processes, thoughts, emotions and attitudes. The growth of realistic self-awareness is a slow and painful process for all of us. It takes the majority of people most of their lives to attain some insight. There is no easy route. One may discover a technique derived from a psychotherapeutic, cognitive or spiritual frame of reference which one finds helpful, but many therapists 'muddle through' in a less structured way.

It is probably more helpful to be aware of the issues than to have some neat prescription for promoting insight or personal growth. The main issue is simple: if you have little understanding of the person you know best – yourself – how can you presume to gain understanding of someone else, or to assist him to gain insight?

People have many motivations for becoming therapists, some altruistic, some not. If the therapist is a person who desperately wants to 'heal the world', she may be storing up a legacy of frustration and disappointment, or even guilt, when she fails to live up to these impossible expectations.

It has to be acknowledged that the position of the therapist is potentially a powerful one. It is important that the therapist should recognize her personal imperatives and the degree of her desire to influence others.

Many therapists have very high expectations of themselves; they frequently transfer these onto other people, including their patients. High expectations are useful if they promote self-development, expertise, high standards and the provision of an efficient and effective service, but are not helpful if they lead to overwork or frustration.

Every person has a mental attic full of accumulated baggage and locked cupboards which he does not care to open. The therapist must strive to avoid inflicting the consequences of her own luggage and 'ghosts' on her patients. She must continually beware of working out her own story, or reliving her own relationships in the lives of others. She must try to notice the danger signs when she starts to over-identify with a particular patient, and ask why.

This is not to suggest a need for in-depth psychoanalysis, only that the therapist may need to recognize that there are some situations, or some types of patients, with whom she will never be at ease. Occupational therapy is a wide world; it is usually possible to choose a different area of work.

The most helpful first stage is to recognize at least some of what is 'locked in the attic', and perhaps where it came from. If possible, open the door, and take a quick look. At the worst, the door will be slammed shut with a vow never to open it again. At best, something may be found which, once confronted, can be dealt with, at least in part. Experiences during training, or practice, may unexpectedly open some of these closed doors. This can be uncomfortable, but is a useful part of the learning process.

The mythology of professionalism includes the assumption that the professional person either feels no emotions, or has them so well under control that they never surface in public. This is incorrect, and attempting to live up to the assumed ideal can, in fact, actually be deeply damaging.

Being a therapist can be a wonderful, rewarding and joyful experience. There is nothing wrong in celebrating with a patient when there is cause, or in taking pleasure in one's share in a successful outcome.

However, the therapist should also be prepared to acknowledge, even if only in private, when the tragedies which a patient has encountered make her want to cry. Some people have lousy lives. Being human, and sensitive, inescapably means taking on other people's loads, and denying this can, in time, lead the therapist to a state of 'burnout'.

One also needs to be aware when a patient has made one angry, tense, or frustrated and to seek the reasons for this. (Is your patient 'refusing to get better'? Are you being reminded of a parent or spouse? Is the patient passing his own emotions on to you? Did you row with someone. There could be a dozen explanations.)

Defense mechanisms can be protective, but can also obstruct as a therapist's work: one must seek to be aware of those which one habitually uses, and of whether these offer effective escape routes or unproductive blind alleys.

It may occasionally be necessary to confront your patient (or even a colleague) with the negative emotions which he has provoked in you, provided one is sure that this is therapeutic for the person concerned, and not just for oneself. Be sure also to communicate positive feelings where appropriate.

When working in emotionally demanding or stressful circumstances it is wise to seek professional support and supervision, and to find someone to share the load.

STRESS REDUCTION

Being a therapist is stressful. There is no easy formula; the actions listed in Box 16.1, which assist the therapist to remain effective and contain personal stress, have been gained through personal experience over many years of practice and are shared on that basis.

Box 16.1   Dealing with stress

1. Resist taking on too much at once, either for one individual or for a caseload. Waiting lists are regrettable, but may be unavoidable. Giving a poor service to many is not preferable to giving an effective service to fewer people. Have approved policies for prioritizing or weighting referrals if necessary.
2. Phase action plans so that stages can be completed. Use personal skills of organization, time management, energy conservation and work-study.
3. Value colleagues; use their support when you need it, and observe when they are under stress and offer yours.
4. Delegate as far as is possible, and use the resources of others effectively and with tact.
5. Take time to build personal networks and 'oil the wheels' so that it becomes easier to obtain resources or services, and so that in emergency action can be taken swiftly, (but do not declare an emergency unless there is one).
6. Make it quite clear – to client, referring agent or anxious relative – when demands are impossible, and make realistic expectations of service provision equally clear. Keep all concerned well informed of progress or lack of it.
7. Avoid making promises unless you can guarantee they can be kept.
8. Keep the paperwork up-to-date; record everything promptly, however briefly.
9. Use supervision actively; check out problems, ensure that managers know what is going on. Pass problems upwards when needed. Acknowledge when a client (or colleague) is worrying you, for whatever reason, and find help to deal with this.
10. Do not continually work a 12-hour day; take coffee breaks and lunch breaks, and take holidays when due.
11. Know when events in your own life impinge on your work as a therapist, and do not disregard this. If you have a personal illness or crisis to cope with it will effect your work. Confide in someone. Seek help for yourself.
12. Arrange treats for yourself when you are under pressure and defend some space in your own life for the activities and people which you value. Use your occupational therapy skills to retain balance in your own life.
13. When frustration reaches boiling point, scream loudly in the privacy of your car, punch pillows, write the scorching letter you would like to send and tear it up afterwards – anything to ensure that you defuse the situation safely and avoid taking it out on colleagues, client, partner or yourself.
14. Remember to find something to make you laugh.

BUILDING A RELATIONSHIP

Two inescapable elements in the healing process are mutual trust and respect. It may even, ultimately, be these feelings which are curative, as much as, if not more than, any prescribed therapy. It is therefore important to understand how these attitudes are engendered and how the therapist can make positive use of them, without falling into the trap of assumed omnipotence.

The two attitudes are linked; we trust more people whom we also respect. We also feel more able to trust and respect people who show the same regard for ourselves. The therapist respects the patient *because he is a patient*, i.e. because he is a person seeking help in order to change some aspect of his life. Respect for the therapist may come initially with the professional title or uniform, but at some point, if it is to continue, it must be earned by effective action.

Why do we instinctively trust some people and not others? At one level, a feeling of trust is simply 'gut reaction'. The other person either looks and feels trustworthy or he does not. It is a primitive response, but gut reaction is not a simple matter. It is a rapid and largely unconscious assessment of social and physical signals.

Confident, upright body language, positive eye contact, appropriate dress, environmental demand and social context all contribute, even before any words have been exchanged. Basic, culturally appropriate, decent manners do help. Reassuring tone of voice, correct speed and content of delivery and even accent can also play a part. Reactions to others are predominantly learned; experience has a role to play. If you happen to remind your patient of the teacher he disliked, or the friend who let him down, or the nationality he despises, you start at a disadvantage.

The therapist, like the actor or salesman can learn to give out the right signals. Some people do this naturally, but it is not dishonest to improve one's technique. A therapeutic relationship always has to be worked at, but the initial contact can make or break subsequent interactions.

Some people have had such unfortunate experiences with others that they are unable to show trust. It may be a slow and difficult process to build a relationship with such a person. Unconditional positive regard may help, but premature opening up of a relationship may put demands on a patient for reciprocation which he is unprepared to make or finds inappropriate.

The skills needed to build a therapeutic relationship are simply those required for any effective interpersonal communication. These have been described in so many texts on communication or counselling that it is unnecessary to go into too much detail here.

SKILLS REQUIRED TO BUILD A RELATIONSHIP

Counselling

'Counselling' is a greatly overused word. Formal counselling involves a continuing relationship in which a counsellor acts to facilitate a process of self-examination or decision-taking with an individual client. Informal counselling is a more spontaneous affair in which basic counselling skills are used to deal with some problem or need. The boundary between the two forms of intervention should be recognized, because formal counselling is a highly skilled process.

Not all clients need counselling; there is still a place for simple, straightforward advice, and an exploration of patient needs and options does not necessarily involve entering into a formal counselling process. Some approaches imply at least a degree of direction on behalf of the therapist, which may not conform with some styles of counselling techniques.

That being said, all therapists need basic counselling skills, because the need for informal counselling may arise unpredictably in the course of a therapy session; it can be damaging to dismiss the need or lose the moment.

Counselling over a long period, or in depth, requires detailed training, practice and expert supervision. It is not a process which it is necessarily appropriate for an occupational therapist to carry out, and it may be preferable to refer the client to a suitable counsellor. Therapists working in settings where counselling is frequently needed should obtain appropriate additional qualifications.

Listening

One of the most important skills is active listening, a skill which, like observation, requires conscious development. The therapist needs to listen to content, analyse and respond to it, and either simultaneously or subsequently be aware of subtexts, and the nuances of what is said and left unsaid. Words may be the main means of human communication, but they are not the only means, nor are they always in harmony with less obvious expressions conveyed by body language.

In order to listen, and to encourage the other person to speak, the therapist must pay attention to positioning, expression and, especially, eye contact. Questions need careful phrasing as closed statements give little scope for gaining information. Verbal cues and prompts may be needed. Small noises of interest or agreement, nods, and echoing or reflecting back what has been said are effective in promoting interaction.

Obtaining and giving information

These are skills which have to be modified to the context and location of the interaction, as well as to the special needs of the patient.

Beginning and ending an interaction

These need careful handling, especially the ending, when important matters may be raised by the patient as an apparent afterthought. It is sometimes necessary to curtail discussion, and body language can be an effective and subtle means of doing this – removing eye contact, leaning back, and shifting position are all accepted social cues that conversation should end. Patients who fail to respond to social cues may need to be tactfully directed towards a conclusion. In some cases it is necessary to set a contracted time-limit with the patient before an interview or session commences; it is then important that both parties adhere to this.

Empathy

The need for empathy in the therapeutic relationship is often mentioned. There is a straightforward distinction between sympathy – sharing someone else's emotions, and empathy, which is knowing how someone else feels, while remaining disengaged from the experience.

Being able to empathize enables a therapist to help the patient to cope with or recognize his emotions. Empathy can be conveyed by words, expressions, gestures and body language which reflect the state of the patient, but often needs to be accompanied by action to help the patient to recognize the emotion, and by support to help him to deal with it.

The therapist, while understanding the emotion, must usually strive to remain detached from it in order to be able to offer appropriate help. Nevertheless, there are rare occasions where some human tragedy is so gut-wrenchingly awful that the therapist can do little else but weep with the patient (or in private), since not to do so would be less than human. Therapists may need, however, to mask their own emotions in public when displaying them would be inappropriate.

Role play

The best therapists are often good actors, especially in psychosocial settings. 'Acting' should not be seen as a contrivance. As actors know, the process of acting often involves offering a part of one's self or one's experience in exaggerated form. In a therapeutic context this may be a means of offering the patient a particular experience or form of relationship.

The therapist may act out many roles – wise advisor, surrogate daughter, clown, fool or competent performer. A patient may be able to use the therapist as a role model for social or other behaviours, and for attitudes and values. It is the therapist's responsibility to ensure that suitable 'scenes' or scripts are constructed and acted out for the benefit of the patient, so that the desired reactions and behaviours can be observed in action.

In more structured contexts, formal role play involving therapist and patient(s) can be a powerful therapeutic tool, especially when it includes playing out personal sociodramas or life events. Indeed, such powerful emotions and memories can be engendered by such techniques that they should never be used without special training and careful supervision.

Feedback

Patients may not be able to monitor accurately the effects of their own actions on objects or people. This may involve physical problems in sensorimotor feedback and perception, in cognitive processing or in social awareness. The therapist may augment and provide feedback so that the patient becomes more aware of himself, his actions and his effects on others.

The therapist may do this by providing verbal feedback, or by using her personal positions, reactions or expressions. Aids such as a mirror or videocamera can provide useful feedback. Selected 'rewards' or 'sanctions' may be needed to reinforce appreciation of behaviours.

In some situations, feedback needs to be accompanied by discussion, rehearsal, role play or other techniques designed to enable the patient to see where an interaction or performance went wrong, and how this could be changed in future.

There has been much emphasis recently on viewing the patient as an open system in which input, throughout, output and feedback are all essential mechanisms. Faulty input or faulty processing of information both affect the appreciation of feedback. A patient who is unable to obtain and analyse feedback from his performances, especially psychosocial ones, may be severely disadvantaged, and will have difficulties in learning and adapting. Therefore, feedback techniques are essential therapeutic tools and must be practised and perfected.

PROMOTING ENGAGEMENT IN THERAPY

Unlike many other forms of treatment, occu-

pational therapy simply cannot be provided to a passive, unresponsive recipient (except in the form of some specialized techniques used on patients with severe brain damage). It requires active engagement and a degree of cooperation from the patient. The more the patient is motivated to take an active part in therapy, the better the results will be.

MOTIVATION

Achieving motivation may sometimes be the primary aim in the early stages of intervention. Because motivation is such an individual concept, it can be hard to promote it. The greatest difficulty is often in discovering why a patient seems unmotivated; sometimes this may be explained by obvious pathology, such as depression, or by fear. In other cases the causes are complex and may relate to personality, experience or unconscious needs or anxieties.

In enabling the patient to be motivated, the therapist may first need to spend time explaining the active, participatory nature of occupational therapy, especially in physical settings. It has been my experience that the first words from a new patient entering a physical occupational therapy department are often 'what are you going to do to me?'. This is to be expected of hospitalized patients who see themselves as the passive recipients of a series of, e.g. nursing procedures, medical or surgical interventions and tests.

Intrinsic and extrinsic rewards

Behaviourally, motivation is related to incentives and rewards. Incentives are perceived goals and purposes, which must be seen as relevant. Rewards can be divided into those which are intrinsic – arising as a direct result of engaging in an activity, and those which are extrinsic – derived from, or contingent to, an activity or situation.

Because occupational therapy is activity-based, it is possible to use intrinsic rewards – from the simple act of drinking the cup of tea which has been made, to pleasure in the production of an artefact or enjoyment of the participation in an event.

The hope of 'getting better' or achieving some desired personal goal as a result of participating in occupational therapy may be a reward extrinsic to the activity. Sometimes it is the only motive: the patient has reached the point where continuing to be 'ill' is so unbearable that he is ready to participate in anything, however threatening or painful, if it will help to promote change.

Other extrinsic rewards may be tangible, such as money or privilege, or, more often, social. Warmth and praise from the therapist or others are often sufficient. Perceptions of added self-worth, status, or personal efficacy are also motivating. Some individuals find altruistic and generative activities which benefit others particularly rewarding.

Again, there is no simple formula. The therapist must make a 'best guess' and if this does not seem to provide the right motivation, must continue to experiment until an effective motivator is found.

Motivational problems

Lack of motivation in a patient can raise ethical problems concerning the degree to which an individual should be cajoled, persuaded, manipulated or coerced into participating in therapy 'for his own good'. Reasoned, and reasonable persuasion is clearly often necessary, but ultimately the patient has the right to refuse to cooperate and must not be 'bullied' into agreeing; this right must not be removed by the expedient of failing to explain to the patient that it exists.

The patient may well agree 'to please the therapist', or even 'for a quiet life', which may be acceptable as a starting point, but will not be sustained unless genuine motivation replaces it. I have not infrequently heard a therapist or assistant say to a patient 'just do it for me'. However, this approach is too manipulative for my personal comfort.

Anxiety, uncertainty or fear inhibit action. In order to benefit from therapy the patient must feel safe and become confident, both in the ability of the therapist to provide the treatment, advice or services which are needed, and in his own abilities to make progress as a result of intervention.

To begin with, the therapist must appear confident in herself and her client. (Appearance is important – one may be inwardly anxious, but must strive not to communicate this). Explanations help, for uncertainty promotes anxiety. Confidence needs to be built, and depends largely on the therapist's use of strong, calm, body language, expression, and verbal reinforcement and encouragement. It is especially important when physically assisting or handling the patient to be steady, competent, and not to fumble. There are, however, times when a patient is over-confident, and the therapist needs to hold him back.

Judicious use of humour can help to take the strain out of threatening situations or failures and make the experience of therapy enjoyable.

Prompts and cues

Prompts and cues help to initiate and sustain motivation. These facilitatory devices may be verbal, physical, sensory or situational and are especially important during developmental or exploratory stages in therapy, being withdrawn gradually as competence is developed.

Prompts and cues are similar in nature, but a cue is used to initiate a performance, while a prompt is used to shape it if it falters when it is under way. Verbal prompts or cues often take the form of questions, e.g. 'what next?', 'what do you need now?' or 'do you remember how you did it last time?' If the response is negative or incorrect, a small piece of information is given to enable the activity to proceed to the next task.

Physical cues can be provided through the position or body language of the therapist, or by providing actual physical contact, such as positioning, touching or holding the patient. It is important that all physical contact is assured and firm, and that trust and a good rapport is developed between therapist and patient. This can be achieved quite rapidly if the patient has confidence in the therapist.

A highly-skilled physiotherapist was observed during a short demonstration to obtain a very rapid rapport with a patient to the extent that once the patient had been established in a good posture small prompts, such as the therapist moving her own head to indicate that the patient needed to straighten his, were all that were needed.

Sensory cues can be provided in many ways – visual, tactile and auditory – and patients with sensory deficits can benefit from these.

Situational cues are provided by ensuring that the environmental demand is compatible with the activity or interaction, and arranged so as to enhance it if required. It is clearly far easier to elicit performance in an appropriate environment, and small changes can make a significant difference. Physical elements in the environment which may be used to provide cues or prompts are usually quite obvious, but social, cultural or temporal elements may be less obvious and may need consideration.

Some patients react very sensitively to situational cues, and can thereby mask quite severe deficits. This is useful when seeking to enhance performance, but may be a problem when trying to assess deficits. I have encountered a number of severely aphasic patients, for example, who, when faced with a smiling therapist holding a teacup and asking 'would you like a cup of tea?', made appropriate responses, with apparent comprehension. If, however, the smile and teacup were removed, and the words were spoken in a neutral voice avoiding social and situational cueing, the patients were unable to understand and respond to the question.

If the therapist can achieve rapport – 'useful communication and harmonious relationship' (COD) – with a patient, the prospects of a successful intervention will be greatly increased.

TEACHING

Teaching is an important form of therapeutic intervention. The therapist needs to have a sound understanding of the psychology of learning, and must acquire and practise a variety of teaching techniques to enable her to instruct, inform, educate or explain in formal and informal settings.

Learning is notoriously difficult to define. A commonly-used definition is: 'a relatively permanent change in behaviour'; however, this is really only a partial description.

It has been suggested that the term learning defies precise definition because it is put to multiple uses. Learning is used to refer to:

1. The acquisition and mastery of what is already known about something.
2. The extension and clarification of meaning of one's own experience.
3. An organisational process of testing ideas relevant to problems.

In other words it is used to describe a product, a process, or a function. (Knowles 1978)

Learning is a complex phenomenon. An individual's ability to learn is affected by internal and external factors (Box 16.2).

The extent to which each factor is significant depends on the perspective of the chosen learning theory. Once the therapist has gained some familiarity with learning theories and teaching techniques, she has a basis for the selection of appropriate methods.

The process of teaching is in many respects similar to that of therapy. A knowledge of the situation, abilities and needs of the learner has to be gained. A decision must be taken about a model or approach. Aims and objectives must be set, by either the teacher or the learner. The educational process must be planned and implemented, and there needs to be some means whereby the effectiveness of learning can be evaluated, either formally or informally.

Box 16.2 Factors that affect learning

Internal factors	External factors
Genetic potential	Opportunity
Readiness to learn	Environment
Motivation	Teaching methods
Emotional state	Stressors
Previous learning (memory)	Disease or trauma
Learning styles, skills and strategies	Social factors
Self-concept	Cultural factors
Age	Rewards

What is to be taught may be categorized as various combinations of knowledge, skill or attitude. These require differing teaching techniques. The learner's readiness to learn is an important prerequisite. If the individual is 'unready' developmentally, cognitively, or in terms of previous learning and experience, or current motivation, a good deal of preparatory work may be needed before the desired learning can take place. Learning will occur most effectively when the therapist can balance the occupational and environmental demand factors with the ability of the learner, so that the learner is at the same time safe and comfortable and yet involved and challenged.

There are many models of teaching, but these can be described as belonging to one or other of two distinct styles of teaching and learning – student-centred and teacher-centred.

In student-centred learning, the teacher takes a humanistic-style role of facilitator, enabling the student to set his own goals, take action to meet them, and decide how to assess whether they have been achieved. Student-centred methods promote in-depth learning which tends to be persistent, but may be slow, and they require careful management. These methods are especially effective with well-motivated adult learners.

In teacher-centred learning, the teacher takes the traditional role of instructor or educator, planning and delivering the instruction or information and designing the means whereby learning is assessed. This style can be effective in terms of time and use of resources, but may result in shallow, less permanent learning.

17

Management of resources

This book has, so far, been concerned with core therapeutic processes. Management of resources provides the material and infrastructure for therapy.

Management at senior level requires specialist training which is beyond the scope of this book. The basic techniques of management are explained well in other books (e.g. Johnson 1992, Perinchief 1993), for management is increasingly a part of every therapist's role. It seems unnecessary to repeat this material in detail.

SOCIAL POLICY

A therapist practises against a background of social policy, as determined by the government of the day. Social policy is derived from a combination of politics, economics and sociology and defines priorities and resource allocation, and the methods, scope and ethos of health care delivery.

Important government policy is often contained not in law, but in documents such as White Papers (policy which is to be carried out), Green Papers (policy which is being considered), or other consultative documents. Reports (usually considering some past or current situation and making consequent recommendations for changes) are often very influential, as are other 'public relations' statements of policy, such as the rights of patients.

Sooner or later the thinking in such documents is likely to filter down to operational level, and will certainly have a considerable effect on the policies of senior managers. Therapists need to keep themselves well-informed on such issues so that they can be appropriately responsive to them, and if necessary make comments on the likely effects on their own service provision.

LEGISLATION

Legislation – the parliamentary process of framing and enacting law – affects every aspect of the delivery of health care, defining both what must be done, and what is illegal.

It is essential for every practising therapist to be fully familiar with the legislation which affects his personal area of work. This, like all education and development, requires continual attention, because legislation is constantly being introduced or revised.

The old legal maxim 'ignorance of the law is no defence' is worth remembering. The therapist is not, of course, expected to be a lawyer, or to have the lawyer's legal memory, but a reasonable familiarity with the important points of legislation has to be attained, with special attention to aspects which impinge on the safety, rights, or well-being of patients.

The therapist must also have a very clear concept of professional ethics and of the actions which might be deemed to constitute negligence or malpractice. All actions must be such that experienced members of the profession would consider them to be justified and reasonable under the circumstances. Negligence is simply acting in a manner which could reasonably have been predicted to breach the therapist's duty of care to the patient, with resulting harm to that person.

It is important that the therapist practises within the limits of his professional competence and experience, and that all therapy given falls within the therapist's individual role and the legitimate remit of occupational therapy.

THE THERAPIST'S ROLE

While there may be a generic concept of the role of the occupational therapist, this is too broad to be of use in specific situations. The role needs further definition by means of an individual job description. This is the summary of personal duties and responsibilities, and shows the therapist's lines of accountability, and the limits of his authority.

Job descriptions, like all other managerial documents should be regularly reviewed and updated, and the therapist should take note of changes in role which may move practice in a direction which is not specified in the existing description.

Such changes should not be taken on without thought, but need to be drawn to the attention of the manager; sometimes the job description needs to be amended and sometimes the additional duties must be rejected as inappropriate or over-burdening.

THE 'THREE Es' OF MANAGEMENT

Enabling, enhancing and empowering are the 'three Es' of therapy. The 'three Es' of management are those attributes of good service delivery which contribute to the provision of therapy, namely: efficiency, economy and effectiveness.

EFFICIENCY

Efficiency is the art of using available resources to maximum effect, with minimum expenditure of time and effort. An efficient system runs on well-oiled wheels and delivers the goods where and when they are wanted. Systems management is an important component of efficiency.

In occupational therapy areas, systems are needed to run many routine aspects of service delivery, e.g. clinics, appointments, timetables, orders for supplies, and transport of people or items. Such systems are notorious for evolving rather than being designed; sometimes an evolved system is efficient but quite often it is not, yet people cease to question it. Frequently, the system was designed at some point in the past for circumstances which have since changed. The system grinds on, but no longer meets the demands of the present.

The most important feature of efficiency is that it has to be continually worked at, and systems need regular review and evaluation. It is also helpful if everyone understands the system, and not personal variations of it! A system must be simple – one so complex that only one or two key people can run it is not of much use, and chaos will erupt rapidly if the key person is unavailable.

ECONOMY

Economy is concerned with careful use of resources, not simply with keeping costs down, important though this is. Everyone knows that to buy the cheapest item is not always economical – it may break or wear out too soon. Being economic means using materials, staff, time, or any other item which has a cost, to good effect, without waste, and keeping correct account of such usage. Economy, like efficiency, has to be worked for and kept under continual review.

Therapists must be prepared to gather data to make justifications for the use of staff time and material resources. Managing a budget in some form is now part of all therapists' role, and detailed costings of services are often required.

Cost-effectiveness is a facet of economy: this is not easy to evaluate, but is very important. If, for example, spending a larger sum on a treatment now can be shown to save money by preventing the need for more prolonged and therefore more expensive treatment later, it is well justified. The use of staff time in relation to patient throughput is often used as a measure of cost-effectiveness, but this needs to be interpreted with care, in relation to the processes, purposes and outcomes specific to occupational therapy. Comparisons between professions are often highly misleading, since like is not being compared with like.

EFFECTIVENESS

Efficiency and effectiveness are closely linked, but they are not identical. A service might be fairly efficient in terms of its processes and procedures, but not very effective in terms of therapeutic outcomes, for example, in a situation where all the patients are processed through the occupational therapy clinic at half-hourly intervals but fail to improve.

Effectiveness is about achieving the purposes of the service to the best possible level. Measurement of effectiveness is not easy, for one needs first a clear idea of purpose (definition of service; individual aims and objectives), and then some means by which one may measure whether this purpose is being achieved (outcome measures).

It is the responsibility of senior management to formulate the purposes of the service (its 'mission') and the definitions or standards for measuring overall effectiveness. The clinician is concerned primarily with personal effectiveness within the service – which means simply, does the outcome of your intervention achieve the objectives which you and your client agreed, in line with set standards of practice?

As has been discussed in Chapter 12, finding appropriate, valid and reliable measures of outcome is difficult, but fundamental to achieving a high quality of service delivery and the development of effective therapy.

POLICIES, PRIORITIES AND PATIENT NEEDS: A MANAGERIAL BALANCING ACT

The process of case management describes how the needs of a patient are determined, goals planned and action taken. Making this process work effectively for each individual is a complex enough matter. However, the problems and pain really begin when the therapist must balance the conflicting needs of a whole caseload, and relate these to the managerial framework of policies, priorities and resources within which he is working. No therapist can find this a comfortable experience, and it may well be one of the major causes of stress and burnout. It is also an ethical and moral minefield.

When resources are finite, but need is continually present and expanding, how can one decide between the competing demands of the individuals referred for therapy? Who shall be seen at once, and who must wait? Even more starkly, in extreme cases, who should be treated, and who should not?

However stressful this may seem, therapists may consider themselves fortunate not to be in the position of doctors or paramedics faced with major disasters, who must engage in 'triage', taking literally life or death decisions about who to treat and who to deal with first. Following the principles of triage, those who are already dying and those who can help themselves are given least attention; efforts are concentrated on people who are seriously injured and for whom rapid treatment can make a real difference.

If transferred into therapy, this practical and utilitarian philosophy produces an apparently simple principle: treatment should be provided where it can do most good; some people will not benefit from therapy, and some will recover without it.

This is, however, not simple but simplistic. In an emergency or during war it may be practical, but these extreme situations sweep aside normal social and ethical considerations. How does one define 'do most good'? To whom? To the patient? To society? Do we treat only people who will thus be enabled to return to being productive contributors to society? Do we ignore people who are elderly, profoundly handicapped or terminally ill because the effort required to care for them is costly and unproductive? This is clearly not morally acceptable.

The difficulty for the therapist is in ethically balancing the therapeutic needs of the patient with the practical, managerial or political constraints placed on the service.

One may wish to argue that such decisions should be unnecessary; resources should be provided for all. This Utopian view, however, ignores day-to-day reality where difficult decisions do have to be taken. The therapist can certainly play a part in national debates about where and how resources are allocated, but at operational level pretending that the problem does not exist, or simply accepting all referrals and coping inadequately with the resulting load, are not options. The therapist must find a strategy for actively managing his caseload.

Policy, like other aspects of management, should be set by senior managers. Criteria which are objective, practical, unprejudiced, and simple to use are helpful, but need careful evaluation.

STRATEGIES

Strategies for caseload management include consideration of case-mix and weighting.

Consideration of case-mix

The mix of patients in a caseload changes continuously. In most situations it is only predictable in very general terms, although analysis of statistics for previous periods may provide data.

There will be numerical peaks and troughs, points at which the majority of the caseload require intensive therapy, and points where the majority require relatively simple and swift interventions. The therapist must consider the effects of these demands on the time, facilities, personnel and space available. Much can be done by intelligent timetabling and appropriate delegation, and the the changing mix must be reviewed continually so that adjustments can be made.

Weighting

This is a formal, or informal, system which allocates 'points' to a client in order to decide priority. It is most often used for managing a waiting list. In a formal system, a senior manager will decide on the basis of weighting, in line with policy decisions about purposes and priorities for the service. In a less structured system, the therapist does not actually allocate points, but undertakes a mental process, considering all the factors which may influence priority.

These factors may include:

- urgency – action now is essential
- severity – the patient has considerable needs or problems
- diagnosis – some conditions are more appropriate to, and responsive to, therapy than others
- complications – factors in the case which affect prognosis and the outcome of therapy

- feasibility – it is possible and practical to provide therapy
- effectiveness – therapy has a high success rate and achieves measurable positive outcomes
- economy – a short, economical input will achieve results; intervention is within the terms of service agreements
- policy – the patient falls within a priority group.

The problem with any weighting system is that it is essentially an artificial way of trying to make sense of uncertainty; weighting systems often have to make assumptions of questionable validity, and the ethical basis may be equally questionable.

Taken to extremes, the biggest danger in a mechanistic application of weighting is that it can lead to assumptions about person A having more right to treatment than person B, which is clearly not the case, since all persons' rights are equal. It is important to try to separate rights from needs: everyone has an equal right to therapy; everyone has not an equal need for it.

This kind of decision-taking requires all the therapist's skills, experience and clinical judgement. Junior therapists require, and should seek, support in taking difficult decisions. Interdisciplinary team discussion and decision-taking also helps to share the burden and ensure that the case is evaluated thoroughly. Use of the ethical grid (see p. 110) may also help to steer equitable service provision.

Nothing, however, will make the therapist's task easy when faced with such judgements as whether to provide intensive therapy over a long period for three patients with complex and serious problems, or whether to provide rapidly successful intervention for 10 patients.

QUALITY OF LIFE

It has already been noted that simple utilitarianism is an insufficient guide to deciding therapeutic priorities. Judgements over whether, and how much, therapy will improve the quality of life of a patient are difficult and delicate since quality of life is an ephemeral, subjective entity.

A person may fail to recognize when it is present, but may only too rapidly feel its loss.

The ethical debate over whether to end treatment which prolongs life without quality – without purpose, enjoyment or meaning – is rightly taken very seriously. Therapists are, fortunately, seldom faced with this decision.

They are faced, however, with making judgements about the effects of their intervention on quality of life, and most therapists would place high priority on interventions which enhance the meaning, pleasure and purpose in a person's life, even if these have little effect on her basic condition.

Dr Alan Williams has proposed a complex and controversial measure called a QUALY (Quality Adjusted Life Years), as an aid to deciding on health care priorities (Seedhouse 1988).

The general idea is that a beneficial health care activity is one which generates a positive amount of QUALYs and that an efficient health care activity is one in which the cost per QUALY is as low as can be. A high priority health care activity is one where the cost per QUALY is low, and low priority where the cost per QUALY is high.

Seedhouse discusses the moral complexities of this measure and concludes that its advocates fall into a logical error: 'They fail to notice the important distinction between the "quality of life" and the 'value of life'.'

He illustrates the fallacy by pointing out that if a better QUALY rating is obtained by treating Fred rather than John, it does not follow that Fred's life has more value than John's. His detailed rebuttal of the idea is well worth studying as an excellent example of how moral reasoning can be applied to health care, but sadly, it fails to resolve the therapist's basic dilemma, except by proposing use of the ethical grid (see p. 110).

Perhaps an overt recognition that case management does have an ethical dimension is itself helpful. Decision-taking is complex, and the most a therapist can do is to use clinical reasoning intelligently and sensitively to enhance, enable and empower his patients, avoiding discriminatory actions and seeking to justify decisions logically, and from a sound moral perspective.

COMMUNICATION

Skilful communication is fundamental to therapeutic use of self, and also to management; it is what makes the difference between an efficient and effective service, and one which is little more than adequate.

Therapists spend a large proportion of their time teaching, explaining, negotiating, requesting, telephoning, writing or typing. It may be argued that some of this is inappropriate and could be delegated, and that therapists should spend their time 'hands on' with patients. There is certainly a need for administrative and secretarial support, but that still leaves much which the therapist must handle himself.

NETWORKING

Each therapist will develop – and it can take months or even years – a network of people whom he can contact for everything from a piece of equipment for a patient to personal support for himself. If an experienced therapist is asked to compile a list of all the people in his own network, this list may be surprising in both length and variety. Other people are one of the therapist's biggest resources; they must be cherished and cultivated with care.

REPORT WRITING

Formal managerial reports (not those concerning patients) require a distinct style of presentation. The basis of skilful report writing is outlined in most texts on management, and yet, regrettably, it seems to be a skill which some therapists are slow to acquire.

Apart from the usual features of good factual writing – clear headings, clarity, brevity, accuracy, logical arrangement and professional presentation – the most important factor in a successful report is consideration of the reader. It is helpful to make some judgements about what the reader wants from the report, her interests or attitudes, and the best 'sales technique' for the ideas which are being communicated. A pragmatic understanding of the pressures affecting the reader, and the inclusion of a clear, concise summary is also helpful.

HUMAN RESOURCE MANAGEMENT

Even junior therapists may manage assistants or clerks. As well as a knowledge of employment legislation and local conditions of service, one would do well to follow the maxim of 'do as you would be done by'. Fairness, consistency and consideration are the foundations of personnel management. The most important skill is that of delegation, which is usually viewed as a downwards distribution of work, but which should also include the ability to pass work upwards, to senior managers, when appropriate.

It is important to remember that work can be delegated but that personal responsibility for it cannot. It is the responsibility of the therapist to give absolutely clear instructions, to ensure that work is delegated appropriately – to the right grade of staff, who have had sufficient training for the job, and whose job description covers it – and subsequently to check that it has been done correctly and to obtain feedback from the person who did it.

AOTA standards (Hopkins & Smith 1993) contain charts indicating how the roles of occupational therapy assistants vary from those of registered therapists; this is useful guidance; there may be local policies to follow.

Managing other people is an active, responsive process which must tread a careful line between autocracy and laissez-faire. A successful manager should be knowledgeable, skilled and creative, with a clear vision of the future; he should be capable of nurturing and developing, and not afraid to redeploy or weed out undesirable or useless elements.

PHYSICAL RESOURCE MANAGEMENT

Physical resources include time, money, equipment, materials, furniture, space, buildings and transport.

Most physical resources have a cost, require active management, and must be accounted for, audited and controlled. Equipment or materials may require continual replacement or planned maintenance. The therapist who can delegate such responsibilities to a competent administrator is fortunate indeed; most therapists have to handle them personally. There are many texts which explain how this should be done.

Cultivating the habit of efficient and economical management of resources can be viewed as a matter of self-preservation, because it promotes effective therapy, and removes frustrations.

The element that is most often overlooked is time. Time *is* money. Time-management is a distinct skill, relying on discipline, organization and a prodigious memory, backed up by a well-kept diary and well-planned systems. The therapist's time is his personal resource; it is unacceptable both to waste time and to be late for meetings, appointments and deadlines.

Far more common than the time-waster is the therapist who overworks, using every coffee break and lunch period, arriving early and staying late. Although acceptable during a short-term crisis, this demonstrates inefficient management of time and resources, and is no more satisfactory than a state of aimless disorganization.

QUALITY

Over the past decade the National Health Service has increasingly taken on the philosophy, language and managerial structures of industry. Taking the lead from industries as diverse as car manufacturers, supermarkets, hotels and fast food, various styles of quality management have been introduced. The patient is now overtly equated with the 'consumer' or 'user'. Consumer satisfaction with the 'products' of health services has become an important measure. Roberts (1992) concludes that:

It is the consumer who ultimately owns quality assurance . . . occupational therapists must increasingly seek the opinions of their consumers in order to monitor satisfaction with the service provided.

Health services have consequently been required to establish standards, define outputs and outcomes, to have valid and reliable methods of audit and, crucially, to ensure that the consumer has information regarding these and a means of exercising personal choice and influence on service development. The result has been a plethora of standards and 'charters' explaining health care provision to the public. While it is possible to argue over the degree to which these changes are politically motivated and cosmetic, they have resulted in a visibly different service culture.

The question of quality is therefore one which must take priority in the mind of any manager. Quality management provides the means whereby systems are monitored, evaluated and continually improved, but quality is also a matter of attitude or culture. Everyone needs to feel involved in, committed to, and able to make positive suggestions towards, provision of a quality service. It is all too easy for quality to become a rather meaningless 'buzzword'. However, the attainment of quality requires perseverance.

To strive for quality is to practise continually with a sense of dissatisfaction; however good one's service, the moment complacency sets in quality diminishes. However, it is implicit that the standards for which one is striving are realistic and appropriate. If they are set too high, staff will feel frustrated at being unable to achieve them; yet if they are too low, there is no incentive; this requires delicate handling by senior managers.

STANDARDS

Standards for professional practice are set in the UK by the College of Occupational Therapists, which publishes standards documents and a statement on professional ethics, and by the Council for Professions Supplementary to Medicine, which sets standards for professional education and deals with cases of negligence or malpractice. The American Occupational Therapy Association also has very well documented standards which are a useful source of reference (Hopkins & Smith 1993).

Wherever a therapist works, one of his first

responsibilities should be to find out what standards are in operation. These should be written and, as described in Chapter 12, quality assurance requires a system whereby service standards can be checked and audited regularly. Standards may lay down procedures to follow, timescales in which action must be taken, formats for documentation, supervisory procedures or methods of receiving and investigating complaints. Audit should lead to action to correct faults or revise and improve standards.

Standards tend to define a level to be attained and relate to a service definition or mission statement, whereas objectives specify in more detail exactly what the purposes of a service are, the action required, and by whom it will be undertaken.

Donabedian's 'structure, process, and outcome' method of service definition (1980), has been mentioned in Chapter 12. Crawford (1989) gives the following definitions:

Structure relates to resources and the organizational aspects of whatever is required to provide the specified care – staff, materials, system, information. Process refers to the actions required for the delivery of care, based on the steps identified as part of care provision. Outcome defines the result which is expected and desirable.

Alternatively, Maxwell (1984) has proposed six dimensions whereby service quality may be specified and measured:

- access to a service not limited by time or place
- relevance of the service to the needs of the population
- effectiveness of the service in meeting its objectives
- fairness of the service that aims to be even-handed
- acceptability of the service meant to satisfy expectations and needs
- efficient and economical use of the service's resources.

Wilson's Relevant Understandable Measurable Behavioural Achievable (RUMBA) (Wilson 1987) acronym is designed to provide a test of the validity of standards statements; the problem is that it is too easy to write standards that include vague terminology such as 'adequate resources', which makes it impossible to evaluate them. Another problem is the use, in statements which are intended for the general public, of language which demands an advanced vocabulary and reading skills.

QUALITY AUDIT

As already discussed, clinical audit is closely linked to quality audit. Apart from formal procedures such as peer review, every therapist should take a regular, critical look at his own caseload, checking the quality of, e.g. case management, use of the process or adherence to a protocol, recording, reporting, achievement of goals, quantity of cases seen and relevant selection of priorities. This should lead to an action plan for areas which can be developed, improved, or changed.

This kind of constructively self-critical review is part of reflective practice and one of the means whereby personal expertise is developed. It is not an optional extra and time must be allowed for it. One advantage of problem-based recording system such as POMR is that they facilitate audit, because it is possible to review very precisely whether objectives have been met.

Supervision of junior staff by more experienced therapists can be a method of quality audit, provided that it is used dynamically and sensitively by both sides. Again, it requires time, which must be regularly allocated and regarded as a priority.

Regular individual performance review (IPR) may also contribute, provided that it is linked to a continuous staff development programme so that skills and professional education can be improved and updated. However, staff development needs to be clearly distinguished from systems of performance related pay.

CONSUMER SATISFACTION

Consumer satisfaction is an important component of quality assurance. In any intervention a contract is evolved and negotiated between therapist and client. This contract – usually specified in the form of aims, goals and objectives –

states what the client hopes to obtain from her participation in the process, and what the therapist will provide in order to help the client to achieve these oucomes. 'Consumer satisfaction' is the measure of the degree to which the individual accepts that the contract has been fulfilled, and the degree to which she feels comfortable with the manner in which this has been undertaken.

Smith C (1992) writes that 'patient satisfaction represents a complex mixture of perceived need, expectations and experience of care.' She offers Pasco's definition of patient satisfaction as 'health care recipients' reaction to salient aspects of the context, process and result of their experience.'

The implication of this is that the client must have been involved in constructing the terms of the contract, must understand the nature of the process of occupational therapy, be capable of evaluating it, and be given the opportunity to do so. None of these aspects is straightforward.

The practice of occupational therapy is predominantly described as client-centred. However, the degree of real control which the client is enabled or empowered to exercise is variable. More 'medical model' frames of reference may constrain client choice and participation and may, in extreme cases, dictate the programme to be used with no input from the client.

Given a client-centred approach, agreement on aims and objectives is still not a simple matter. Participation in goal setting implies that the client is developmentally, physically, socially, cognitively, and educationally prepared and able. Some clients are, and are able to take on responsibility for their own therapy with relatively little facilitation and guidance from the therapist.

The majority, however, by the very nature of the problem or circumstance which has brought them into the process of therapy, are unable to some degree to take this form of control. Indeed, the denial of a problem, or the inability to take action to define or solve it, may *be* the problem, especially in the early stages of intervention. Austin & Clark (1992) describe the problem of having 'moving goal-posts' because of the need to continually redefine objectives.

Perceptions at the start of intervention may differ substantially from those at the end; furthermore, perceptions at some further point in time may differ from those at the end point of therapy, whch is when the expression of satisfaction is most often sought.

Occupational therapy is difficult to explain, and is widely misunderstood. In order for a client to say whether or not she was satisfied, she must have some concept of what service, in an ideal situation, she should have received. This has to be presented in user-friendly, jargon-free terms. A person cannot express dissatisfaction with some deficiency, if she was unaware that the service should have been provided.

Some of the goals of occupational therapy may be met by actions of the therapist on behalf of the client. These are relatively easy to evaluate: the adaptation was provided and used; the visit happened and the advice was carried out. However, occupational therapy is essentially a process in which the patient/client must play an active part.

Unless the nature of occupational therapy is clearly explained, the client may not perceive her own input as being contributory to achieving an outcome, and even if she does, evaluating personal participation as an element of satisfaction is extremely difficult.

As shown by McAvoy (1992), the client may even be unaware that occupational therapy services have been provided. McAvoy found that, in a sample of 75 patients, 24 were unaware of having been seen by an occupational therapist. Again, this indicates the need for information and explanation.

This is not only a question of the information being provided, but relies also on the capacity of the client to evaluate the results of intervention objectively. This may not be a reasonable expectation, because knowledge may be insufficient, and also because the client is enmeshed in an intensely personal perception of her experience which she may have difficulty in expressing. In some cases – severe learning disability, psychosis, brain damage – the client may be capable of expressing satisfaction in only the most basic ways.

The client's level of dependence on the therapist, and her personal feelings towards him, may also prejudice her ability to be critical. Complaining may be considered as impolite. Being a patient can make the individual feel powerless and vulnerable. It may seem much safer to give an impression of satisfaction, or at least to say nothing negative.

Flaws in the system

The major flaw in the system is frequently that, even when the consumer understands the nature and purpose of the service and is capable of evaluating it, the means of doing this are either defective or absent. Consumer satisfaction surveys may be seen as 'one-off' research tools, rather than on-going evaluations of the service. Alternatively, they may simply become routine procedures which give the impression of being client-centred, but which in reality have little real effect on service provision.

A further problem is the difficulty of designing an objective and valid method of capturing what is essentially 'soft' subjective data. As consumer surveyors know well, it is a simple matter to design a questionnaire which produces the results which the commissioner of the survey would like to obtain; this may be done inadvertently by inexperienced questionnaire designers.

The above difficulties are not arguments for ignoring consumer satisfaction, for this is a major part of quality assurance; it becomes difficult to justify the provision of occupational therapy if clients remain dissatisfied, and satisfaction cannot be assumed. Smith C (1992) notes pragmatically that a satisfied client is also more likely to be a compliant client; compliance implies that the individual will gain more benefit from intervention.

Methods of ascertaining consumer satisfaction

There is a need for more accessible and more valid methods of ascertaining consumer satisfaction. Banta (1992) states that 'evaluation of patient satisfaction is still in its infancy. What is relatively clear is that patients are more qualified to judge the interpersonal aspects of quality than the technical aspects.' He quotes a review of 23 studies of patients' assessments of care which found that 17 contained evidence of the validity of patients' assessments.

Informal, structured and formal methods may be used to ascertain consumer satisfaction. Informal methods include group discussion and interviews. More structured methods include semi-structured interviews, quality circles in which both clients and staff participate, and regular, critical review of complaints. Formal methods typically involve surveys and questionnaires. Formal methods, although time-consuming, are likely to provide more quantifiable results than informal methods, but may miss the nuances of personal experience and opinion; combining techniques may produce a more comprehensive view.

SERVICE AUDIT

Quantitative methods of service audit are widely used because they are relatively easy, if time-consuming, to collect, and can be processed by computer.

It has been learned from research methodology that in the case of complex situations with many interrelated factors, quantitative measures alone are relatively poor descriptors. Therapists are well aware that measures such as numbers of patient attendances, throughput and staff hours are of little practical use when it come to making judgements about therapeutic efficacy.

These measures can become seriously misleading when misinterpreted by managers who mistakenly try to compare services. If, for example, an occupational therapy department's output ratio of patients to staff time is compared with that of a physiotherapy department using a system of 15-minute treatment slots, the comparison might, at face value, seem to indicate that occupational therapists provide a costly and inefficient service.

Performance indicators are statistics which are used as measures of 'the three Es'. These can include statistics such as numbers of patients treated, percentage success rates, or unit costs, and may be compared with some regional or local 'norms', or with figures from previous periods. They are intended to be interpreted in the light of local circumstances, and not to be used simply on a 'league-table' basis.

All therapists are obliged to keep detailed records of work carried out, both to monitor service contracts and costs and to provide statistics concerning throughput, and the nature of intervention.

These statistics can be useful tools when managed properly, but in the past, while systems were developing, the data took too long to collect, was often not collected in a form which was relevant to the therapist, or simply disappeared into a computer and was never seen again. Systems developed in isolation are frequently incompatible, and much effort and money has been wasted in 'reinventing the wheel' in terms of software and systems.

INFORMATION TECHNOLOGY

As information technology in the NHS becomes more sophisticated and responsive, sytems for gathering and interpreting managerial data will improve. At the time of writing the NHS Executive is considering a national strategy on information management and technology (IMT), utilizing a standardized 'language of health', and five key principles have been suggested (NHS Information Management Group 1994):

- person-based information
- information collected by systems built into the day-to-day work of health care professionals
- restricted access to information so that it will remain confidential and secure
- information shared across the NHS; all systems should be compatible
- information should focus on health: it should

look further than the incidence of illness and provision of treatment. Evaluation should be outcome related.

A person-centred, outcome-related strategy for IMT should be more compatible with the practice of occupational therapy, provided that therapists are able to contribute to the design of the system.

THE NEED FOR MULTIPLE OUTCOME MEASURES IN ASSESSING QUALITY

It may be that measures developed for qualitative research may be more appropriate to occupational therapy than quantitative measures which have to meet strict criteria of validity and reliability. One useful technique may be triangulation, where a number of different measures can be used and compared to show themes and trends.

If outcomes for a department show that objectives are being met, functional indices, where appropriate, demonstrate improvement, client satisfaction is expressed in positive terms, patient throughout is maintained at a realistic level in relation to staff hours, and standards of service provision are seen by systematic audit to be met, one might with some justification state that the department is working efficiently and effectively and is producing a quality service.

It would, however, be difficult to undertake a comparison with other occupational therapy departments, unless they were very similar and were using comparable measures. It would be equally problematic to identify whether the unit could become even more efficient, and if so, how this could be achieved. For this we will have to await the development of far more sophisticated and sensitive outcome measures than we currently possess.

PART 3

Perspectives and processes

18

Postscript: perspectives and processes

In the preface to this book I described the contents as a travelogue: the journey is now over, at least for the present. Having looked at various aspects of the occupational therapy scene, from a variety of angles, it now seems useful to try to obtain an overview of the terrain which has been covered, and especially of those parts of it which I have reinterpreted as I went along.

I have reached the conclusion that occupational therapy is a complex entity which cannot be explained by a single model. It is necessary to define the principles, possessions, purposes, processes and products of occupational therapy as a profession, to define the occupational nature of human beings, to define the nature of occupational competence and the role of occupational therapy in relation to this, and to define one or more models for the therapist's provision and practice of therapy.

In plainer language, it is necessary for ourselves, our clients, and our referring agents and managers to understand what occupational therapy is, why people need it, what occupational therapists do, why and how occupational therapy is effective, and what scientific rationale or accepted theory underpins it.

THE CORE OF OCCUPATIONAL THERAPY

I have presented a multi-layered view of the core of occupational therapy (Fig. 18.1). In the centre are the defining components: the 'occupational therapy triad' – person, occupation and therapist,

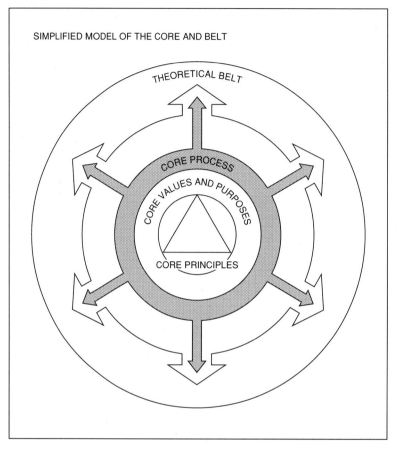

Figure 18.1 The central core and theoretical belt.

surrounded by the environment. These produce the principles and philosophy of the profession, delimit its scope and 'possessions' and give rise to the knowledge, skills and values on which practice is based.

The three purposes of occupational therapy – enabling, empowering and enhancing – are put into practice by means of six core processes: clinical reasoning, intervention, assessment and evaluation, occupational analysis and adaptation, environmental analysis and adaptation, and therapeutic use of self and resource management. These are coordinated by the problem-based process of case management. The products are expressed in terms of the outcomes of intervention for an individual.

The core is surrounded by a theoretical belt containing options for practice. Therapists may adopt one of these options and become theory-driven (see Fig. 18.5), or may choose to be driven by the problem-based process of case management, subsequently an appropriate approach from the belt (see Fig. 18.6).

The central triad can be used to integrate four aspects of the profession: a model of the occupational nature of the individual, a model of the nature of occupational competence and the ways in which the occupational therapist may intervene to restore this, a theory-driven pattern for practice, and a process-driven pattern for practice (Fig. 18.2).

There are, at this stage of our knowledge, variations on concepts concerning both the exact nature of the core, and also of the other supporting conceptual or practice models. In this text some new models have been suggested.

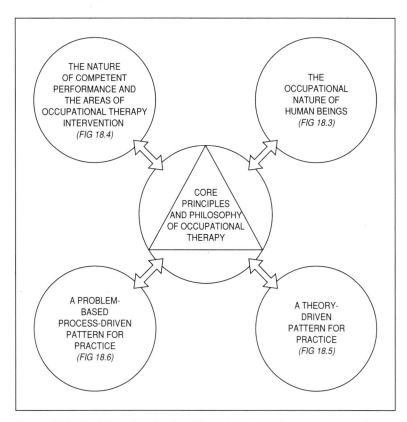

Figure 18.2   Models to describe the philosophy and practice of occupational therapy.

THE OCCUPATIONAL NATURE OF HUMANITY

The occupational nature of humanity is explained through the model of the productive self (Fig. 18.3). In this model, the individual is seen as functioning within two separated worlds, the potent sector and the patent sector. The former consists of the private self and the inner, physiological and psychological environment; the latter contains the public self and the external, physical and social environment.

THE NATURE OF OCCUPATIONAL COMPETENCE

Skills, in the sensorimotor, psychosocial and cognitive–affective domains, are used in the performance of roles, occupations, activities and

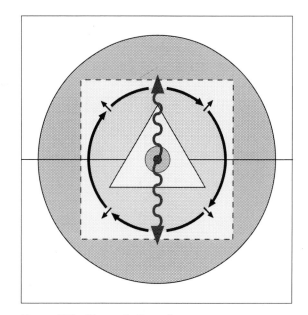

Figure 18.3   The productive self.

tasks within an ever-shifting life space within each sector. Life space is constructed by the person's perceptions and interests. Occupational performance links the two worlds in the experience of the individual, and makes it possible for him to have a personal effect on the environment, and consequently to gain a concept of self as an effective and competent actor within the world.

For competent performance, three components have to be in harmony: the knowledge, skills, attitudes and motivation of a person, the performance demand of an activity, and the demand of the environment. When any one of these factors becomes out of balance, dysfunction results. Dysfunction renders the individual in some way less able to cope with occupational demands.

THE ROLE OF OCCUPATIONAL THERAPY

Occupational therapy involves the therapist's intervention to balance the interaction between the person, the environment and the occupation, in order to enable, enhance and empower competent performance (Fig. 18.4).

The therapist can remedy dysfunction by working on the aspect (or aspects) which contribute to it. Since people function in complex and highly integrated ways, and since activities involve coordinated action, reaction, and inter-action, and link the patent and potent sectors, they have especial potential for therapeutic use.

It is possible to study and analyse occupations in order to understand them better. Occupations

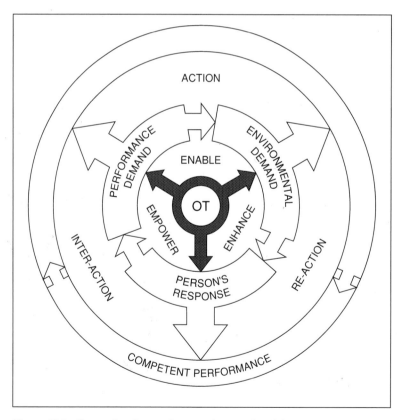

Figure 18.4 Occupational competence and occupational therapy.

and processes occur at the organizational level of performance, activities at the effective level and tasks at the developmental or proto-occupational level. Analysis can take place at each level; macroanalysis is concerned with the nature of occupations, activity analysis with the structure, context, and performance of activities, and micro-analysis with the detailed sequence and skills of a task. The environment can also be analysed at various levels and for various purposes.

Similarly, it is possible to assess and evaluate a person's occupational performance, from the building blocks of skill components, to his patterns of performance, his functional competence, and his existential experiences.

PATTERNS FOR PRACTICE

The therapist uses clinical reasoning to identify the nature of the problem and plan intervention. This process may be conducted with reference to a theory, by means of which the situation is interpreted and explained, elements are included or excluded from consideration, and actions can be taken. This is the theory-driven pattern (Fig. 18.5).

Alternatively, the process-driven pattern has been presented as a method of person-centred problem-framing, involving a choice of four causational explanations of the problem (Fig. 18.6), leading to a view of the individual as benefiting

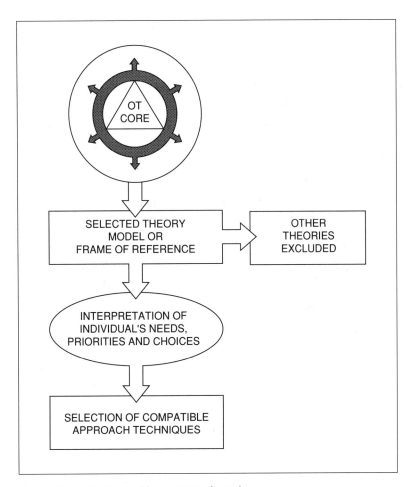

Figure 18.5 The theory-driven pattern of practice.

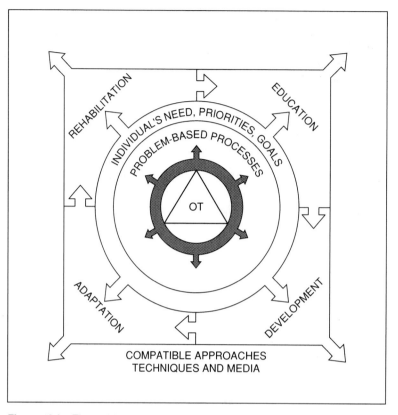

Figure 18.6 The problem-based, process-driven pattern.

from one or more of the problem-based models: development, education, rehabilitation or adaptation. Goals can then be set in partnership with the patient, and a relevant approach can be selected from the options within the theoretical belt.

These are hypotheses in search of researchers. The reader may decide to dip into the more established content of the book, and to disregard the rest. However, it is hoped that some therapists will find echoes of their own practice in these concepts, and will want to take them further, so that they may assist in unravelling the complexities of each individual's situation, and may help therapist and patient to embark jointly on a 'new beginning'.

References and bibliography

Allen C K 1985 Occupational therapy for psychiatric disorders: measurement and management of cognitive disabilities. Little Brown, Boston

AOTA Representative Assembly Minutes 1981 American Journal of Occupational Therapy 13: 792–802

Atkinson R L, Atkinson R G, Smith E, Benn D 1993 Introduction to psychology, 11th edn. Harcourt Brace Jovanovich, Florida

Austin C, Clark C R 1993 Measures of outcome: for whom? British Journal of Occupational Therapy 56(1): 21–24

Ayres A J 1972 Sensory integration and learning disorders. Western Psychological Services, Los Angeles

Bandura A 1977 Social learning theory. Prentice Hall, New Jersey

Banta D 1992 Developing outcome standards for quality assurance. Quality Assurance in Health Care 4(1): 25–32

Barnitt R 1993 What gives you sleepless nights? Ethical practice in occupational therapy. British Journal of Occupational Therapy 56(6): 207–212

Baron R A, Byrne D 1987 Social psychology, 5th edn. Allyn & Bacon, Massachusetts

Bigge M 1987 Learning theories for teachers, 4th edn. Harper & Row, New York

Blom Cooper L 1989 Occupational therapy: an emerging profession in health care. Duckworth, London

Bloom B S (ed) 1956 Taxonomy of educational objectives handbook: cognitive domain. McKay, New York

British Association of Occupational Therapists 1990 Code of professional conduct. British Association of Occupational Therapists, London

Bruce M A, Borg B 1987 Frames of reference in psychiatric occupational therapy. Slack, New Jersey

Buckminster-Fuller R 1969 The artist–scientist–inventor. In: The arts and man. Prentice Hall, New Jersey

Burke J P, DePoy E 1991 An emerging view of mastery, excellence and leadership in occupational therapy practice. American Journal of Occupational Therapy 45(1): 1027–1032

Campbell P H 1989 Using a single subject research design to evaluate the effectiveness of treatment. American Journal of Occupational Therapy 42(11): 732–738

Carlson M E, Clark F 1991 The search for useful methodologies in occupational science. American Journal of Occupational Therapy 45: 235

Caulton R 1993 Occupations and healing. Otago Polytechnic occupational therapy department. Occupation 1(1): 6–17

Concise Oxford Dictionary of Current English, 7th edn. J B Sykes (ed) 1982 Oxford University Press, Oxford

Clark F, Larson E A 1993 Developing an academic discipline: the science of occupation. In: Hopkins H, Smith H (eds) Willard and Spackman's occupational therapy, 8th edn. Lippincott, Philadelphia

Clark et al 1993 Dangers inherent in the partition of occupational therapy and occupational science. American Journal of Occupational Therapy 47(2): 184–186

Cohn E S 1991 Clinical reasoning: explicating complexity. American Journal of Occupational Therapy 45(11): 969–971

College of Occupational Therapists 1989 Occupational therapy: an emerging profession in health care: report of a commission of enquiry. Duckworth, London

College of Occupational Therapists 1994 Core skills and a conceptual foundation for practice: a position statement. COT, London

Colson J H C 1944 The rehabilitation of the injured. Cassell, England

Council for Professions Supplementary to Medicine 1990 Statement of professional conduct. Council for Professions Supplementary to Medicine, London

Crawford M 1989 Setting standards in occupational therapy. British Journal of Occupational Therapy 52(8): 294–297

Creek J (ed) 1990 Occupational therapy and mental health; principles, skills and practice. Churchill Livingstone, Edinburgh

Creek J 1992 Why can't OTs say what they do? Hong Kong University. Proceedings of Hong Kong International occupational therapy conference 17–25

Csikzentmihali M 1993 Activity and happiness: towards a science of occupation. Occupational Science 1(1): 38–42

Cynkin S, Robinson A M 1990 Occupational therapy and activities health: towards health through activities. Little Brown, Boston

Deitz J C 1993 Research: a systematic process for answering questions. In: Hopkins H, Smith H (eds) Willard and Spackman's occupational therapy, 8th edn. Lippincott, Philadelphia

Donabedian A 1980 The definition of quality and approaches to assessment. Health Administration Press, Michigan

Dutton R 1993 In: Hopkins H, Smith H (eds) Willard and Spackman's occupational therapy, 8th edn. Lippincott, Philadelphia

Dyck I 1992 The daily routines of mothers with young children: using a socio-political model in research. Occupational Therapy Journal of Research 12(1): 16–34

Eakin P 1989a Assessments of activities of daily living: a critical review. British Journal of Occupational Therapy 52(1): 11–15

Eakin P 1989b Problems with assessments of activities of daily living. British Journal of Occupational Therapy 52(2): 50–54

Eakin P 1993 The Barthel index: confidence limits. British Journal of Occupational Therapy 56(5): 184–185

Fidler G, Fidler J 1954 Introduction to psychiatric occupational therapy. Macmillan, New York

Fidler G, Fidler J 1963 Occupational therapy: a communication process in psychiatry. Macmillan, New York

Finlay L 1988 Occupational therapy practice in psychiatry. Croom Helm, London

Fish D, Twinn, Purr 1991 Promoting reflection. West London Institute of Higher Education, London

Fisher A G 1990 Assessment of motor and process skills. Unpublished test manual. Department of occupational therapy, University of Illinois, Chicago

Fisher A G, Liu Y, Velozo C, Pan A W 1992 Cross-cultural assessment of process skills. American Journal of Occupational Therapy 46(10): 876–885

Fleming M H 1991a The therapist with the three-track mind. American Journal of Occupational Therapy 45(11): 1007–1014

Fleming M H 1991b Clinical reasoning in medicine compared with clinical reasoning in occupational therapy. American Journal of Occupational Therapy 45(11): 988–996

Fleming M H 1993 Aspects of clinical reasoning in occupational therapy. In: Hopkins H, Smith H (eds) Willard and Spackman's occupational therapy, 8th edn. Lippincott, Philadelphia

Fondiller E D, Rosage L J, Neuhaus B E 1990 Values influencing clinical reasoning in occupational therapy: an exploratory study. Occupational Therapy Journal of Research 10(1): 41–55

Foster M 1992 The occupational therapy process and assessment. In: Turner A, Foster M, Johnson S (eds) Occupational therapy and physical dysfunction: principles, skills and practice, 3rd edn. Churchill Livingstone, Edinburgh

Francella F 1982 Psychology for occupational therapists. Macmillan (British Psychological Society), London

Fricke J 1993 Measuring outcomes in rehabilitation: a review. British Journal of Occupational Therapy 56(6): 217–221

Friedman P J, Leong L 1992 The Rivermead perceptual assessment battery in acute stroke. British Journal of Occupational Therapy 55(6): 233–237

Gagné R M 1977 The conditions of learning and theory of instruction, 3rd edn. Holt Saunders, UK

Glaser B L, Strauss A L 1967 The discovery of grounded theory. Strategies for qualitative research. Aldine Publishing Co. New York

Grandjean E 1988 Fitting the task to the man. Taylor & Francis, London

Hagedorn R 1969 Our apparatus and techniques are often out of date. British Journal of Occupational Therapy 18–19

Hagedorn R 1987 Therapeutic horticulture. Winslow Press, Bicester

Hagedorn 1992 Occupational therapy: foundations for practice. Churchill Livingstone, Edinburgh

Hargie O, Saunders C, Dickson D 1994 Social skills in interpersonal communication. (3rd edn) Routledge, London

Haralambos M 1985 Sociology themes and perspectives, 2nd edn. Bell & Hyman, London

Hasselkus B R 1992 The meaning of activity: day care for persons with Alzheimer's disease. American Journal of Occupational Therapy 46(8): 199–206

Hopkins H, Smith H (eds) 1993 Willard and Spackman's occupational therapy, 8th edn. Lippincott, Philadelphia

Illich I et al 1987 Disabling professions. Marion Boyars, London

Jay P, Mendez A, Monteath H 1992 The diamond jubilee of the professional association 1932–1992: an historical review. British Journal of Occupational Therapy 55(7): 252–256

Jeffrey L H 1993 Aspects of selecting outcome measures to demonstrate the effectiveness of comprehensive rehabilitation. British Journal of Occupational Therapy 56(11): 394–400

Johnson S 1992 Management. In: Turner A, Foster M, Johnson S (eds) Occupational therapy and physical dysfunction: principles, skills and practice, 3rd edn. Churchill Livingstone, Edinburgh

Jones M 1967 An approach to occupational therapy. Butterworth, London

Jongbloed L, Morgan D 1991 An investigation of involvement in leisure activities after a stroke. American Journal of Occupational Therapy 45(5): 420–427

Kielhofner G (ed) 1985 A model of human occupations. Williams & Wilkins, Baltimore

Kielhofner G 1992 Conceptual foundations of occupational therapy. F A Davis, Philadelphia

Kielhofner G 1993 In: Hopkins H, Smith H (eds) Willard and Spackman's occupational therapy, 8th edn. Lippincott, Philadelphia

Kings Fund Centre 1988 The problem orientated medical record (POMR): guidelines for therapists. Kings Fund Centre, London

Knowles M 1978 The adult learner: a neglected species. Gulf, Houston

Krefting L 1991 Rigor in qualitative research: the assessment of worthiness. American Journal of Occupational Therapy 45(3): 214–222

Krefting L, Krefting D 1991 Leisure activities after a stroke: an ethnographic approach. American Journal of Occupational Therapy 45(5): 429–436

Kuhn T 1970 The structure of scientific revolutions, 2nd edn. University of Chicago Press, Chicago

Laver A J, Huchison S 1994 The performance and experience of normal elderly people on the COTNAB. British Journal of Occupational Therapy 57(4): 137–142

Law M et al 1990 The Canadian occupational performance measure: an outcome measure for occupational therapy. Canadian Journal of Occupational Therapy 57(2): 82–87

Law M, Letts L 1989 A critical review of scales of activities of daily living. American Journal of Occupational Therapy 43(8): 522–528

Lewin K 1936 Principles of topological psychology. McGraw Hill, New York

Lewin K 1951 Field theory. In: Social science. Harper & Row, New York

Llorens L A 1970 Facilitating growth and development: the promise of occupational therapy. American Journal of Occupational Therapy 24: 93–101

Lloyd C, Maas F 1993 The helping relationship: the application of Carkhuf's model. Canadian Journal of Occupational Therapy 60(2): 83–89

Long A P, Haig L 1992 How do clients benefit from snoezelan? An exploratory study. British Journal of Occupational Therapy 55(3): 103–108

Lovell R B 1987 Adult learning. Croom Helm, London

McAvoy E 1991 The use of ADL indices by occupational therapists. British Journal of Occupational Therapy 54(10): 383–385

McCulloch D 1991 Can we measure 'output'? Quality adjusted life years, health indices and occupational therapy. British Journal of Occupational Therapy 54(6): 219–221

MacDonald M 1964 Occupational therapy in rehabilitation, 2nd edn. Bailliére Tindall & Cox, London

Maslin Z 1991 Management in occupational therapy. Chapman & Hall, London

Maslow A G 1970 Motivation and personality, 2nd edn. Harper & Row, New York

Matthey S, Donnelly S, Hextell D 1993 The clinical usefulness of the Rivermead perceptual assessment battery: statistical considerations. British Journal of Occupational Therapy 55(10): 365–370

Mattingly C 1991a What is clinical reasoning? American Journal of Occupational Therapy 45(11): 979–986

Mattingly C 1991b The narrative nature of clinical reasoning. American Journal of Occupational Therapy 45(11): 998–1005

Mattingly C, Fleming M H 1994 Clinical reasoning. Forms of enquiry in a therapeutic practice. F A Davis, Philadelphia

Maxwell R J 1984 Quality assessment in health. British Medical Journal 288: 1471

May K 1994 Abstract knowing: the case for magic in method. In: Morse J M (ed) Critical issues in qualitative research. Sage Publications, London

Mocellin G 1988 A perspective on the principles and practice of occupational therapy. British Journal of Occupational Therapy

Mocellin G 1992a An overview of occupational therapy in the context of American influence on the profession: part 1. British Journal of Occupational Therapy 55(1): 7–12

Mocellin G 1992b An overview of occupational therapy in the context of American influence on the profession: part 2. British Journal of Occupational Therapy 55(2): 55–59

Mosey A C 1981 Occupational therapy: configuration of a profession. Raven Press, New York

Mosey A C 1986 Psychosocial components of occupational therapy. Raven Press, New York

Mosey A C 1992 Partition of occupational science and occupational therapy. American Journal of Occupational Therapy 46(9): 851–853

Mosey A C 1993 Partition of occupational science and occupational therapy – sorting out some issues. American Journal of Occupational Therapy 47(8): 751–754

Moustakas C 1990 Heuristic research. Design, methodology and applications. Sage Publications, London

Murdock 1992a, A critical evaluation of the Barthel index. Part 1. British Journal of Occupational Therapy 55(3): 109–111

Murdock 1992b A critical evaluation of the Barthel index. Part 2. British Journal of Occupational Therapy 55(4): 153–156

Murphy J 1984 Perspectives on socialization. Course D307, Social psychology, unit 4. Open University Press, Milton Keynes

NHS Information Management Group 1994 OT briefing: focus on information management and technology. NHS Executive, London

O'Donnell M 1992 A new introduction to sociology, 3rd edn. Thomas Nelson, Walton-on-Thames

O'Sullivan E 1955 A textbook of occupational therapy. Lewis, London

Pahl R E 1984 Divisions of labour. Blackwell, Oxford

Parker S 1971 The future of work and leisure. Prager, New York

Pedretti L (ed) 1985 Occupational therapy: practice skills for physical dysfunction, 2nd edn. Mosby, St Louis

Pedretti L W, Zoltan B 1990 Occupational therapy practice skills for physical dysfunction (3rd edn) Mosby, Philadelphia

Perinchief J M 1993 Service management In: Hopkins H, Smith H (eds) Willard and Spackman's occupational therapy, 8th edn. Lippincott, Philadelphia

Piaget J 1952 The origins of intelligence in children. International Universities Press, New York

Piajet J, Inhelder B 1969 The psychology of the child. Basic Books, New York

Polatajko H J 1992 Naming and framing occupational therapy: a lecture dedicated to the life of Nancy B. Canadian Journal of Occupational Therapy 59(4)

Polgar S, Thomas S A 1991 Introduction to research in the health sciences. Churchill Livingstone, Edinburgh

Pollock N et al 1990 Occupational performance measures: a review based on the guidelines for the client-centred practice of occupational therapy. Canadian Journal of Occupational Therapy 57(2): 77–81

Reed K L 1984 Models of practice in occupational therapy. Williams & Wilkins, Baltimore

Reed K L 1993 The beginnings of occupational therapy. In: Hopkins H, Smith H (eds) Willard and Spackman's occupational therapy, 8th edn. Lippincott, Philadelphia

Reed K L, Sanderson S R 1983 Concepts of occupational therapy 2nd edn. Williams & Wilkins, Baltimore

Reilly M 1962 Occupational therapy can be one of the great ideas of twentieth century medicine. American Journal of Occupational Therapy 16(1) 1–9

Roberts A E K 1992 Who owns quality in the occupational therapy profession and how do we assure it? British Journal of Occupational Therapy 55(1): 4–6

Robertson L 1988 Qualitative research methods in occupational therapy. British Journal of Occupational Therapy 51(10): 344–346

Rogers J C 1983a Freedom to learn for the 80s. Merrill, Ohio

Rogers J C 1983b Clinical reasoning: the ethics science and art. Eleanor Clark Slagle Lectureship. American Journal of Occupational Therapy 37(9): 601–616

Rogers J C, Holm M B 1991 Occupational therapy diagnostic reasoning: a component of clinical reasoning. American Journal of Occupational Therapy 45(11): 1045–1053

Roos L, Brazauskas R 1990 Outcomes and quality assurance: facilitating the use of administrative data. Quality Assurance in Health Care 2(1): 77–88

Rowntree D 1985 Developing courses for students. Harper and Row, London

Schell B A, Cervero R M 1993 Clinical reasoning in occupational therapy: an integrative review. American Journal of Occupational Therapy 47(7): 605–610

Schon D 1983 The reflective practitioner: how professionals think in action. Basic Books, USA

Schon D 1987 Educating the reflective practitioner. Jossey-Bass, San Francisco

Schwartz K B 1991 Clinical reasoning and new ideas on intelligence: implications for teaching and learning. American Journal of Occupational Therapy 45(11): 1033–1036

Schwartzburg S L 1993 Therapeutic use of self. In: Hopkins H, Smith H (eds) Willard and Spackman's occupational therapy, 8th edn. Lippincott, Philadelphia

Seedhouse D 1988 Ethics: the heart of health care. Wiley, Chichester

Sexton D 1992 Kirton companions, the clients assess: evaluating a community mental health day facility. British Journal of Occupational Therapy 55(1): 414–418

Shah S, Cooper B 1993 Commentary on 'a critical evaluation of the Barthel index'. British Journal of Occupational Therapy 56(2): 70–72

Shah S, Cooper B, Maas F 1992 The Barthel index and ADL evaluation in stroke rehabilitation in Australia, Japan, the UK and the USA. Australian Journal of Occupational Therapy 39: 5–13

Simon C J 1993 Use of activity and activity analysis. In: Hopkins H, Smith H (eds) Willard and Spackman's occupational therapy, 8th edn. Lippincott, Philadelphia

Skinner B F 1938 The behaviour of organisms. Appleton-Century-Crofts, New York

Slater D Y, Cohn E S 1991 Staff development through the

analysis of practice. American Journal of Occupational Therapy 45(1): 1038–1044

Smith C 1992 Validation of a patient satisfaction system in the United Kingdom. Quality Assurance in Health Care 4(3): 171–177

Smith H D 1993 Assessment and evaluation: an overview. In: Hopkins H, Smith H (eds) Willard and Spackman's occupational therapy, 8th edn. Lippincott, Philadelphia

Smith R O 1992 The science of occupational therapy assessment. Occupational Therapy Journal of Research 12(1): 3–15

Stewart A 1990 Research. In: Creek J (ed) Occupational therapy and mental health. Churchill Livingstone, Edinburgh

Stewart A M 1992 The Casson Memorial Lecture: always a little further. British Journal of Occupational Therapy 54(8): 297–300

Sweeney G M, Nichols K A, Kline P 1993 Job stress in occupational therapy: an examination of causative factors. British Journal of Occupational Therapy 56(3): 89–93

Trombley C A (ed) 1989 Occupational therapy for physical dysfunction, 3rd edn. Williams & Wilkins, Baltimore

Turner A (ed) 1981 The practice of occupational therapy: an introduction to the treatment of physical dysfunction. Churchill Livingstone, Edinburgh

Turner A 1992 In: Turner A, Foster M, Johnson S (eds) Occupational therapy and physical dysfunction: principles, skills and practice, 3rd edn. Churchill Livingstone, Edinburgh

Unsworth C A 1993 The concept of function. British Journal of Occupational Therapy 56(8): 287–292

Vercruyesse B 1994 Proceedings of the congress of the World federation of Occupational Therapists

Warren I 1993 An introduction to protocols for occupational therapy. British Journal of Occupational Therapy 56(1): 25–27

Whalley Hammell K R 1994a Establishing objectives in occupational therapy practice. Part 1. British Journal of Occupational Therapy 57(1): 9–14

Whalley Hammell K R 1994b Establishing objectives in occupational therapy practice. Part 2. British Journal of Occupational Therapy 57(2): 45–48

Wilcock A A 1991 Occupational Science. British Journal of Occupational Therapy 54(8): 297–300

Wilson C R M 1987 Hospital wide quality assurance models for implementation and development. B Saunders, London

World Health Organization Regional Office for Europe 1988 Quality assurance of health services, 38th session. Technical discussions, Copenhagen (Doc no. EUR/RC38/Tech. Disc.)

Yerxa E J, 1980 Audacious values: the energy source for occupational therapy practice. American Journal of Occupational Therapy 38: 15–23

Yerxa E J 1987 Research: the key to the development of occupational therapy as an academic discipline. American Journal of Occupational Therapy 41(7): 415–419

Yerxa E J 1983 In Kielhofner G (ed) Health through occupation: theory and practice in occupational therapy. F A Davis, Philadelphia

Yerxa E J 1990 Some implications of occupational therapy's history for its epistemology values and relation to medicine. American Journal of Occupational Therapy 46(1): 79–82

Young M, Quinn 1992 Theories and practice of occupational therapy. Churchill Livingstone, Edinburgh

Glossary and Appendices

Glossary

Activity

An integrated sequence of tasks which takes place on a specific occasion, during a finite period, for a particular purpose. A completed activity results in a change in the previous state of objective reality or subjective experience. An activity is commonly identified by a short phrase indicating the primary action and objective.

Activities may be chained to form processes; in any chain an *antecedent activity* is one which precedes that which achieves the primary objective, while a *consequent activity* is one which must be performed as a result of the primary activity.

Aim

A brief, general, statement of the agreed intention of intervention.

Applied analysis

Describes and analyses an activity or task in order to use it as therapy; or identifies tasks, sequences and performance skills, to enable the individual to function more effectively.

Approach

Ways and means of putting theory into practice. (Hagedorn, Creek, Foster & Turner 1993)

Basic analysis

To describe an occupation, activity or task in order to understand its nature and the basis for engagement.
Macroanalysis. Basic analysis of occupations and processes.
Activity analysis. Basic analysis of activities.
Microanalysis. Basic analysis of tasks.

Cognitive component

Involves learning and the application of knowledge, and interpretation of perceptions.

297

Competence

Skilled and adequately successful completion of a task, routine or activity.

Core components

The person, therapist and occupation, interacting within an environment for the purpose of therapy.

Developmental level

The level at which skill and knowledge is evolved and tasks and routines are performed. (Syn: *proto-occupational level.*)

Dysfunction

A temporary or chronic inability to cope with, and engage in, the roles, relationships and occupations expected of a person of similar age and culture.

Effective level

The level at which a complete activity or chain of activities is performed, with some effect, product or consequence. (Syn: *productive level.*)

Environment

'The aggregate of phenomena that surrounds the individual and influences his development and existence. It includes physical conditions, things, other individuals, groups and ideas.' (Mosey 1986)

The environment may be described as consisting of: the *sociocultural environment*, e.g. people, social structures, beliefs, values: and the *physical environment* – non-human organic and inorganic features; human constructs and artefacts.

Environmental analysis

The process of describing the environment and its effects on people, and the needs for adaptation to elements within it to enable or enhance performance.

Environmental demand

The combined effect of elements in the environment to produce expectations for certain human actions and reactions. (Syn: *press.*)

Expertise

Consistently exceptional performance of a process or occupation.

External environment

The physical and psychosocial environment; the world and universe.
Outer resource area.   The area of the external environment containing the objects, constructs, tools and materials which the individual customarily uses, the people he knows and the places he usually goes to.
Outer exploratory area.   The rest of the world.
Outer closed area.   The unknown universe.

Frame of reference

'A system of theories serving to orient or give particular meaning to a set of circumstances, which provides a coherent conceptual basis for therapy.' (Hagedorn, Creek, Foster & Turner 1993)

Functional

Having the ability to perform competently the roles, relationships and occupations required in the course of daily life.

Functional analysis

To describe an individual's engagement in occupations at all levels. (Syn: *functional assessment.*)
Participation analysis.   Deals with patterns of engagement.
Performance analysis.   Describes how competently an individual can perform activities or tasks.
Existential analysis.   Describes how an individual thinks and feels about his roles and activities.

Generic process

Describes a typical kind of performance which is part of an occupation, e.g. cooking: baking, boiling, frying.

Goal

A concise statement of a defined outcome to be attained at a stage in intervention. Goals may be long-term or short-term.

Integrative occupational therapy model

One which gives an explanation of humans as occupational beings in relation to their environments, and of the therapeutic benefits of occupation.

Integrative process

Draws together a sequence of activities and generic processes for a purpose.

Internal environment

The abstract area in which the individual experiences his inner personal existence and actions. (Syn: *psychological environment*.)

Inner resource area. The area in which the individual has stored memories, knowledge and patterns of action.

Inner exploratory area. Contains repressed and suppressed material, e.g. dreams, symbols and buried memories.

Inner closed area. Equivalent to the unconscious. Material of which the individual is unaware and cannot reach.

Intervention

A generic description of all forms of action taken by a therapist during the process of case management.

Action taken by a therapist in conjunction with, or on behalf of the client.

Level of occupation

A hypothetical hierarchy of organization and action.

Life space

A changeable area defined by the person's perception, interest and attention at any given moment. The person acts and interacts within life space.

Mastery

Fluent and faultless performance of an activity or process.

Metaprocess

Organizes a chain of processes within an occupation, over an extended timescale, e.g. manufacturing sequence.

Model

'A simplified representation of the structure and content of a phenomenon or system that describes or explains the complex relationships between concepts within the system and integrates elements of theory and practice.' (Hagedorn, Creek, Foster & Turner 1993)

Objective

A very precise definition of an outcome, including a statement of what action will be taken, by whom, by when, and a means of evaluating the degree to which it has been effective.

Occupation

'The dominant activity of human beings that includes serious, productive pursuits and playful, creative and festive behaviours.' (Kielhofner 1993)

'Activities or tasks which engage a person's resources of time and energy, specifically, self-maintenance, productivity and leisure.' (Reed & Sanderson 1983)

'Any goal-directed activity that has meaning for the individual and is composed of skills and values.' (Creek 1992)

'That which occupies us between birth and death and may be classified into occupations related to play, leisure, work and self-maintenance.' (Young & Quinn 1992)

'Specific chunks of activity within the ongoing stream of human behaviour which are named in the lexicon of the culture.' (Yerxa et al)

Occupation is a generic term encompassing all aspects of a person's engagement in roles, processes, activities or tasks in the course of daily life.

An occupation is an organized form of endeavour which provides longitudinal organization of time and effort in a person's life and provides the person with a role.

An occupation is an organized form of human endeavour having a name and associated role title. It may be described as a sociocultural phenomenon having attributes including: principles, positions, possessions, and purposes. It may also be defined by observable attributes including: products, processes, patterns, practical requirements and performance demands. A participant engages in an occupation over an extended period of time.

Occupation analysis

A generic term indicating various forms of analysis and description of occupations at all levels.

Occupational therapy

'The use of purposeful activity with individuals who are limited by physical illness or injury, psychosocial dysfunction, developmental or learning disabilities, poverty and cultural differences, or the aging process in order to maximise independence, prevent disability and maintain health.' (AOTA 1981)

'The treatment of physical and psychiatric conditions through specific activities to help people to reach their maximum level of function and independence in all aspects of daily life.' (WFOT 1989)

'The restoration of optimum function and life satisfaction through the analysis and use of selected occupations that enable the individual to develop the adaptive skills required to support life roles.' (Creek 1990)

'The prescription of activities, interactions and adaptations to enable the individual to regain develop or retain the occupational skills and roles required to maintain personal well-being and to achieve meaningful goals and relationships appropriate to the relevant social and cultural setting'. (Hagedorn 1992, amended)

'Intervention by an occupational therapist to adapt and balance the interactions between a person and the demands of his/her environment and occupations, in order to enable, enhance and empower competent performance in, and satisfaction with, relevant aspects of his/her daily life.' (Hagedorn 1994)

Occupational therapy core

A statement of the core components, values, assumptions, knowledge, purposes and processes of occupational therapy.

Occupational therapy paradigm

'The paradigm consists of the basic assumptions, values and perspectives that unify the field. It defines and gives coherence or wholeness to the entire profession. It speaks to the nature and purpose of occupational therapy. It gives therapists a common understanding of what it means to be an occupational therapist.' (Kielhofner 1992)

'An agreed body of theory, explaining and rationalizing professional unity and practice, that incorporates all the profession's concerns, concepts and expertise and guides values and commitments.' (Creek 1992)

Organization level

The level at which occupations and processes can be described. (Syn: *occupational level*.)

Outcome

An agreed, predetermined, clearly defined result of therapy.

Outcome measure

A means of evaluating the degree to which an outcome has been achieved.

Patent sector

The area of human knowledge, experience and observable action which exists in the physical world, of which people have some shared perceptions and which is open to view by the individual and others.

Performance demand

The intrinsic features of an activity or task which require the participant to possess certain physical or psychological characteristics, and certain forms of knowledge, skill or attitude for competent performance.

Potent sector

The area of human knowledge and experience which exists within the mind of an individual and can be known only to that individual.

Private life space

The individual's area of awareness of his internal environment.

Private self

The part of personal identity which is partly known to the individual, but unknown to others.

Problem-based model

One which gives a causational explanation of the origins of problems in social or occupational performance, and indicates consequent action. The four problem-based models are: development, education, rehabilitation, adaptation.

Procedure

A rigidly structured task sequence which must be followed to achieve the desired result.

Process

A process is a description of the means whereby the purposes and products of an occupation may be carried out.

Process-driven pattern

One in which the therapist employs the problem-based structure of case management in order to define the problem, and subsequently selects an appropriate model/approach.

Product

Any change in the nature of objective reality or subjective experience, brought about as a result of engagement in activity.

Psychosocial component

Required for communication and interaction with others, including awareness of self in relation to others.

Public life space

The individual's area of awareness of his external environment.

Public self

The part of personal identity and appearance which is observable by others, and known to a variable extent by the individual.

Routine

An automated and habitual chain of tasks with a fixed sequence.

Sensorimotor component

Required for the execution of movement and for the appreciation of position, and the reception of input from the environment.

Skill

The ability to put skill components together in smoothly integrated and sequenced, competent, performance.

Skill component

A single, identifiable, part-skill.

Task

A self-contained stage in an activity. Tasks chain to form an activity

Task segment

The smallest piece of performance which can be identified separately.

Task stage

A completed act which forms part of a whole task.

Theoretical belt

Theories associated with the practice of occupational therapy which are available to the therapist as options, additional to those contained within the core.

Theory-driven pattern

One in which the therapist selects a theory (or model) before commencing intervention and uses it to direct all subsequent clinical reasoning and action.

Therapy

Treatment of the patient by the therapist.

Appendix 1

Experiential and reflective exercises

The purpose of these exercises is to enable people who wish to do so to explore the processes described in this book and to relate these to their own experiences and practice.

It is not envisaged that anyone will want to work their way through the entire set – it might be very instructive, but I suspect that time will not permit. If you feel it may be useful, choose an area of interest to you, try an exercise, and see where it leads you.

For each process a number of 'tasks' are suggested. These are particularly suited to students on placement – several of them have been used successfully as student assignments – but some may be equally useful to an experienced practitioner who wishes to evaluate her own practice and to reflect upon it.

Reflection is the most important part of the exercise: the outcome of the task is not really important, nor does it really matter whether it seems 'successful', for even 'unsuccessful' experiences have value when thought about in retrospect. There are no 'right answers'.

Exercises are given code numbers for ease of identification.

CASE MANAGEMENT: CLINICAL REASONING AND PROBLEM ANALYSIS

CM 1

Select a recent case which caused you to give it some extra thought. See if you can detect instances when various forms of clinical reasoning were used: hypothetical (it might be . . ., if so . . . then . . .); interactive reasoning (listening, and directing the course of the interaction as it occurs); narrative reasoning (the patient's story, and how it might continue); pattern recognition (I have come across this before . . ., it is likely that . . .); procedural reasoning (this is what I will do, in this order . . .).

What does this tell you about the way you approach a case? How difficult was it to unravel your thought processes?

CM 2

Take a sample referral – the next one which lands on your desk will suffice. Before you see the patient or client, sit down with the referral information and generate as many ideas or hypotheses as possible about the case, and consider what you are likely to find when you meet the client, what you think the client's needs are, or what your intervention might be. Simply 'empty your head', making notes or jotting down key words as rapidly and uncritically as possible.

When you have done this, look back through your notes and decide what you will accept or reject – you may find you have an open mind with many hypotheses, or that you have come to a conclusion.

Now go and interview the client, and obtain the usual information which will enable you to start intervention. How far did your gut reaction ideas hold up in practice? Were there any automatic assumptions and biases which proved unfounded?

(It is worth repeating this exercise a few times to obtain an overview of the way in which you generally tackle a case.)

CM 3

This is an exercise for therapists who work in interdisciplinary teams.

Take a sample case and analyse whether or not the different team members have differing perceptions of it, and whether these differ from your 'occupational therapy view'. Include the patient and relative or carer in this exercise. It may take some time to obtain the different views; simply observe and make mental notes; it is not necessary to ask specific questions unless you want to create a more formal exercise.

If there are different attitudes and opinions, why do you think this is? How do these different views contribute to the intervention?

CM 4

Complex cases can be interpreted in different ways. If you have a suitably complex case (yours or someone else's) to use as an example, see whether different occupational therapy theories (models, frames of reference, approaches) could be used to frame the problem. If there are different ways of framing it, does this illuminate the situation and suggest ways of tackling it, or does it simply confuse the issue? Has a particular model or frame of reference been used in this case?

INTERVENTION

INT 1

How is the cycle of intervention applied in sample cases? Identify stages and repetitions of the cycle.

INT 2

Critically review a selection of the aims, goals or objectives which you have for your current caseload. Are you happy with these or could they be improved? Do they give you scope to measure outcomes?

INT 3

If you are using an action plan or goal-planning system, take a sample case which has recently been discharged and review the implementation of the plan. With hindsight, did it work out as you expected, and if not, how might you have altered it?

INT 4

Is there a clinical question which might give you the opportunity for a small research project in your area? If there is, try to formulate the question, and compile some notes about how might you tackle the project, and circumstances which might help or hinder your research.

INT 5

Keep a diary about your practice for 1 month; it is not necessary to give a detailed account of every day, just note very briefly what you did which you would like to remember or which might be useful later, problems, solutions, things which worked, and things which did not. At the end of the month evaluate this diary. Was it a useful exercise? Did it take more time than was justified by the results? If it had value, could it be built into your practice as a regular feature, perhaps with suitable modifications?

ASSESSMENT AND EVALUATION

AE 1

Identify the types of assessment used in your area of work. Are assessments standardized or not? Criticize them for suitability, validity and reliability.

AE 2

Check a recent assessment report for, e.g. clarity, accuracy, precision, predictive validity, presentation. Reflect on whether it could be improved.

AE 3

Do you undertake:

- skill analysis
- performance analysis
- participation analysis
- existential analysis.

If so, how? If not, why not? Is it inappropriate, or might it be useful in some cases?

AE 4

If you assess performance of daily living tasks (personal,

domestic, social), review the way in which this is done in relation to the realities of the individual's circumstances and environment. Is your assessment comprehensive, and how far is it adapted to the needs and priorities of the client?

AE 5

Carry out a participation/existential analysis for yourself or a friend. Reflect on the value of this exercise and the insights gained.

ANALYSIS AND ADAPTATION OF OCCUPATIONS

OCC 1

Choose any occupation and conduct a general macroanalaysis using the '10P' headings. Did this enlarge your understanding of the occupation?

OCC 2

Choose any occupation (other than a profession). Consider how, in different circumstances, this might be viewed by the participant as work, leisure or self-care. What affects the classification? Does this matter to the participant or affect his performance? If one of these classifications is inappropriate or if the selected occupation does not seem to fit any of these classifications, or requires an additional one, consider why this may be. Does it matter in occupational therapy terms?

OCC 3

Take an activity which has a visible end-product and is commonly used by occupational therapists for therapeutic purposes. Conduct an activity anlaysis using the headings given for stable and situational factors Table 14.2 (p. 224).

OCC 4

Take the above activity, and conduct an applied analysis for a particular individual for whom you consider this activity to be therapeutic. Use Box 14.1 on page 233 and Fig. 14.1 (p. 234) as a guide.

OCC 5

Undertake a microanalysis of a task; break the task into stages, and subdivide a sample of the stages into task segments. Analyse the skill components required to complete the task segments.

Was this exercise simple or complex? How easy was it to define the stages?

Was it necessary to change your initial definition of the task?

OCC 6

How do you maintain a focus on the occupations and activities of your clients? Is the focus generic, or slanted in some way? How easy or difficult is it to maintain this focus?

OCC 7

How far do you incorporate activities into your therapy programmes? Reflect on the relevance of what you use, or the reasons for not using activities.

ENVIRONMENTAL ANALYSIS AND ADAPTATION

This is a process which can be learned satisfactorily only through experience and practice in real environments; these exercises are therefore more detailed than those in other sections.

ENV 1

Design a checklist for a comprehensive environmental observation.

This task is in preparation for ENV 2, which is an observation of a public area – indoors or external. The checklist will serve as a means of noting the observations and making conclusions. As with other types of checklist, there is no single, perfect example. It is suggested that you use the following headings, and then decide what to list under each:

* physical features
* users
* Sociocultural features
* occupations and purposes for which environment is used
* environmental demand.

Discuss your checklist and, if possible, compare it with those of others. Identify the difficulties which you encountered in making the checklist, and reflect on the design process. When you have a satisfactory format, you are ready to tackle ENV 2.

ENV 2

Select an easily accessible public environment. You may need to seek advance permission from a company or local manager, in order to avoid being regarded with suspicion! Spend at least 30 minutes observing your selected environment and completing your checklist and any other notes.

Analyse your observations: what did you discover about the environment? Make a few summary notes under each heading, paying particular attention to any obvious or 'hidden' sociocultural aspects, suitability for purpose, and level of demand in relation to use and users. If possible, discuss your findings with others who have done the same exercise.

ENV 3

Personal environments are often very revealing. For this exercise, you should choose one room in someone's home, which both the owner and you feel is an area which she has consciously designed in some way to suit her own tastes, interests, activities or needs. Your task is first to observe the content, and secondly to discuss with the owner the uses of the area and the personal significance of selected items which attract your interest and attention as being potentially revealing about the inhabitant. You may like to use, or modify, the observation checklist for this visit. Do not let your questioning become intrusive – sensitive material can sometimes be uncovered unexpectedly, and it would be inappropriate to pursue this unless the owner is obviously willing to do so.

For this exercise you must, of course, begin by asking permission. You need a person who is prepared to select one room in her home, let you take a detailed look at it, and be open about discussing the features, purposes and history of its contents. It is suggested that you do not select someone with special needs for this exercise. It should be a person whom you do not know well – otherwise you will make assumptions rather than observations; a friendly acquaintance, neighbour or colleague would be ideal. Arrange a convenient time and allow $1\frac{1}{2}$–2 hours; it is surprising how long this exercise can take; you must also allow a little time for being sociable.

Following the visit, review the information obtained and reflect on the process and what was discovered.

ENV 4

It is difficult to understand the practicalities and complexities of home adaptation without a real home and a real client. In order to gain some experience of this, the following simulation is suggested.

Obtain a 'dummy' referral for a disabled or handicapped client, preferably following the format for referral that is in local use in the community. The client may be fictitious or based on a real person. The situation and diagnosis should represent some commonly encountered, typical problem which might be expected to require a significant alteration to the home. It is not necessary to over-elaborate the history, but the essential information about the client's abilities, difficulties and preferences, and those of any carer or relative, should be given.

Using this referral as a basis, make a domiciliary visit to a real home – preferably a friend's, although it could be your own; choose a standard house, flat or bungalow typical of the area. Imagine that the client lives there. What problems will this client encounter in the home? What alterations or adaptations can be made? Draw up draft plans. Write notes on these recommendations and discuss them with an experienced colleague. How could the alterations be provided?

Reflect on the impact of the environment on the abilities of the client. Consider the implications of any alterations for other members of the family. (In using this exercise with students it was noted that where the role play was taken seriously, the owner of the home sometimes found himself emotionally involved in the proposals. If this should occur, take note of such reactions, for this may aid the understanding of those of future clients).

ENV 5

Using Mosey's list of activity groups (Box 15.1, p. 251), and the room layouts illustrated in Fig. 15.2 try the following exercises:

1. Decide which layout would be appropriate for each group.
2. Decide what kind of activities might be used with this type of group.
3. What environmental factors would you consider in organizing this?

THERAPEUTIC USE OF SELF

TS 1

List the aspects of being a therapist which you most enjoy and value, and the aspects which you find frustrating or unrewarding. How can you make the most of the positive elements? Can you take any action to minimize the negative elements?

TS 2

Identify experiences with clients in your training or professional practice which were especially difficult for you as a person. Why did they cause a problem? What does this tell you about your own personality or coping skills?

TS 3

Identify your personal 'danger signs' and your strategies for coping with stress. Where do you go for support?

TS 4

What personal attributes help you in your work as a therapist? Are there any which hinder you? How do you compensate for these?

TS 5

The therapeutic relationship tends towards an unequal balance of power between therapist (in control) and client; how do you consciously compensate for this inequality, and ensure partnership with your clients? Are there factors in your service provision which deliberately, or unintentionally, contribute to removing control or choice from the client?

TS 6

Identify a time when you have consciously acted out a role to help a client. Reflect on the process and outcome.

TS 7

Identify ways in which you give feedback to your clients.

TS 8

Think of a client who was difficult to motivate. What strategies did you use to try to motivate this person. Were these successful? In hindsight, was there any other strategy you could have used?

RESOURCE MANAGEMENT

RM 1

Review your job description (or someone else's). How well does it reflect your (their) role?

RM 2

Find the mission statement, or equivalent document, for your area and critically review its contents and usefulness.

RM 3

Identify the degree to which your area is constrained by resource problems. Can you identify a single change which would improve the service *without* necessitating an increase in resources?

RM 4

Is there a system, formal or informal, of prioritizing cases in your area? How does this stand up to ethical examination?

RM 5

Discuss the management of a caseload with an experienced therapist. What strategies does he use? Is he aware of conflicts and compromises?

RM 6

List the ways in which you communicate and the people in your own network. Ask an experienced therapist to list the people in her own network.

RM 7

How is quality assurance managed in your area? Identify policies, standards and methods of audit.

RM 8

If you have written service standards, review the standards for one aspect of your service. What were your conclusions?

If there are no written standards, try to write some for just one aspect of your work, and see if it is possible to put them into practice. Include some means of evaluating whether these standards have been achieved.

RM 9

Describe one aspect of your service under the headings: structure, process, outcome. How helpful was this exercise?

RM 10

Critically review the data collection system. Whose needs does it meet? Does it provide useful information for the therapist? If not, could it be made to do so?

Appendix 2

Standardized assessments

I stressed in Chapter 13 that it is important for therapists to use standardized assessments when available. It seems clear from the literature that there are many such instruments, and also that therapists in the UK are not, on the whole, using these, despite being frequently urged to do so.

There are probably many reasons for this, but it seems likely that the primary difficulty is a very practical impediment; with the exception of the few which have been published or marketed in the UK, it is extremely hard to obtain copies of these assessments. Therapists who wish to find and use an assessment, especially one produced in another country, must therefore be prepared to spend an amount of time and effort which is likely to deter all but the most determined inquirer.

ADVICE ON SOURCES

Suppliers

In the UK, assessments published specifically for occupational therapists are supplied by Nottingham Rehabilitation. Other suitable tests may be found in catalogues of psychological tests, e.g. NFER-Nelson. However, the more specialized of these usually demand additional training before you are permitted to use them.

Journals

If you look back through the British Journal of Occupational Therapy or other occupational therapy journals to find articles on assessment, you should be able to find references to original publications from which sufficient details of the assessment can be gleaned to enable it to be used. Assessments connected with rehabilitation are often described in medical journals, rather than in occupational therapy journals.

However, this type of search is unsatisfactory because of the time involved, and also because the information may be incomplete, or out-of-date. More fundamentally, the assessment may need to be re-standardized for your intended population. Nevertheless, it is informative to read the literature, and this will be helpful if, in the absence of a standardized test, you decide to design your own assessment instrument or procedure.

Books

Some books include assessment procedures, forms or check-lists; these are, however, protected by copyright, and should not be used unless permission has been obtained from the publisher. Although publishers are often slow to reply, it is worth writing to request permission. Willard and Spackman's Occupational Therapy (Hopkins & Smith 1993) is particularly useful as a source.

The original author

Detective work may be required to discover the author, but, where the article describing the assessment is relatively recent, it will give the name and, usually, the work location of the author. Try sending a letter.

College of Occupational Therapists

The Disability Information Service may be able to provide information on British assessments, but may not be able to be of much help with sources for those from abroad.

Other occupational therapy associations

Details of American, Canadian and Australian assessments may be obtained from the appropriate national occupational therapy association.

Occupational therapy colleges

If you have access to a sympathetic lecturer or librarian, he may be able to give you information or samples which the college uses for training purposes. However, it is not the primary function of colleges to act as such a resource, and too many inquiries would be likely to overwhelm them.

LIST OF SOURCES (Tables A2.2, A2.3)

Where a source is known it is listed, or alternatively one or more references are given. Some additional assessments and checklists are included.

CHECKLIST (Box A2.1)

A useful checklist for selecting or designing an assessment is given in Box A2.1.

Table A2.1 List of standardized assessments available in UK

Title	Available from
Rivermead perceptual assessment battery (Rivermead)	NFER-Nelson
Chessington occupational therapy neurological assessment battery (COTNAB)	Nottingham Rehabilitation
Allen's Assessments of cognitive disability	Nottingham Rehabilitation
Functional independence measure (FIM) Functional assessment measure (FAM)	State University of New York at Buffalo, School of Medicine and Biomedical Sciences, The Centre for Functional Assessment Research, Uniform Data System for Medical Rehabilitation, 232 Parker Hall, SUNY South Campus, 3435 Main Street Buffalo, New York 14214–3007, USA or Northwick Park Hospital, Regional Rehabilitation Unit, Northwick Park Hospital, Watford Rd, Harrow, Middlesex HA1 3UJ, UK (For research information/workshops)
Assessment of motor and process skills (AMPS)	
Canadian occupational performance measure (COPM)	The Canadian Association of Occupational Therapists, 110 Eglinton Avenue West, 3rd Floor, Toronto, Ontario, M4R 1A3, Canada Or may be available from College of Occupational Therapists

Table A2.2   Sources and references

Assessment	Source	Main author	Title	Notes
AMPS	AJOT 46(10)	Fisher et al	Cross-cultural assessment of process skills	Refs listed include other papers by Fisher/Kielhofner (And details of assessments available in USA – see list below.) Publisher MUST provide approval before use of any printed material
	Willard & Spackman's occupational therapy, 8th edn AMPS form and score sheet, p. 214 Fisher	Hopkins & Smith (eds)		
Barthel index	BJOT 55(3) BJOT 55(4) BJOT 56(2)	Murdock Shah	A critical evaluation of the Barthel index: parts 1 and 2 Commentary on A critical evaluation of the Barthel index	Critical reviews of validity
	BJOT 56(5)	Eakin	The Barthel index: confidence limits	
	BJOT 56(6)	Fricke	Measuring outcomes in rehabilitation: a review	
COTNAB	BJOT 57(4)	Laver	The performance and experience of normal elderly people on the COTNAB	Elderly found to perform differently
COPM	CJOT 57(2)	Law, Pollock et al	Occupational performance measures; a review based on the guidelines for the client-centred practice of occupational therapy	Reviews measures listed: justifies COPM development
	CJOT 57(2)		The Canadian occupational performance measure: an outcome measure for occupational therapy	Second paper describes COPM development
FIM and FAM		Hall, Hamilton Wayne Zasler	Characteristics and comparisons of functional assessment indices: Disability rating scale, FIM and FAM (Journal of head trauma rehabilitation 1993 8(2) 60–74)	
Rivermead	BJOT 55(6)	Friedman	The Rivermead perceptual assessment battery in acute stroke	Compares RPBA with Barthel; shortened RPBA recommended
	BJOT 56(10)	Matthey et al	The clinical usefulness of the Rivermead perceptual assessment battery; statistical considerations	Reviews use and validity
Functional limitations profile	BJOT 54(6)	McCulloch	Can we measure 'output'? Quality-adjusted life years health indices and occupational therapy	Concludes FLP useful
Idiosyncratic activities configuration	Little, Brown & Co, Boston	Cynkin & Robinson	Occupational therapy and activities health	Obtain permission from publisher
Occupational questionnaire	Churchill Livingstone, Edinburgh	Creek	Occupational therapy and mental health	Sample form and source (page 77)
General reviews	BJOT 54(10)	McAvoy	The use of ADL indices by occupational therapists	Reviews content of non-standardized indices
	BJOT 56(8)	Unsworth	The concept of function	Reviews content of 23 ADL indices
	BJOT 56(11)	Jeffrey	Aspects of selecting outcome measures to demonstrate the effectiveness of comprehensive rehabilitation	Critical review of those listed
	AJOT 43(8)	Law & Letts	A critical review of scales of activities of daily living	Review of 6 indices
	BJOT 52(1)	Eakin	Assessment of activities of daily living: a critical review	Two very useful articles
	BJOT 52(2)	Eakin	Problems with assessments of activities of daily living	

Table A2.3   Recommended texts

Hopkins H, Smith H (eds) 1993 Willard and Spackman's occupational therapy, 8th edn. Lippincott, Philadelphia
'Willard and Spackman' is a widely used occupational therapy text, which contains many sample ADL forms and assessment checklists. Some of these have already been listed but others which may be of particular use are listed below. Permission *must* be obtained from the publisher before any printed material is used.

Item	Page(s)
Lists of USA published tests with sources	
Table 7–1	173–181
Manual dexterity and motor function tests	
Developmental tests	
Sensory integration tests	
Sensory integration and praxis tests	
Intelligence tests	
Psychological tests (e.g. adaptive behaviour, social maturity, cognition, projective tests)	
Stress tools	
Tests for young children and their families	
Tests for geriatric patients	
Table 13–11 Selected assessment tools for birth–3 years	464–465
Table 13–12 Selected assessment tools for evaluating family needs	466
Forms and checklists for nonstandardized assessments	
Joint range measurement forms and checklist	183–186
Manual muscle evaluation form	187–188
Sample self-care assessment form	195
Sample home recommendations checklist	225
Environmental control systems needs assessment	334–338
Table 8–7 The Jacobs prevocational skills assessment	236–237
Formats for displaying results of play and game evaluation (child functional assessment)	513–514
Formats for displaying results of social intervention and task performances (child interactive assessment)	515
Evaluation record for mildly neurologically impaired (schoolchild)	805
Evaluation record for young moderately to severely handicapped child	807
Time use record	594
Sample daily pain diary (adults)	599
Sample occupational therapy worksheet (functional checklist, suitable for domiciliary use)	617
PIZZI assessment of productive living for adults with HIV infection or AIDS	720–721
Hospice assessment of occupational function	858–859

Allen C K 1985 Occupational therapy for psychiatric disorders: measurement and management of cognitive disabilities. Little Brown, Boston, provides information on Allen's cognitive theories.
Cynkin S, Robinson A M 1990 Occupational therapy and activities health: towards health through activities. Little Brown, Boston
Creek J (ed) 1990 Occupational therapy and mental health: principles, skills and practice. Churchill Livingstone, Edinburgh
Pynsent, Fairbank, Carr 1993 Outcome measures in orthopaedics. Butterworths, London.
Standardized checklists for orthopaedic assessment, including measurement and functional evaluation. Reviews and gives examples of available assessments.

Box A2.1   A checklist for selecting or designing an assessment

---

Aim
- What is the purpose of the assessment? Descriptive, evaluative, predictive, to provide feedback to patient? Other?
- At what occupational level is it to be focused?
- Is it general or specific?

Form/method
- Is it a single event or sequential?
- Does it involve an individual alone, or in a group?
- Does it involve:
  interview: unstructured or structured?
  questionnaire: self-rated or assessor-rated?
  checklist or inventory: with or without scoring?
  general observation of behaviour and/or performance?
  structured observation or sampling?
  — event recording?   — duration recording?
  — time sampling?   — critical incident analysis?
  — interval recording?
  performance of task or activity?
  completion of product – is there a set standard?
  projective tests?
  specific tests of skill components?
  physical measurement?
  self-evaluation?
- Is there a clear instruction sheet or manual?

Layout
- Is it clear, using plain language, well-designed and 'user-friendly'?
- Will the recipient of the report understand it, and feel that it is a professionally produced document?

Rating or scoring
- Standardized or not?
- Numerical or descriptive?
- Graded?
- Weighted?
- Is a baseline required for reassessment and evaluation?
- Is data to be converted into visual form?
- Is data to be transferred to a computer? How?

Validity and reliability
- Standardized or unstandardized? On relevant population?
- Is the procedure formal and rigid, or informal? Is it written down?
- Is it valid – in what ways?
- Is there evidence of intra-rater and inter-rater reliability?

Participation from patient
- What is the patient required to do?
- Is the patient aware of being assessed?*
- Is the patient to be made aware of the results?*
(*These have ethical implications.)

Environment
- Where should this assessment be carried out?
- Does the task/test require a distinct environmental demand to facilitate performance?
- How realistic is the environment? If it is specially designed or safeguarded, in what way does it differ from normal?
- Is it free from unwanted distraction or interruption?
- Is it safe?

Practical requirements
- What is needed for the patient to undertake the assessment tasks? This may include furniture, materials, tools and equipment.
- What is needed for the therapist to carry out and record the assessment?
- How long will it take?

Personnel
- Who will perform the assessment? Does this person have the necessary information and skills?
- If the assessment is to be repeated, will this be by the same person or different people? If different, is the assessment standardized?

Index